I0056601

Hospital and Clinical Pharmacy

Second Edition

Hospital and Clinical Pharmacy
Second Edition

A Textbook for Graduate Students in Pharmacy

Prof. S. Balasubramanian

M.Pharm.

Professor and Head of the Department,
C.L. Baid Metha College of Pharmacy,
Chennai.

Dr. N. Narayanan

M.Pharm., Ph.D.

Director, Jaya College of Pharmacy, Chennai,
(Formerly Joint Director of Medical Education (Pharmacy) &
Principal, Govt. College of Pharmacy, Madras Medical College, Chennai.)

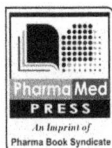

PharmaMed Press

An imprint of Pharma Book Syndicate

A Unit of BSP Books Pvt. Ltd.

4-4-309/316, Giriraj Lane,
Sultan Bazar, Hyderabad - 500 095.

PharmaMed
PRESS
An imprint of
Pharma Book Syndicate

Hospital and Clinical Pharmacy - *Second Ed.* by *Prof. S. Balasubramanian and Dr. N. Narayanan*

© 2014 *by Publisher*

All rights reserved. No part of this book or parts thereof may be reproduced, stored in a retrieval system or transmitted in any language or by any means, electronic, mechanical, photocopying, recording or otherwise without the prior written permission of the publishers.

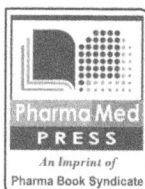

Published by

PharmaMed Press

An imprint of Pharma Book Syndicate

A Unit of BSP Books Pvt. Ltd.

4-4-309/316, Giriraj Lane, Sultan Bazar, Hyderabad - 500 095.

Phone: 040-23445605, 23445688; Fax: 91+40-23445611

E-mail: info@pharmamedpress.com

ISBN: 978-93-85433-46-7 (HB)

PREFACE TO THE SECOND EDITION

More than two decades has passed after the introduction of Hospital and Clinical Pharmacy subject in pharmacy curriculum. During these period not only new subjects but also new pharmacy courses have been introduced. Apart from the M.Pharm course with Pharmacy Practice specialization, a six years Pharm.D course was introduced to elevate the Indian Pharmacists to global standards. Recently Pharmacy Council of India has proposed to introduce a 2 years condensed course of Bachelor of Pharmacy Practice for working D.Pharm pharmacists, in which only clinical oriented subjects will be thought, it has announced. Hence this edition of our book is expanded with additional chapters to cover the entire syllabus of Pharm.D course, as well to meet the future requirements. This is in addition to all HCP topics, prescribed by many Indian universities for under graduate course in pharmacy, already present in this book.

We hope this book will be of much use to pharmacy students of India to study a wide range of topics in Hospital and Clinical Pharmacy. Sincere attempt has been made to present the subject in a simple and relevant manner to Indian conditions.

Our heartfelt thanks go to M/s BSP Books Pvt. Ltd, Hyderabad for publishing this book in such a nice manner and at affordable price. Also we wish to thank and acknowledge many websites like Pubmed, WHO, Wikipedia, etc and authors of reference books listed at the end. Any omission or error in the subject matter of the book can be brought to our knowledge which will be appreciated.

CHENNAI- 91   *- Authors*

1ˢᵗ January 2015

PREFACE TO THE FIRST EDITION

Clinical Pharmacy is one of the new subjects introduced in the syllabus of graduate course in pharmacy around the beginning of 1990's. Since there was no single book available for the students to cover the entire portions of the syllabus, we thought, it will be of great help to the students, if we prepare materials for them to study, from the available resources some 12 years back. Thus began the foundation work for this book and with more than a decade of experience in teaching the subject, a book like the present one if written and published will be much use to the students as well as, teaching fraternity, we believe.

This book is written in accordance with the syllabus prescribed for undergraduate students in pharmacy by many Indian universities. We hope it will be useful to the students of Pharm. D. course also to certain extent.

Sincere effort has been made to present the subject as simple as possible, so that the students can make a bright future with this strong foundation, when they complete their postgraduate specialization in clinical pharmacy or pharmacy practice.

We wish to record our appreciation to M/S BSP Books Pvt. Ltd., Hyderabad for bringing out this book in a palatable manner. We also wish to acknowledge and thank the pioneer authors of this subject and request the students and teachers of pharmacy to bring to our notice any improvement, they think, to be useful.

Constructive criticisms are always welcome to improve the content and correct any error crept in.

CHENNAI   *- Authors*

1ˢᵗ December 2012

CONTENTS

PART - I
HOSPITAL PHARMACY

CHAPTER 1

Hospitals – an Introduction

CHAPTER 2

Hospital Pharmacy

CHAPTER 3

Pharmacy and Therapeutic Committee

CHAPTER 4

Hospital Formulary

CHAPTER 5

Hospital Committees

CHAPTER 6

Therapeutic Guidelines

CHAPTER 7

Pharmacy Procedural Manual

CHAPTER 8

Budget of Hospital Pharmacy

CHAPTER 9

Manufacturing in Hospitals

CHAPTER 10

Total Parenteral Nutrition and Intravenous Admixture

CHAPTER 11

Pre-packing and Repacking in Hospitals

CHAPTER 12

Purchase and Inventory Control

CHAPTER 13

Organization and Management of Drug Store

CHAPTER 14

Drugs Distribution System

CHAPTER 15

Central Sterile Supply Department

CHAPTER 16

HOSPITAL ACCESSORIES

CHAPTER 17

Nuclear Pharmacy

CHAPTER 18

Records and Reports

CHAPTER 19

Professional Relations and Practices

PART - II
CLINICAL PHARMACY

CHAPTER 20

Clinical Pharmacy

CHAPTER 21

Medication History Interview

CHAPTER 22

Medical Abbreviations and Terminologies

CHAPTER 23

Ward Round Participation

CHAPTER 24

Rational Drug Therapy

CHAPTER 25

Pharmacotherapy

CHAPTER 26

Pediatric Pharmacy

CHAPTER 27

Geriatric Pharmacy

CHAPTER 28

Use of Drugs in Pregnancy and Lactation

CHAPTER 29

Pharmacogenetics

CHAPTER 30

Patient Compliance

CHAPTER 31

Drug Therapy Review and Therapeutic Drug Monitoring

CHAPTER 32

Patient Data Analysis

CHAPTER 33

Drug Utilisation Evaluation and Review

CHAPTER 34

Individualization of Dose and Pharmacist Intervention

CHAPTER 35

Adverse Drug Reactions

CHAPTER 36

Drug Interactions and Drug Induced Diseases

CHAPTER 37

Pharmacovigilance

CHAPTER 38

Pharmaceutical Care

CHAPTER 39

Patient Counselling

CHAPTER 40

Drug Information Center and Role of Pharmacists in Education and Training

CHAPTER 41

Poison Information Center and Treatment of Poison Cases

CHAPTER 42

Communication in Pharmacy and Presentation of Cases

CHAPTER 43

Critical Evaluation of Biomedical Literature

CHAPTER 44

Medication Errors

CHAPTER 45

Clinical Trials

PART - I

HOSPITAL PHARMACY

CHAPTER 1

HOSPITALS – AN INTRODUCTION

Definition

Hospital is an organization of public health. It is an institution which takes care of the health and diseases of people with the help of sophisticated equipments and instruments, by a group of specially trained persons.

As many people think, hospital is not only a place where sick people are given care, it also looks after the health or well being of the people and maintains it. It tries to keep them in good health and disease free by undertaking immunization, educational program and by teaching personal and social hygienic practices.

Classification

Hospital can be classified according to their

- I. Size
- II. Ownership
- III. System of treatment and
- IV. Specialization.

I. Size Basis

Hospitals are classified more conveniently as per the size that is the number of beds available to admit and treat patients. Thus there are hospitals with,

A. Less than 20 beds

B. Between 20 to 100 beds and

C. Above 100 beds (up to 1000 and more)

They can be referred as small, medium and large hospitals. Many hospitals run by private practitioners fall under the first category of small hospitals, where there may be one or two general wards available.

A couple of doctors may be working here and these hospitals may not have much diagnostic facilities like clinical lab, x-ray, scan etc. They send the patients to outside agencies for these services. Primary health centers (PHC) run by government can be classified under this category and they are all aptly called as primary care hospitals, where majority of patients go to get treatment first for their illness. Many of these hospitals are not open at nights.

Medium size hospitals are those opened in small towns like Taluk head quarters. Here 5 to 10 doctors may be working including one or two specialists. Some diagnostic facilities are available in these hospitals. From primary level hospitals, little complicated cases are sent to these secondary care hospitals for treatment. Upto 100 beds are available here in few essential wards like, medical ward, surgical ward, paediatric ward and maternity ward. These hospitals work day and night.

Large hospitals are highly specialized hospitals with almost all facilities and they have bed strength of 100 to 1000. District head quarter hospitals, Teaching (Medical College) hospitals and big private, corporate hospitals fall under this category. They are also called as tertiary hospitals or referral hospitals because more complicated cases from first two types of hospitals are referred here for further treatment. More than 50 doctors and 300 or so Paramedical professionals are working here in 3 shifts throughout the day.

II. Ownership Basis

Hospitals can also be classified according to the ownership. There are two broader categories.

1. Government owned hospitals and
2. Private hospitals

1. Government Hospitals

Starting from Primary Health Centers in small villages to Taluk, District and Medical college hospitals in cities, large number of hospitals are owned by State Governments. There are many quasi/semi Government hospitals, also called local body hospitals like municipal hospitals, (municipal) corporation hospitals and panchayat union hospitals. These are run by local bodies which are getting financial aid from Government for this purpose.

Central Government also owns some hospitals like Central Government Health Scheme (CGHS) hospitals, All India Institute of Medical Sciences (AIIMS) etc. Many hospitals are being run by central government under takings or corporations to serve a particular group of people like, railway hospitals, port trust hospitals, military hospitals, ESI hospital, etc.

2. Private Hospitals

There are many private hospitals of same size, if not bigger than Government hospitals. They are established by trusts, societies, and families or by individuals. They have all sophisticated instruments, facilities and doctors with different specializations. They are also called corporate hospitals. e.g.: Apollo Group of Hospitals. Medium and small private hospitals are also available in all the cities and towns of our country. These private hospitals are having facilities and standards equivalent to that of Western countries and hence lot of patients from abroad are coming to India to have medical treatment at very less expenses (medical tourism).

III. System of Treatment Basis

These groups of hospitals are those in which different systems are followed for treatment. They are Ayurveda Hospital, Siddha Hospital, Unani Hospital or Homeopathy Hospitals. The physicians in these hospitals are educated and/ or having experience in these systems and they are using medicines of these systems for treatment. These hospitals or physicians are popular in rural areas because they are there, even before allopathic system was introduced by British Rulers in our country.

IV. Specialization Basis

Hospitals can also be classified according to the specialized services offered in a particular hospital. For example there are few hospitals which treat only a particular part of the body or a particular disease. Thus we have two groups:

Group I

   A. Eye hospital

   B. Dental hospital

   C. ENT hospital

   D. Chest hospital and

   E. Skin hospital

Group II

   (i) Psychiatric hospital

   (ii) Orthopedics hospital and

   (iii) Communicable and infectious diseases hospital.

This apart, there are some other hospitals for giving treatment to special group of patients like Children's hospital, Maternity hospital etc. In all these hospitals doctors who are qualified in particular specialization are employed.

Thus in a big country like India there are varieties of hospitals and practices. Government of India has recently brought legislation, by name, Clinical Establishments Registration Act, which envisage, registration of all types of hospitals and clinics. Hence hereafter, they can also be classified according to the facilities available in them, into Grade I, II, III etc.

Organization

The nature and size of organization of a hospital differ according to the need. The organization of a big hospitals have two separate wings, one for the clinical administration another for office administration. The structure of these wings is given below:

The clinical administration and office administration both have many divisions or departments and each of this section are headed by qualified persons with specialization in the particular subject and experience. Needless to point out large administrative bodies require persons with special training and education in hospital administration.

Flow chart of a Hospital Organization

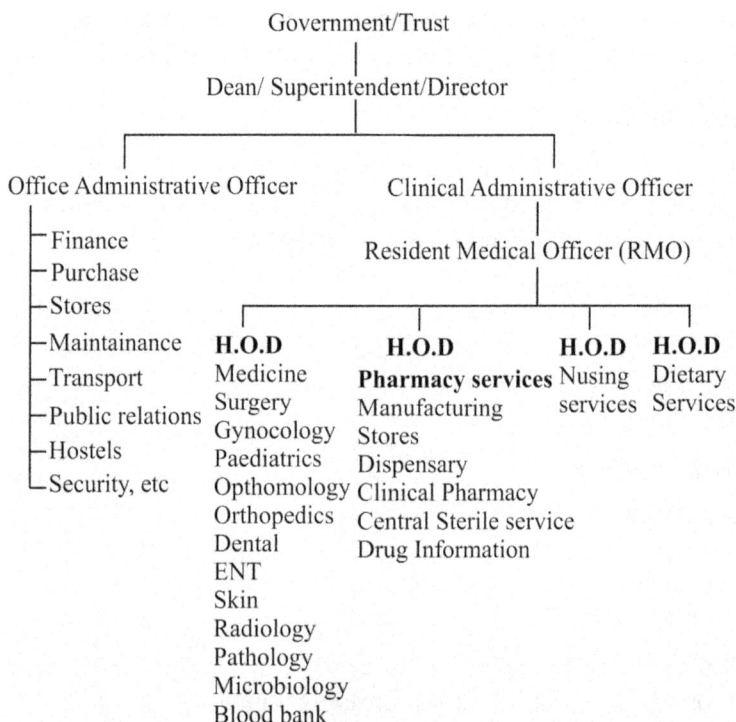

Government/Trust

Dean/ Superintendent/Director

Office Administrative Officer

- Finance
- Purchase
- Stores
- Maintainance
- Transport
- Public relations
- Hostels
- Security, etc

Clinical Administrative Officer

Resident Medical Officer (RMO)

H.O.D
Medicine
Surgery
Gynocology
Paediatrics
Opthomology
Orthopedics
Dental
ENT
Skin
Radiology
Pathology
Microbiology
Blood bank

H.O.D
Pharmacy services
Manufacturing
Stores
Dispensary
Clinical Pharmacy
Central Sterile service
Drug Information

H.O.D
Nusing
services

H.O.D
Dietary
Services

Medium size hospitals like Taluk hospitals and hospitals in small towns differ in the above organizational set up, that some of the sections may not be available with them. They are added whenever necessary. Because these hospitals are too big to control by an individual, the Government or trust constitutes various committees to assist Dean, in his administration.

These committees are called Governing council or Board of Directors. They have members from the trust and various departments of the hospital and even outside. People's representatives like MLA, MLC, MP or MC are given membership in Government Hospital Councils to function effectively and to meet the aspirations of the people.

Apart from this, various subcommittees are also formed at various levels of the hospital for the same reason e.g.: finance committee, purchase committee, development committee, ethical committee etc. Thus big hospitals are organized.

Administration

The above committees regularly conduct meetings and forward their recommendations to the Governing Council or Board of Directors, where these recommendations are considered, approved, modified or rejected. The approved decisions are then implemented by the Dean, either through his office administrative or clinical administrative wing.

Only policy matters and/or decisions involving huge sum of money are thus routed through the governing council, other small issues and day to day affairs are decided by the Dean himself and implemented. However, Dean reports all the important matters to the Council or Trust or Government through periodical reports.

Functions

The major functions of a hospital are,

1. Treatment of patients
2. Prevention of diseases and
3. Education of public

As pointed out above, hospitals are not only treating the patients but also preventing the disease from occurring and spreading. They undertake large scale immunization programs by vaccination drive and other programs like oral polio drops campaign, health camps to identify and/or prevent diseases in particular area and population etc.

As we know, prevention is better than cure, Government of India gives more importance to this and many public health programs like mosquito eradication, chlorination of drinking water etc, are promoted through various Government bodies.

In order to achieve the aim of 'Health for all', prevention and treatment alone are not sufficient unless general public are aware and cooperating with schemes. Hence large scale education campaign is carried out to create awareness among people, about diseases, preventive methods, nutrition and personal and social hygienic practices, by posters, cinema, TV and other Medias, by hospital and public health authorities.

Questions

Short Answer Questions

1. Define hospitals.
2. Draw a flow chart of Hospital Administration.
3. What are secondary care hospitals?
4. Why the referral hospitals are called so?

Long Answer Questions

5. Classify hospitals and explain each one of them in detail.
6. What are the functions of a hospital? Briefly Explain.
7. How big hospitals are administered? Enumerate the role of various committees formed in hospitals.

CHAPTER 2

HOSPITAL PHARMACY

Definition

"Hospital pharmacy is an organ of a hospital, where drugs are manufactured and/or purchased, stored, dispensed and its uses monitored and also, drug information, education and training are provided to inpatients, outpatients as well as to fellow health professionals by a team of highly qualified pharmacists".

Origin and Development

Long ago, a pharmacy inside the hospital was called 'Hospital Pharmacy', just like a pharmacy among the community is called 'Community Pharmacy'. These pharmacies were merely managed the job of 'Dispensing drugs' to the patients coming with a prescription.

But modern 'Hospital Pharmacy' is different. Its services are broader and almost covering the entire range of services with respect to the drugs. Thus starting from manufacture to Therapeutic Drug Monitoring (TDM) and beyond a modern pharmacist is expected to perform all services in relation to drugs at patient level. Earlier there was no other responsibility for a pharmacist, once dispensing was over. But now, a great deal of services awaiting him, after dispensing-viz-the clinical pharmacy services, where he has to obtain medication history of the patient, advice the doctors in selecting suitable drugs to the patient, monitor the therapy, intervene if necessary to correct the course of treatment and offer counselling to the patient either during treatment or at the time of discharge of the patient.

Thus hospital pharmacy and its organization, objectives and functions has widened enormously because of its transformation from product oriented service to patient oriented service.

But at the outset one must be clear that in India the above mentioned modern hospital pharmacy services are not available at present, in all the hospitals, with few exemptions like Christian Medical College Hospital, Vellore in Tamil Nadu and Trivandrum Medical

College Hospital, Trivananthapuram. Nevertheless these services have to be introduced sooner or later in India, as and when people realize their rights and requirements.

Hence a pharmacy student should study about this ideal hospital pharmacy set up and be familiarized with its requirements and services expected from him as and when it is established in India. He must strive to achieve this, in his own interest, as well as that of the society he lives in.

The following pages describe the ideal hospital pharmacy set up to be established in India, on the lines of those already exists in developed countries.

Organisational Structure

The organizational set up of a hospital pharmacy starts with fully qualified and experienced Head of the Department. He must have necessary education, specialization, training and experience in majority of the functions of a Hospital Pharmacy. Thus an M.Pharm graduate with Ph.D and specialization either in Pharmacology, Pharmacy Practice or Clinical Pharmacy is suitable for the job. Alternatively a 'Pharm D' graduate with experience is also apt for the job, as these graduates have adequate exposure in hospital works, they are given preference over others in western and developed countries.

The head of the department is supported by various section heads with experience in relevant fields of specialization. For example, pharmacy postgraduates and graduates with experience and endorsement by Drugs Control Administration are appointed in the Drugs Manufacturing sections of the Hospital Pharmacy.

Similarly Pharmacy Graduates with experience in the analysis and quality control of drugs and formulations are given charge of the quality control section.

The medical stores of the hospital are given control to pharmacy graduates with experience in dispensing of drugs. In both these sections D. Pharm holders are also appointed in adequate numbers to assist the works.

The Central Sterile Service Department of the hospital which supplies the required materials in sterile condition to various departments is also given in charge of a pharmacy graduate assisted by D. Pharm holders.

Once dispensing is over, the highly skilled and professional service namely clinical pharmacy services has to start. These services are also referred to as 'Pharmaceutical Care' which is defined as the responsible provision of drug therapy for the purpose of achieving definite outcomes that improves quality of life of the patient. The success of pharmaceutical care lies in determining or anticipating drug related problems and taking measures to improve outcomes thereby resulting in a better quality of life for the patient. Hence this section of hospital pharmacy require highly qualified pharmacist with experience in relevant works. M. Pharm graduates in pharmacology, clinical pharmacy or pharmacy practice specialization or Pharm. D graduates are appointed in this section. Adequate numbers of assistants are provided to carry out the enormous works involved.

The remaining services of a hospital pharmacy like, Drug Information Services, Education and Training are also suitably manned by appointing pharmacy persons with relevant qualification and experience. Thus an organization of modern 'Hospital Pharmacy' consists of at least 9 sections, as described below in the form of flow chart.

Flow Chart of a Modern Hospital Pharmacy Organization
(With Technocrats and their Qualifications)

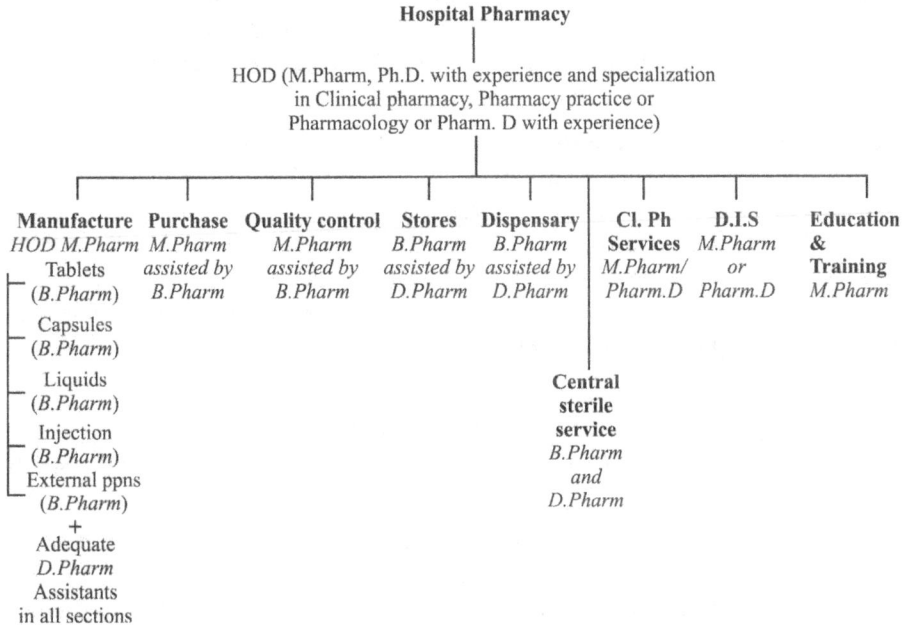

Hospital Pharmacy

HOD (M.Pharm, Ph.D. with experience and specialization
in Clinical pharmacy, Pharmacy practice or
Pharmacology or Pharm. D with experience)

Manufacture	Purchase	Quality control	Stores	Dispensary	Cl. Ph	D.I.S	Education
HOD M.Pharm	M.Pharm	M.Pharm	B.Pharm	B.Pharm	Services	M.Pharm	&
Tablets	assisted by	assisted by	assisted by	assisted by	M.Pharm/	or	Training
(B.Pharm)	B.Pharm	B.Pharm	D.Pharm	D.Pharm	Pharm.D	Pharm.D	M.Pharm
Capsules (B.Pharm)							
Liquids (B.Pharm)				Central sterile			
Injection (B.Pharm)				service B.Pharm			
External ppns (B.Pharm)				and D.Pharm			

+
Adequate
D.Pharm
Assistants
in all sections

Staff, Infrastructure and Work Load Statistics

Staff

From the above organizational flow chart, we can easily list the number of staff required for a Modern Hospital Pharmacy. It is obvious that this number depends on the work load or volume of activity of each section of the Hospital Pharmacy. Hence the first and foremost thing before deciding on the number of staff required is to fix the services which the Hospital Pharmacy is required or indented to provide.

In a full pledged hospital pharmacy like the one charted above there are nine sections each require persons with some sort of specialization or experience in the relevant area. Thus starting with director or HOD of the Hospital Pharmacy experienced staff are required to head each section. The director or HOD of the hospital pharmacy must have overall knowledge of each section of his department. Hence an M.Pharm, Ph.D or Pharm.D with minimum 10 years experience in various activities of Hospital Pharmacy will be an ideal person. He is supported by few associate or deputy directors with same qualifications but less experience of say 5 or 6 years.

Manufacturing section of the hospital pharmacy requires not only experience persons but also the person should have approval or eligibility to get the approval from the Drugs Control Department for the manufacture of the formulation concerned. Similarly the quality control section, where the hospital manufactured or procured drugs are tested for its quality, need to have experienced and approved analytical pharmacists. He should able to independently handle and operate the sophisticated modern analytical instruments and equipments. Pharmacists with experience in the manufacture and analysis of injectable especially in Large Volume Parenterals [LVP] are very much essential for hospital pharmacy manufacturing units as these LVPs are the single largest drug used daily in almost all the wards of the hospitals.

Next important section of a hospital pharmacy is clinical pharmacy services section, where pharmacists who can provide advisory and consultancy services to the treating physicians are essential. Hence Pharm.D graduates with experience must be appointed in this section. The clinical pharmacist also has to carryout, patient's medication history interview, therapeutic drug monitoring and patient counseling in this section. Hence few fresh Pharm.D or M.Pharm pharmacy practice graduates should be trained in this important area of hospital pharmacy service.

Other sections like medical and surgical stores, purchase, dispensary, central sterile service and drug information centre should be provided with regular staff with experience. Education and training section on the other hand require well experienced staff.

Thus all sections of hospital pharmacy should be manned with suitable pharmacists, which are easier said than done. Hence the man power requirement of the hospital pharmacy should be thoroughly studied and planned accordingly. Experienced people for each section is hard to get, hence suitable training program should be developed simultaneously where fresh pharmacy graduates should be recruited as 'Resident pharmacists' similar to Resident Doctors or 'House Surgeons' of medical field. These resident pharmacists should be appointed in all the sections of hospital pharmacy in rotation where senior hands are available to train, supervise and evaluate their work. Thus suitable man power can be created in the due course of time.

Infrastructure

In order to provide proper and effective service to the patients, good infrastructure must be provided for the hospital pharmacy. These infrastructure facilities can be as per the following requirements:

(a) All equipments and instruments for the manufacture and analysis of formulation as per schedule M for Drugs and Cosmetics acts and rules of govt of India. These are necessary to follow GMT and GLP as per WHO and USFDA standards.

(b) All the necessary equipment for compounding, repacking and dispensing in the main, satellite and ward pharmacies as per medical and pharmacy manuals and orders of Governments

(c) Proper storage facilities including refrigerators and air conditioners with adequate, cubboard, storage space, flour space and lightings in the medical and surgical stores of the hospital. These stores as well as dispensaries should have separate cubboard with lock facilities for narcotics and other controlled substances.

(d) Central sterile service section should be equipped with latest sterilization facilities and storage area free from contamination with laminar work bench, airlock ante room etc.

(e) As all above area are continuous processing and /or storage areas and midway stopping of which may create huge problems they must be provided with un interrupted power supply using generators, invertors etc.

(f) A library with adequate latest books and online and data base resources should be available both for use by pharmacists and doctors. There should be necessary facilities for data retrieval, storage, copying and recording. New edition of Pharmacopoeias, Text book on Pharmacology, toxicology, therapeutics biochemistry, microbiology, and drugs indexes should be available in this library apart from professional periodicals (journals) on the above subjects.

(g) In order to mountain above facilities, adequate clerical and non-clerical services should be provided. Hence a well equipped office with stenographic, book keeping people must be available. Needless to mention furniture and fixtures necessary for all the above activities must be in place.

Work Load Statistics

While calculating work load for the entire hospital pharmacy organization, each of its section's specific needs should be taken into account. For example, in order to calculate the number of pharmacists required to man the outpatient counter for dispensing prescriptions, average number of outpatients per day has to be arrived at. Then average time in minutes required to dispense prepackaged medicines for a prescription has to be calculated and then number of counters to be opened and manned by pharmacists can be arrived at. It was estimated usually 4 minutes are required to dispense prepacked medicine and upto 14 minutes if compounding and packaging are required. If sufficient manpower is provided, the waiting time by the patient in front of the dispensary and the crowd can be minimized.

As per medical/ pharmacy manual published by state governments in India, a pharmacist has to dispense around 60 patients per day of 6 hours shift, allotting 6 minutes per patient. But in practice, due to various reasons like, huge crowd in government hospitals, disproportionate pharmacists appointed in our hospitals, a Govt. Hospital pharmacist is dispensing to 100 patients per day and he is forced to work more than 10 hours a day. This makes the quality of services provided by a pharmacist to a patient to go down, resulting in friction, quarrel, dissatisfaction and disappointment to patients as well to the pharmacist.

Hence correct calculation of work load and its statistics assume importance to determine the manpower requirement. The work load has to be calculated for other sections of hospital pharmacy, for example, in the case of clinical pharmacy services, at least one clinical pharmacist should be appointed for two wards and to provide round the clock service 3 of them are needed. Similarly to provide these services to outpatients 2 or 3 clinical pharmacists are needed during OP hours. Other sections like central sterile services, drug information centre, stores and purchase require a minimum of one PG pharmacist and 2 or 3 graduate pharmacist as assistants.

If a manufacturing section is available in hospital, it requires elaborate production program and planning as in Pharma industry. It may need the services of experts in material management and finance which are dealt below separately.

Pharmacists required for a 500 bed hospital with full Hospital Pharmacy and 1200 outpatients per day:

Table 2.1 Work Load Statistics- Manpower Requirement

S. NO	SECTION/ DESIGNATION	NUMBER OF M.PHARM OR PHARM.D	NUMBER OF B.PHARM	NUMBER OF D.PHARM	TOTAL
1.	H.O.D/ DIRECTOR	1 [M.PHARM OR PHARM.D, AND PH. D]	-	-	1
2.	DEPUTY DIRECTOR [PRODUCTION, Q.C, CSS]	1[M.PHARM]	-	-	1
3.	DEPUTY DIRECTOR [CL.PH, DIC, EDUCATION]	1[PHARM. D]	-	-	1
4.	DEPUTY DIRECTOR [PURCHASE, STORES, DISPENSARY]	1[M.PHARM]	-	-	1
5.	MANUFACTURE	1[M.PHARM]	5	12	18
6.	QUALITY CONTROL	1[M.PHARM]	2	-	3
7.	CENTRAL STERILE SERVICE	--	1	2	3
8.	CLINICAL PHARMACY SERVICE	12[PHARM.D]	-	-	12
9.	DRUG INFORMATION CENTRE	1[PHARM. D]	3	-	4
10.	PURCHASE AND STORES	1[M.PHARM]	3	6	10
11.	DISPENSARY	-	3	20	23
	TOTAL	20	17	40	77

Functions

As described in the flowchart above, each section of the modern hospital pharmacy perform specific function assigned to it. The following are some of the functions of each section.

1. Manufacturing Section

(i)   It estimate the annual demand for each drug used in the hospital.

(ii) Plan the production schedule.

(iii) Manufacture the required items as per plan after purchasing needed raw materials, packing materials etc.

(iv) Carryout any special work entrusted to it like, preparation of IV admixture, total parental nutrition etc.

(v)   Check the standards of formulations by QC and QA department.

2. Purchase Section

(i)   Estimate the demand or the quantity of drugs required.

(ii) Specifications for the needed drugs are arrived at, in consultation with departments concerned. This includes quality, quantity, packing, strength, etc.

(iii) Follow the approved purchase procedure like calling for tenders, quotations and identifying the supplier to place orders.

(iv) Receive, verify and dispatch the drugs to quarantine area and then to stores after approval by quality control section.

(v)   Settle the bills and be ready for any emergency purchases.

3. Quality Control Section

(i)   It keeps ready the methods of analysis, equipment, chemicals and other requirements for almost all drugs either manufactured or purchased by the hospital.

(ii) Draw sample from manufacturing section or quarantine area if purchased from outside.

(iii) Analyze and submit its report to the people concerned. Thus certifying the quality of drugs used in the hospital.

(iv) Undertake research and development studies with respect to the drugs manufactured in the hospital in order to improve its efficacy as well as to reduce the cost.

(v)   Send samples to outside laboratories, if it cannot be analyzed by it.

4. Stores Section

   (i)   It receives drugs from either manufacturing section or purchase department.

  (ii) Store them properly until issued to the dispensary and other places, according to specified storage conditions, so as to preserve its efficacy and potency.

 (iii) Issue drugs to dispensary and other departments as per their approved indents.

 (iv) Keep account for all input and output as well as stock on hand (inventory control).

  (v) Monitor the drug use pattern to inform and assist the authorities and manufacturing section in production plan or purchase plan.

 (vi) Look for expiry date of all items stored, periodically and physically and bring to the notice of people concerned, about near or short expiry items, so as to either use them earlier or return to the supplier.

5. Dispensary

   (i)   Receive the drugs required for dispensing to outpatients, in sufficient quantities from the stores of the hospital.

  (ii) Be ready with prepacking or repacking of drugs for dispensing.

 (iii) Dispense them to patients by following high standards of dispensing like auxiliary labels, proper packing and instructions written on the envelope apart from clear and louder oral instructions.

 (iv) Maintain account for the drugs issued on daily basis.

  (v) Provide clean, neat and comfortable environment for the patients waiting to get their drugs.

6. Central Sterile Supply Department

   (i)   Procure, install and maintain all the required sterilization equipments.

  (ii) Prepare, update, stock and maintain an inventory of items, equipments and instruments required by various departments of the hospital.

 (iii) Sterilize the required items, as per the SOP prepared earlier and supply to needed departments.

 (iv) Prepare and circulate educative literatures to all the departments concerned on infection control as well as on maintenance of sterility and sterile area up keeping.

  (v) Always keep ready the emergency ward supplies.

7. Clinical Pharmacy Services

   (i)   Adequate numbers of clinical pharmacists are engaged, wherever needed, including outpatient department and all wards.

(ii) Conduct medication history interview for all or specific patients admitted in the hospital and forward the relevant details to the treating physician or surgeon.

(iii) Identify the drugs brought to the hospital by the patients and give guidance either to use or discard them or forward to doctor.

(iv) After diagnosis, the clinical pharmacist is required to give his expert opinion on the suitable drug formulation and dose for the particular patient to the treating doctor, if solicited.

(v) Once treatment commences, he has to monitor the patient for the effects of drugs by conducting necessary pharmacokinetic tests on his blood, body fluids and other samples. Based on these tests he can recommend to the doctor, to change the medicine or reduce or increase the dose or altogether stop the medicine. Adverse drug reactions are particularly monitored on the patients who are on long time treatment.

(vi) He has to counsel the patients, as and when necessary during the course of treatment or at the time of his discharge from the hospital. Provide the patient with necessary medicines and instructions to follow, to continue the treatment or recovery at home.

(vii) Receive and maintain the feedback sent by patients after discharge.

8. Drug Information Services

(i) Pharmacist in charge of this service is required to collect, arrange and provide whatever drug information needed by public or health care professionals or research students.

(ii) Update the information available with him, periodically.

(iii) Prepare and circulate literatures, brochures, bulletins or circulars on all important matters with respect to the drugs use to all the people concerned.

9. Education and Training Services

(i) Provide education and training to student pharmacists, student nurses, student doctors and even to other health care employees of the hospital.

(ii) Undertake educational programs for the public.

(iii) Accept and deliver lectures in professional associations and other clubs like Lions club, Rotary club etc., on the drug related matters and also on public health issues.

Management of Materials and Finance

Materials Management is an art, not science because it differs from organization to organization depends on the importance given to it. It has no set standards as in science subjects, because of company's perception about it differs according to the need and policies of the company. However in a hospital pharmacy set up we have to define it, as the hospital pharmacy is dealing with life saving job.

Experts of management define it as follows: "Materials management is all about planning, organizing and controlling all activities concerned with flow of materials in to an organization"

Another western expert define it as "the function of business that is responsible for the co ordination of planning, sourcing, purchasing, making, storing and controlling materials in an optimum manner, so as to provide service to the customer at a pre determined level at a minimum cost"

The second definition reveals all about the functions of materials manager. Simply speaking his job is to maintain supply chain without interruption in the production or normal function of the department. It is a challenge to maintain consistent flow of materials as it depends on various external factors which are not directly under our control. It is actually about maintaining control over the inventory which is dealt in detail in a separate chapter on 'Purchase and Inventory control'

One may be inclined to believe materials management begins only after its procurement or purchase and its arrival. But the reality is it starts even before that. Materials manager has to first identify the right source for the supply of the materials and then gather information about its quality, price, reliability, transportability etc, before purchase. Thus he has to purchase the materials at right time, of right quality, in the right quantity, from the right source at right price—the five 'R's. Even if one R goes wrong, it will have great impact on the services by the materials management department. Hence the department should set the following goals or aims:

1. To purchase correct quality material at lowest price.
2. To maintain flow of materials without break.
3. To have three or four suppliers for the same goods thereby promote competition among them.
4. To maintain good relationship with suppliers, so that up to date information about materials are shared or conveyed.
5. To follow good 'inventory turn over rate' thereby avoiding excess stock and consequent carrying cost and damage to the materials.

If the above goals are achieved by hospital pharmacy department, then the cost of production or purchase of drugs will be cheaper than other supplies, which automatically leads to less cost of distribution and maximum satisfaction about the organization to the higher authorities and patients.

Finance Management

It is the efficient and effective management of finance of the organization in order to achieve the goals of it. It deals with the subjects like how to get or raise capital or how to allocate it to various activities so that the organizations functions are carried out smoothly and correctly. It is defined differently by different experts. Let us look at few of them:

"Financial management is the area of business management devoted to the judicious use capital and a careful selection of source of capital in order to able a business firm to move in the direction of reaching its goals' – J.F. Bradlery.

"Financial management may be defined as that area or set of administrative function in an organization which relate with arrangement of cash and credit so that organization may have the means to carry out its objective as satisfactory as possible"—Haward and Option.

"Financial management can be defined as the management of finances of a business or organization in order to achieve financial objectives" The objectives are

1. To create wealth for the business
2. Generate cash and
3. Provide an adequate return on investment bearing in mind the risks the business is taking and the resources invested –Jim Riley

Though a pharmacist is not completely involved in hospital management, at least he must be familiar with his department's income and expenses. He cannot plead ignorance about the subject and hence a junior pharmacist on joining the department should be involved in hospital pharmacy's budget preparation and related works. The basic aspects of these works are explained in Chapter 8 – Budget of Hospital Pharmacy. If the hospital pharmacy choose to undertake manufacturing of drugs an elaborate set up is needed with people having experience in accounts, purchase, billing, correspondence etc., The HOD or director must be in a position to control and supervise above people. These works can be learned by experience in the department; hence the students and junior pharmacists are advised to show interest in these activities of hospital pharmacy from the beginning of their career.

As most of the functions of financial management like estimation of capital requirement, composition of capital, choice of source of funds, investment of funds etc, are taken care of by the top hospital management, a HOD or Director of hospital pharmacy has to assist them in arriving at the decisions and conclusions in those matters. Minor functions like, management of cash of the department etc, has to be carried out by the department head and he must be in a position to avoid wastage of funds and find out methods to generate income by any of the services of the department.

Strictly speaking financial management is about income and expenses of the department. But as far as a hospital is concerned income is negligible and all expenses only. Hence hospitals and health care sector is always considered as 'white elephants' by the finance ministry of the Govt, meaning thereby they 'eat too much and produce nothing.' Though this image is hard to break, the hospital pharmacy can minimize the burden on the government by generating some income or by reducing expenses on drugs. Hospital Pharmacy manufacturing unit offer such a golden chance to the pharmacists, as drugs and formulations can be manufactured in it, often at one fourth or one third of its cost by outside suppliers. This aspect should be focused to finance ministry officials, so that they start supporting drug manufacturing units in hospitals, which the author [S.B] personally witnessed during his student days.

Role and Responsibilities of Hospital Pharmacist

Role of a Hospital Pharmacist

The primary role of a Hospital Pharmacist was to dispense drugs to the outpatients. This was the major and almost only role played by him traditionally till a few decades ago. But after the concept of modern hospital pharmacy was evolved, where the functions of it is widened he has multiple role to play. Now a modern hospital pharmacist to undertake manufacturing and analysis of drug formulations, provide clinical pharmacy services to patients, educate and train student pharmacists, nurses and doctors, provide drug information to medical practitioners, research scholars and general public, procure, store and distribute drugs and surgical items, apart from sterile equipments to wards and operation theaters through central sterile services.

Though all these roles are assigned to a hospital pharmacists, in practice, many of these roles are denied to him or yet to be developed in poor countries. However today's budding pharmacists may have to shoulder these roles and responsibilities sooner or later, once our governments decided to go for full pledged hospital pharmacy.

Responsibilities of Hospital Pharmacists

(a) **Chief pharmacist:** He is overall in charge for the functioning of the department. Hence he must have some working knowledge about each and every section of his department and that is the reason why only experienced pharmacists are promoted and appointed as chief pharmacists. A highly academically qualified pharmacist without experience in day to day functioning cannot be directly appointed to the post as he cannot do justice to the post.

The chief pharmacist has the responsibility to plan, organize and control all activities of the hospital pharmacy. He should be able to guide, motivate and supervise works of all sections of hospital pharmacy. As he is included as a member of many hospital committees, he is expected to participate and contribute meaningfully to functions of those committees.

Manufacturing of drug formulations require constant supervision and vigilance on the part of higher authorities otherwise a simple mistake there can lead to huge losses and problems to the hospital. He must periodically inspect those facilities, often without prior intimation. He has similar responsibilities in the proper functioning of central sterile services, clinical pharmacy services and dispensary. All these services have great impact with functions of various departments of hospitals and in patients safety and their satisfaction about pharmacy services.

The chief pharmacist is also responsible for organizing training for pharmacy students and staff. He should organize and participate in public health camps periodically or as and when necessary and should publish news letters, bulletins etc. He should maintain cordial relationship with other HODs, so that a smooth functioning of hospital is ensured and also pharmacy department will get needed support and services from other departments whenever needed.

(b) **Other pharmacists:** These are given as functions of different sections of hospital pharmacy elsewhere in this chapter. One important responsibility common to all these pharmacists is to learn the works of other sections also, so that, on transfer or in case of emergency, the department can function effectively without interruption. Senior pharmacists in charge of each section have to give training to student pharmacists and newly appointed junior pharmacists in their section. Thus future man power requirement of hospital pharmacist will be fulfilled.

Supportive Services

In any hospital apart from the clinical or medical departments there are many other departments or services which are essential to provide efficient and complete therapy to the patients. They are generally known as supportive services. In India these services are together called by the name 'Paramedical Services' derived from the word 'parallel.' As a train requires two parallel rails to run, hospital services also require both these medical and paramedical services on equal plain for its functioning, thereby emphasizing their co-operation.

Various Supportive Services

There are many services which support a clinician in his task of providing safe and effective treatment to the patients. They are

1. Pharmacy services,
2. Nursing services,
3. Dietary services,
4. Laboratory services,
5. Medical record services and
6. Other services.

Under lab services there are many sub divisions like, Pathology, Radiology, and Blood bank etc. Apart from the above there are few other departments like Central Sterile Service department and medical social service department. If students in pharmacy undergo a training program in hospitals, they can come across all these services, for that they have to be posted in other areas like wards. Even otherwise, they should try to know about these services on their own interest. They should not confine themselves within the four walls of dispensary or Medical stores of the hospital where only they are usually trained. To help them in that endeavor a brief introduction about these services are given below:

1. ***Pharmacy services:*** This is elaborately dealt in the chapter on 'Hospital Pharmacy.' The services of Central Sterile Service department also explained there, as they are under Pharmacy department in many hospitals.

2. ***Nursing services:*** There are two types of nursing services in any hospital, outpatient services and inpatient services. Nurses are posted in all clinical department's outpatient sections or in wards. In outpatient department [OPD] they assist the doctors in physical examination of the patients and then guide them to either Clinical lab for tests or to dispensary for collecting medicines prescribed. In most of the OPD they administer injections to patients though they are not supposed to. As the doctors are busy with large number of patients in crowded Govt hospitals, they are not administering injections to the outpatients even though 'Medical Manual' rules insist.

    Services of nurses are well recognized only in wards, where they are providing an appreciable service in patient care. They look after almost all needs of each patient admitted in the ward. They help in diagnostic tests, medicine administration, diet and even personal cleanness. These services were offered single handedly by nurses earlier but now-a-days a team of nurses including trainees are performing these tasks round the clock. As anything may happen to any patient at any time they are vigilant and active throughout their duty hours and beyond. Emergency situations in wards are managed by them till the doctor arrives to take over.

    Nurses are educated and trained for varying number of years from one year to four years after school finals. Thus we have Midwives, Nursing assistants, Health Visitors, Diploma nurses and B.Sc and M.Sc nurses. Usually a nursing school or college is attached to big hospitals to train student nurses who are posted in all wards and OPD to help and learn nursing services. A senior nurse [Matron, lecturer or professor] will be teaching them in ward settings. In rural Primary Health Centers apart from the above, nurses are providing medical and MATERNITY services to village peoples via sub centers or by directly visiting patient's home. Thus nursing services are one of the best supportive services of health care sector.

3. **Dietary services:** These services are organized only in big hospitals to provide special diet needed for patients admitted in wards. A post graduate senior dietician will be in charge of these services assisted by a team of junior dieticians, cooks, suppliers and helpers. They prepare the menu for day-to-day supply. They provide hygienically prepared food to all in-patients three or four times a day. These supplies include milk, fruits, eggs and even gruel or liquid diet for patients who require special diets. In small and private hospitals mostly food is not supplied but one or two dieticians will be appointed to advice and counsel the patients or their caretakers. This service is given in big hospitals also while the patients undergoing treatment in the ward or at the time of discharge. They also note down any food allergy the patient has, in patient medication chart or record. Thus dietary services are unique in nature and well received by all concerned.

4. **Laboratory services:** In olden days these services were provided by lab technicians with diploma qualification. Now B.Sc and M.Sc Biochemistry or Microbiology or Lab technology graduates have taken over the service as clinical laboratories are equipped with modern sophisticated electronic instruments. Their service starts from collecting samples like body fluids from the patients either in the lab itself or by visiting wards on the orders of clinicians and after conveying it to them by nurses. These samples are analysed or tested immediately to provide the results as early as possible to the doctors who ordered them, so that they can start or modify the treatment given to the patients. Hence they too work round the clock in a hospital.

There are dozens of tests to carry out from tests on blood, urine, sputum, stool etc to liver function, kidney function, thyroid function and pulmonary function tests. To perform these complicated tests more special sections of lab service department are opened. They are Pathology, Radiology and microbiology sections where specialist doctors and technologists of respective fields are appointed. Thus doctors with M.D Pathology or Radiology are providing yeomen service to the patients through this department. As these departments use latest computer controlled electronic equipments like MRI scan, CT scan etc, Electronic engineers and technicians are also appointed in these sections for operation and maintenance. Sometimes the company which manufactured, supplied or erected the costly, imported machine is given maintenance contract.

As the blood bank too performing same function as clinical laboratories, most of the time they are under the control of Department of Lab services. Now-a-days blood banks are not only collecting, store and supply the blood but also separate the components of blood like platelets and supply them to needed hospitals. Hence graduates specialized in blood bank technology are appointed in this department. As with any health care department this department also functions through day and night.

5. *Medical record services:* In this department medical records of all inpatients are stored for future reference. Records of deserving, chronic and essential outpatients also kept here. These services were once maintained with papers, files etc which make it difficult for up keeping and retrieval after few years as thousands of cases are treated every year in big hospitals. But after the arrival of computers it has become less onerous job.

    In this section complete detail about the patient is maintained starting from his identification, medication history, case diary with day-to-day physical examination results, lab tests results including x-ray, scan reports, patient medication profile and discharge summary. In the unfortunate event of patient's death in hospital his post mortem report also filed. Hard copies of all these records are maintained in separate files or folders. As it has become voluminous and unmanageable mass, now-a-days all these records are scanned and entered in computers. This requires a skilled person to do the work and hence Medical Record Stores keeper courses are conducted and persons with this qualification are given preference over others with just clerical qualification. The medical records not only help the doctors to understand the patients' body condition in future, if they come back to hospital but also serve as a proof or defensive document in court litigations, if any to save the health care team and the hospital. Thus medical record services also acquire importance in a hospital's supportive services.

6. *Other services:* In developed countries a separate medical social record services section function to focus on the social aspects of patient and his family. They follow-up the patients if it is not all, at least critical cases. They record home environment of the patients, help if any from the community agencies, rehabilitation or risk of relapse of disease etc and convey to health care authorities for necessary actions including framing of national health policy. In India separate medical social services are not established though some of the above functions are carried out by various members of health care team like Health Visitors [Nurses], Health Inspectors, Sanitary inspectors and Non Governmental organizations. Any how a coordinated service is lacking. Let us hope this will be established in future.

'Medical Tourism'

As drug therapy given to a patient is monitored, evaluated and adjusted to suit the needs of individual patient by clinical pharmacists, he is considered as an authority for safe and rational use of drugs by law enforcing and insurance authorities in developed countries. Hence when patients from foreign countries come to India for treatment, they expect such services from Indian hospitals also. This leads to appointment of clinical pharmacists by big corporate Indian hospitals, thus, they ensure continuous flow of foreign patients.

In 'Medical Tourism' as it is named recently, people coming to India as tourists, utilizes their trip to treat their illness. It is a growing sector that is expected to achieve an annual growth rate of 30% to reach a turnover of Rs 10 Lakhs crores by 2015. There are many reasons for this. Major among them is raising cost of treatment in developed countries. Other reasons are long waiting period to get treatment or surgery in their countries and availability of high class facilities in India.   Hence every year near about 1,50,000 persons come to India for treatment in areas like cosmetic surgery, heart surgeries or bypass surgeries, bone marrow transplantation, hip replacement etc.

To attract more such patients, Indian Government is taking steps to improve infrastructure facilities available in India. In order to raise the health care standards to international level, appointment of post graduate clinical pharmacist in every hospital, is important. As the cost of treatment in India is approximately one tenth of that in developed countries, appointing clinical pharmacist and charging the patients for his services may not be a big problem. Thus big development prospects are waiting for pharmacists of India.

Questions

Short Answer Questions

1. Define hospital pharmacy.
2. Write briefly about origin and development of hospital pharmacy.
3. Write a note on the responsibilities of Hospital Pharmacist.

Long Answer Questions

4. Enumerate the organizational structure of a modern hospital pharmacy.
5. Explain the functions of various sections of a hospital pharmacy.
6. Describe the works of a hospital pharmacy with qualification of persons appointed to carry out those jobs.
7. What are the duties a pharmacist is expected to perform after dispensing in a modern hospital pharmacy set up?
8. Explain the staff requirement, infrastructure and work load of a modern hospital pharmacy.
9. Enumerate the management of materials and finance of a hospital pharmacy.
10. Discuss the role of supportive services of a hospital.

CHAPTER 3

PHARMACY AND THERAPEUTIC COMMITTEE

Introduction

Spurt in the growth of scientific knowledge and availability of sophisticated electronic instruments and equipments, in the last few decades lead to thousands of new drugs being introduced into the market. It is estimated that there are more than 70,000 formulations available in India for prescribing by doctors. It is obviously impossible for anybody to remember so many formulations and their uses or merits.

Hence it is necessary for the hospital to establish a system to bring the best medicine to the attention of the staff and this assists them in the proper selection of drugs for the treatment of patients. This educational programme is achieved through 'Pharmacy and Therapeutic Committee' formed in the hospitals.

It is a committee of the medical and Paramedical staff and serves as a liaison between the medical staff and the pharmacy service on all matters pertaining to the use of drugs in the hospital.

Definition

Hassan defines Pharmacy and Therapeutic Committee as "a policy framing and recommending body to the medical staffs and the administration of the hospital, on matters related to the safe and rational use of drugs".

Objectives

There are three major roles for the Pharmacy and Therapeutic Committee:

1. Advisory
2. Education and
3. Safe and rational use of drugs

1. **Advisory**

   As seen earlier, the primary role of PTC is to assist the physician in the proper selection of drugs. Hence PTC is advising on the formulation and adaptation of policies regarding evolution, selection and therapeutic use of drugs in hospitals. Thus its main objective is to serve in an advisory capacity to the medical staff and hospital administration in all matters related to the use of drugs including investigational drugs. It also advises the pharmacy department regarding effective drug distribution and control.

2. **Education**

   PTC helps the administration of hospitals in formulating programs to meet the educational needs of all the staff concerned like Physicians, Nurses, Pharmacists and other health care professionals to update their knowledge on matters related to drugs and their use. Towards this objective PTC is entrusted with the function of selecting staff for continuing education program and also preparation and updating of Hospital formulary – a valuable reference book for hospital staff.

3. **Safe and rational use of drugs**

   As present day medicines are highly potent and powerful one has to take extra care while handling, administering and using the drugs. If the advises of PTC and its educational supports are correctly followed safe use of drugs can be ensured. But in reality medical staff, nurses and pharmacists are overlooking the guidelines given by the PTC, resulting in irrational and dangerous use of drugs. When an adverse incident involving the use of drugs happened and reported outside, everybody starts blaming each other for whatever happened. Hence PTC is repeatedly warning the staff not to ignore its guidelines on matters pertaining to the safe and rational use of drugs. Thus the first two objectives of advice and education are to achieve the final objective of safe use of drugs.

Organization

The organization of the committee may vary from hospital to hospital. However the following composition is generally followed:

1. A minimum of 3 physicians from among the medical staff of the hospital.
2. A Pharmacist (usually the HOD or chief pharmacist)
3. A Nurse and
4. An Administrator

One among the above physician is appointed as the chairman of the committee. The pharmacist is designated as the secretary.

PTC also constitutes many sub-committees, which are either permanent or formed for a specific purpose temporarily. In these sub-committees, specialists are included either as president or as member in order to utilize their knowledge and experience in the particular field. Thus there may be sub-committee on Antibiotics, cardio vascular drugs, hormones and corticosteroids, narcotics and other CNS drugs.

PTC can also invite persons from within or outside the hospital to its meetings, who can contribute their specialized knowledge and judgments. The committee must meet regularly at least six times in a year, or more times if necessary. As it is usual with any committee, the secretary should maintain minutes of the meeting with all necessary other documents. The decisions of the committee are communicated to the people concerned and implemented or executed by the secretary. These works are reported by him to the committee members, in the next meeting of the committee.

Primary Functions

Though PTC has advisory and educational objectives, the primary or ultimate aim of the PTC is safe and rational use of drugs in the hospital. In order to fulfil that objective, PTC plays important role in:

1. Adverse Drug Reaction (ADR) monitoring
2. Drug product defect reporting
3. Psychotropic drugs use
4. Emergency drugs use
5. Drug utilization review and
6. Safe use of all drugs.

Each of the above functions is meticulously carried out by PTC by issuing necessary regulations and guidelines to the staff concerned. Let us have a look at these guidelines in detail.

1. *Adverse drug reaction monitoring (PTC and ADR):* Adverse drug reaction is defined as a reaction that is noxious, unintended and occurs at *normal* doses used in human. Though it occurs less frequently, the cause for it must be thoroughly investigated to prevent such reactions in other patients, or at least to be vigilant on all patients given the drug in question.

   Hence, some organization in the hospital must be given charge of this responsibility. PTC takes up this responsibility and monitors the therapy throughout the hospital. Its main aim is to prevent ADR and if occurred, to take follow-up action, including treatment to the particular patient, reporting to authorities concerned and avoids such ADR in future.

   In order to do that effectively PTC issues a set of guidelines to the medical and Para-medical staff of the hospital, including ADR reporting form, to report in the unfortunate event of its occurrence without hiding. The model ADR reporting form is given below:

Name of the Hospital and Location
Adverse Drug Reaction Report

Ref. No: Date: ………..

Patient's Name:

Age/sex:

Hospital O.P/I.P/Regn. No.:

Disease reported/diagnosed

Details of treatment given:

Drug suspected to have produced ADR:

Detail about that drug (B. No, Mfg. Date, Exp. date, Manufacturer's Address):

Reaction Detail:

Step taken to treat ADR:

Drug in question prescribed by:

Administered by:

Other drugs concurrently administered or taken by patient, if any:

Any other relevant information:

Department/   *Signature of treating*
Ward   *physician with date*

N.B: The packing or container or balance of the suspected drugs should be retained for further reference and investigation.

On receipt of ADR report from the department or ward where it occurred, PTC starts its investigation to find out the reason for that particular ADR. If necessary it calls for further information from the reporting physician, nurse or patient. At the end of investigation by its sub-committee specially assigned this duty, PTC submit its report to authorities whoever concerned. Usually it is reported first to the Dean or Director of the hospital and then to ADR reporting authority of the State and/or Central Government and to State Drugs Control Authorities. Depends upon the seriousness and frequency of this ADR, the drug in question may be withdrawn from the market, on the orders of Drugs Control Department or it issues warning to the medical fraternity to be vigilant while using the particular drug through press or media.

2. ***Drug product defect reporting (PTC and drug's defect):*** Though everybody concerned with the use of drugs, especially patients and doctors expect a zero error or 100% defect free product, it is not always possible. Due to machine error or human error, occasionally drug reaches the user point with some or other noticeable defect. Such defects should be detected by the pharmacist or nurse or doctor, before it reaches the patient. If detected, they are duty bound to report the same to the PTC of the hospital.

Reportable defects include, inadequate packing, confusing or inadequate labels, deteriorated, contaminated or defective dosage forms, inaccurate fill or count of a drug product, faulty drug delivering apparatus, etc. Obviously, the health care professionals should report anything which in their professional opinion, is considered to be defective or undesirably associated with the drug product.

The model form for reporting the defective drug product is given below:

PTC on receipt of the above report, initiate investigation and take possession of the suspected drug product from the reporter. It reports the matter, after verification, first to the manufacturer and then to other authorities concerned, if necessary. It also orders physical inspection of the entire lot or batch of the product supplied to the hospital and take necessary action.

By this program, a sense of vigilance and duty consciousness is instilled in the minds of health care professionals and ultimately patients are getting defect free products.

3. ***Psychotropic drugs use (PTC and dangerous drugs):*** Psychotropic drugs are those drugs which on longer use produce dependence or addiction and hence it is dangerous to the patient as well as the society. Hence they are also called dangerous drugs. PTC develops guidelines, whereby dangerous drugs are purchased, stored, dispensed and properly administered under control.

The procedure for this is no different from the Psychotropic Substances Acts and rules. PTC ensures strict adherence to the above Act by the hospital staff. In some hospitals, automatic stop orders are in force whereby "all drug orders for narcotics, sedatives and hypnotics shall be automatically discontinued after 48 hours, unless

1. the order indicates the exact number of doses to be given
2. an exact period of time for the medication is specified or
3. the attending physician records the medication."

In some other hospitals, the automatic stop orders require, "all orders for narcotics, sedatives and hypnotics must be rewritten every 24 hours". Thus the PTC takes care of the use of psychotropic drugs and the patients of the hospital.

NAME OF THE HOSPITAL
ADDRESS
DRUG DEFECT REPORT

Ref No: Date:

1. Name of the drug:

2. Dosage form and strength:

3. Batch No. ------ Dt. of Mfg ----- Expiry Date: ----------

4. Manufacture's Name and Address:

5. Date of Purchase:

6. Name of the supplier and address:

7. Defects noted or suspected:

8. Reported by (Name and Designation)

9. Signature

10. Department/ward

N.B: The suspected defective drug should be preserved for further investigation.

---

4. *Emergency drugs use (PTC and emergency drugs):* As time factor is very important during emergency cases, PTC prepares a list of drugs and other supplies to be made available in emergency boxes. These boxes are kept in all important places of the hospital and given charge to some pharmacist or nursing supervisors of the hospital.

As these medicines are available literally by the side of the beds of the emergency cases, they are referred to as 'Bed side Pharmacy'.

After the emergency cup boards have been placed on the wards and other places like emergency procedures room of the department of radiology, it is mandatory that a program be developed whereby they are checked daily either by the hospital pharmacist or by the nursing supervisor responsible for the ward. The drug used on the day is replenished, as early as possible, so that, constant amount of drugs are available in the emergency cup-board, always.

Usually, some 30 items of important, life saving drugs and about 10 to 15 items of surgical instruments and dressings including syringes and needles are kept in the emergency boxes. The list may vary depends on the need of a particular hospital which may decide to add or delete some items in the emergency box. Overall, the PTC of the hospital is responsible for preparation and up-keeping of the emergency Drugs kit or 'Bed side Pharmacy'.

The following list of content is given to serve as a guide

Emergency Drugs

1. Aminophylline 0.25 gm/10 ml
2. Amphetamine sulphate 20 mg/ml
3. Amyl nitrite inhalation
4. Atropine sulphate 0.4 mg/ml
5. Caffeine sodium benzoate 0.5 gm/2 ml
6. Calcium gluconate 1 gm/10 ml
7. Chlorpheniramine maleate 10 mg/ml
8. Digoxin 0.25 mg/ml
9. Diphenyl hydantoin sodium 50 mg/ml
10. Epinephrine HCl 1:1000
11. Heparin 10,000 units/ml
12. Hydrocortisone 100 mg
13. Isoproterenol 1:100
14. Magnesium sulphate injection 10% and 50%
15. Mannitol injection 25%

16. Nalorphine HCl 10 mg/2 ml
17. Neostigmine Methylsulphate 0.25 mg/ml
18. Nor. epinephrine Injection 0.2%
19. Pentobarbital 50 mg/ml
20. Phenobarbital 120 mg/ml
21. Phenylephrine HCl 10 mg/ml
22. Picrotoxin injection 3 mg/ml
23. Procainamide 100 mg/ml
24. Protamine sulphate 10 mg/ml
25. Saline for injection 30 ml
26. Sodium molar Lactate solution
27. Water for injection 50 ml

Other Items

1. Syringes of all sizes – each 2
2. Needles of all sizes – each 2
3. Venous cannulatization set
4. Oxygen catheters
5. Sterile suction catheters
6. Razor with blades
7. Sterile gelatine sponge
8. Resuscitation tube & cart
9. Oxygen equipments
10. Burn sheets and
11. Other surgical instruments like scissors, forceps etc.

5. *Drug utilization review: (PTC and drugs use)*: Drug utilization includes prescribing, dispensing and administration of prescription drugs. Though there is no drug utilization review outside a hospital, such a review can be organized in a hospital by PTC. Providing "Hospital formulary" is one of the institutional authorities to control the drug utilization, as well as a mechanism for continuing education of physicians, nurses and pharmacists.

Obtaining 'Medication History' of the patient and maintaining 'Patient medication profile' are the other two programs, useful for a pharmacist to monitor drug utilization within the hospital.

Medication histories are taken by clinical pharmacist of required patient admitted to the hospital or seen in the outpatient department. This is accomplished by personal interview or through a computerized questionnaire specifically designed for the purpose and if the patient is in a condition to answer those questions.

If not, the interview is conducted at appropriate time, but at the earliest, with the help of patient's helpers or family members. During the interview, details regarding medicines taken during the recent past, at the time of admission and OTC drugs taken if any, are collected.

Also information about known drug allergies, idiosyncrasy towards food products and about lab tests anything conducted using diagnostic agents are also recorded. This information is passed on to the treating physician for early correct diagnosis and prescribing.

Once this is over, the patient's medication profile is prepared in the following format:

NAME OF THE HOSPITAL

ADDRESS

PATIENT MEDICATION PROFILE

No: Date:

Patient's Name

Age/sex

Address

Hospital OP/IP Regn. No.

Date of Admission

Diagnosis on Admission

Other pathology

Drug Profile

Date	Name of the Drug	Dose	Route	Started on	Stopped on	Remark	Ph. initial

Discharged on:

Signature of Chief Pharmacist

The patient medication profile can be prepared and maintained by both hospital pharmacists and community pharmacists, because drug utilization review is not possible without medication history of the patient. Community pharmacists can maintain patient medication profile of the patients who frequent their pharmacy for getting medicines for themselves and their family members. Their services will be much useful in the case of patients requiring long time therapy and those who continue treatment from their home as outpatients such as diabetes, hypertension, asthma, epilepsy and TB patients.

Modern community pharmacies, with graduate pharmacists and computer systems in their pharmacy are offering such services to the patient

6. *PTC and safe use of drugs:* Day by day lots of new drugs are introduced by hundreds of pharmaceutical manufacturers throughout the world. Consequently the responsibilities of health care professionals in general, pharmacists in particular, also increased many fold. Possibilities of error in prescription writing, dispensing and administration of these new drugs poses great problem to the pharmacist especially when the chances for Drug interaction, ADR and other problems are relatively unknown for the new drugs.

Hence PTC formulates many policies and guidelines to be followed by all concerned while handling, not only new drugs, but even the existing drugs. The following are some guidelines:

1. The hospital should appoint a qualified pharmacist to supervise the entire pharmacy services. He must be at least a graduate in pharmacy with adequate experience.

2. All dispensing operations must be carried out by qualified registered pharmacists. Non-pharmacy people should not be engaged for dispensing.

3. Adequate number of pharmacists must be appointed proportionate to the work load and round the clock service.

4. Hospital must provide adequate and safe work space and storage facilities for the pharmacy.

5. Hospital should have a hospital formulary and it should be updated every now and then or at least once in a year.

6. The pharmacist must follow all the rules regarding the storage and dispensing of narcotics, poison, and external use preparations.

7. In the hospital manufacturing section, the drugs should be manufactured according to Current Good Manufacturing Practice (CGMP) and other rules by Drugs Control Department. Strict quality control and quality assurance measures must be followed.

8. All wards and Nursing stations should be periodically checked for expired drugs, deteriorated drugs, legibility of labels etc.

9. The pharmacy should have a small library with reference books on pharmacology, toxicology, posology and pharmacopoeia, hospital formulary, drug index, etc.

10. Periodical continuing education programs should be conducted by the hospital for the staff and attendance for those programs must be compulsory.

If the above guidelines and any other guide line issued from time to time by PTC are followed in letter and spirit, safe use of drugs in the particular hospital can be ensured by and large.

Other Functions of PTC

1. The manufacturing unit of the hospital is inspected by the PTC for quality production.

2. PTC visits outside manufacturing units also before approving their products for inclusion in hospital formulary or purchase list.

3. Prepares written policies and procedures for the evaluation, selection, purchase, storage, dispensing and use of drugs.

4. Prepare the Hospital formulary and updates it periodically.

5. Forms sub-committees as and when necessary on the subjects considered essential by it.

6. Establishes procedures for cost effective drug therapy.

Questions

Short Answer Questions

1. Define PTC.
2. What are the objectives of PTC?
3. Name the composition of members of PTC.
4. Write a note on PTC and emergency drugs.
5. What are the other functions of PTC.

Long Answer Questions

6. Enumerate the functions of PTC.
7. Explain the role of PTC in the safe use of drugs.
8. Justify the need for forming PTC in hospitals.
9. How PTC controls ADR in hospitals?

CHAPTER 4

HOSPITAL FORMULARY

Introduction

Hospital formulary is nothing but hospital's own pharmacopoeia. Why a hospital needs its own pharmacopoeia as the Government publishes Pharmacopoeia for the entire country? There are many reasons.

1. A national Pharmacopoeia is a very big volume, which contains monographs for lot of drugs for which the government fix standards. Such a long list of drugs is not necessary for a hospital.

2. It cannot be used as a ready reference in a hospital set up, where information about a drug may be required on the spot and it cannot be made available to everybody.

3. The Pharmacopoeia does not contain all the formulations used by hospital, which are separately published in books like National Formulary, Pharmaceutical codex etc.

4. Pharmacopoeia does not contain all the information required by different health care professionals of a hospital like nurses, dieticians and laboratory technicians.

5. Since India was part of British Empire in the last two centuries, British pharmacopoeia was official in India and it has to be imported to India. Naturally it was not available throughout our country and hence hospitals have no other choice but to prepare its own pharmacopeia, in those days.

6. Due to tremendous growth of science in early 20th century, there came thousands of drug formulations into the market, with claims of unproven efficacy and safety. Doctors were confused with this claims and counter claims and also with aggressive marketing technique adopted by pharmaceutical manufactures. There arises a need for someone to verify the claim, find a worth and safe formulation, and recommend to the physicians. Hospital managements also found it very difficult to stock all the formulations prescribed by all its doctors.

Hence Hospital formulary, which contains the list of drugs approved by the hospital concerned, was prepared by expert members of the committee formed by the PTC of the hospital. The objective, content and other details about the hospital formulary are discussed below.

Objectives

The ultimate aim of publishing hospital formulary is to give the best treatment to the patient at less cost. Hospital formulary as a book has the following objectives.

It provides information on:

1. The name and other details about the drugs approved by the Hospital (to be prescribed to the patients of the particular hospital).
2. Hospital policies and procedures on the use of above drugs.
3. General Information such as dosing rule, abbreviations etc.

Content

The contents of the formulary are arranged under three main sections:

Section 1: Introduction (Policies and Procedures)

Section 2: List of Drugs and

Section 3: Additional Information

Section 1: Introduction (Policies and Procedures)

In this section, detail about the Pharmacy and Therapeutic Committee, name of its members and their designation and official addresses are given. Then the detail of sub-committee or the special committee which prepared the formulary and duties and responsibilities given to the various members of the sub-committee are detailed. It is followed by the guidelines on how to use the formulary and interpretation, meaning and legal limitations of its content. Reference to sources of detailed information on formulary drugs, such as Pharmacopoeias, National Formularies and Hospital's own Drugs Information services, are given here.

As the formulary is binding in nature to the medical and paramedical staff of the hospital, it contains all the policies of the hospital with reference to the use of drugs. For example, it describes, hospital regulations governing the prescribing, dispensing and administration of drugs. It also explains the rules regarding the prescription of controlled (Narcotic) drugs, automatic stop order, verbal drug orders, use of drug samples, reporting ADR and medication errors etc.

Pharmacy operating procedures, like working hours of various pharmacy wings of the hospital, outpatient services, inpatient services, pharmacy charging system, Drug information services etc, are also included in this premier of the hospital formulary so as to ensure a tussle free, smooth functioning of the hospital.

Section 2: List of Drugs

This section is the heart of the formulary. It lists the entire range of drugs and formulations approved by the hospital for prescribing to the patients of the hospital. They can be arranged under any one of the following methods.

1. Drugs under generic names, arranged alphabetically.
2. Drugs under generic names, arranged alphabetically but within the therapeutic classification.
3. Combination of the above two methods, in which, majority of the drugs are arranged under first method and few therapeutic classes like ophthalmic drugs, otic drugs, dermatological preparations etc are separately printed and drugs under generic name listed alphabetically in each of the above special sections

As the elaborate information about each drug is not possible and will defeat the very purpose of a book for ready reference, the formulary contains minimum essential information on each drug. They are:

1. Generic Name, if not available, as in the case of formulations, common name or even trade name.
2. Synonym, if any.
3. Dosage forms, strengths, packages and sizes, commonly stocked in the hospital's pharmacy.
4. Formula, if it is a combination product.
5. Dose (adult, children and pediatric).
6. Special instructions/precautions.

Section 3: Additional Information

The hospital formulary is prepared to guide and help the entire health care team of the hospital. Hence it contains information useful for nurses, dieticians, Lab. technicians and other public health workers. The following are the wealth of information available in a hospital formulary:

1. Posology (including methods of calculating doses)
2. Pediatric doses
3. Poisons and antidotes
4. Important laboratory values
5. Nutrition and calorific values
6. Height and weight chart

7. Immunization schedule
8. Diagnostic and pathological reagents
9. List of hospital approved abbreviations and
10. General and pharmacological index

Guiding Principles to Include or Exclude a Drug in the Formulary

The very difficult task of Pharmacy and Therapeutic committee is the selection of drugs to include in the formulary. This is more difficult because no member of the sub-committee formed for the purpose of preparation of formulary, is experienced enough in all the fields of therapy. Hence the committee always invites specialists from particular field to its meetings to take decision about the group of drugs used or available in the particular field. Thus the expert's as well hospital staff's own experience is the very first, undisputable guideline to include or exclude a particular drug in the formulary.

The second criterion is the inclusion of particular drug or formulation in other books of standard like Pharmacopoeias, National formularies etc.

The third one is the manufacturer of a particular drug must have proven integrity, dependability and track record.

The fourth one is the product in question must be approved, accepted and in market for a long time.

The fifth one is the drug or formulation must declare all its content in the label and no secret composition is acceptable to the committee.

The sixth principle is the drug or formulation must comply with all legal requirements of Drugs and Cosmetic Act and Rules, etc.

If the drug, after approval and inclusion in the formulary is found to be deficient in any one of the above principles, it will be deleted from the formulary by suitable notification or circular by the PTC.

The above principles may be published in the hospital formulary itself and/or circulated among the staff of the hospital, so as the staff to acquire an understanding, why a particular drug is not found or left out from the formulary. Also it encourages staff concerned, to recommend particular drug to the PTC if it meets all the above guiding principles.

Preparation of the Formulary

PTC of the hospital as and when decided to prepare and adopt a formulary for the hospital concerned, constitute a subcommittee for the purpose. The director or chief of pharmacy services of the hospital is given responsibility for preparing the formulary with the active participation and co-operation of all the members of the sub-committee.

The sub-committee is briefed on the series of rules or guidelines (refer above) to evaluate drugs for admission to the formulary and also on the content, format etc by PTC. If the PTC decides to have only a drug list or catalogue for use in the hospital, instead of a full formulary that is conveyed to the subcommittee which prepare the one desired. However there are many differences between a formulary and mere drug list.

A formulary is more informative in nature, as described above, its contents range from generic name of the drugs to posology, poisons and antidotes, and data required by nurses, dieticians and lab technicians, whereas the drug list or catalogue contains only the name of the drug and dose range.

Thus the formulary has an informative, educative role and hence is useful to trainee doctors, nurses and pharmacists. However the preparation, maintenance and updating the drug's list or catalogue are easier, compared to formulary. Additions and deletions are easily made to the list, whereas it requires lot of efforts, time and cost to update a formulary.

Additional information if any required about a drug in the list can be obtained only by referring to suitable sources like books, manufacturer's literature or internet or drug information centers. But the formulary gives adequate, essential information about each drug in a nutshell.

Format and Appearance

As the formulary is for ready reference on daily basis, its format is very important. Looking at the previously published formularies of other hospital within the country or abroad will give an idea to develop the one suitable for local conditions. Thus the formulary published by Vellore Christian Medical College (CMC) hospital in Tamil Nadu, offer a very good model for others. The National formulary of India (NFI) published by Government of India is equally useful as a forerunner.

Size: Experience has shown that a formulary which is sufficiently small in size to fit into the apron or clinical/lab coat will enjoy the acceptance of all concerned. Thus it can be in the size of 4″ × 7″ or 10 cm × 18 cm.

*Appearance***:** Each section of the formulary can be printed in different colour papers, thus helping the user to locate the particular section quicker. Thus poisons and antidotes section, for example, can be printed on pink colour paper and pediatric section on light green colour paper, laboratory values on blue colour paper and so on. Additionally or alternatively 'edge index' can also be used, but which make the production cost to go up marginally.

Since the formulary is to be used often and carried daily, good bound volumes should be prepared with covers ranging from paper and card board to plastic or leather binding. At the same time formulary should be printed on good quality paper in order to reduce its overall weight to carry in coat packets, easily.

Moreover hospital formulary must be updated and revised as often as possible or necessary. Usually formulary is updated once in a year. In the meanwhile if required, supplements may be published in between the editions.

Distribution of Formulary

Formulary should be distributed to the following people or places of the hospital.

1. All the Doctors employed in the hospital
2. All the wards of the hospital
3. All the Heads of the Department who are related to patient care.
4. Outpatient Department (OPD) and emergency room (causality)
5. All the sections of hospital pharmacy including stores and Drug Information Center and
6. Administrative office of the hospital.

The hospital formulary copies can be sent to the higher authorities like Pharmacy Council of India, State Pharmacy Council, Director of Medical Education, Director of Medical and Public Health Services, Director of Drugs Control and to the Library of University of Health Sciences.

Advantages and Disadvantages of Hospital Formulary

Advantages

1. Patients are assured of safe and rational drug therapy.
2. The treatment given to them costs less, compared to treatment with irrational and expensive drugs or drugs with doubtful benefits.

Disadvantages

1. It restricts doctor's freedom to prescribe drugs of their choice.
2. If the formulary is not updated regularly new and effective drugs arrived cannot be prescribed to patients.
3. If the guiding principle for including or excluding a drug in the hospital formulary is not followed strictly, there are chances of unwanted drugs entering into the formulary or deserving drugs left out of the formulary, which results in the defeating the very purpose of hospital formulary.

Nevertheless, by and large hospital formulary system is a most useful system to large country like India.

Questions

Short Answer Questions

1. What is Hospital formulary?
2. What are the objectives of Hospital formulary?
3. Discuss the advantages and disadvantages of Hospital formulary.

Long Answer Questions

4. Explain the content of Hospital formulary.
5. What are the criteria for selecting a drug to include in Hospital formulary?
6. What are the guiding principles to prepare a Hospital formulary?
7. How Hospital formularies differ from Pharmacopeia? Explain the format and appearance of the Hospital Formulary.

CHAPTER 5

HOSPITAL COMMITTEES

Introduction

There are many committees formed in a hospital for efficient functioning and administration of the hospital. Some are formed for a specific purpose, whenever necessary and known as ad-hoc committee. They are temporary and as and when the purpose of the committee is over they get dissolved. Such committees may be formed not only at hospital level but department and unit level too. In contrast to these committees, what we are referring to hospital committees in this chapter are permanent and standing committees formed in a hospital.

Definition

Hospital committees are regular, permanent or standing committees formed as prescribed by regulatory agencies and considered essential by hospital administration in formulating policies, coordinating and monitoring all hospital activities that are considered important to deliver quality health care services.

Various Committees

In a large hospital like medical college hospital and district head quarters hospitals, various committees are formed for the hospital's effective function and to monitor various activities of it, because of their sheer size and inevitability. The following are some of these committees.

1. Pharmacy and Therapeutic Committee (PTC).
2. Antibiotic committee.
3. Infection control committee.
4. Research and Ethics committee.
5. Purchase committee etc.

Organization

These committees are formed by the top hospital administration in consultation and consent of Board of Directors or Trust or Government. They report to and supervised by a person higher in rank and whose main responsibility is related to that of committee he supervises. He must be in a position to assist in the performance of the particular committee. Usually he, in turn report to the Dean or Medical Director or Hospital Superintendent of the hospital on behalf of the committee he supervises.

Members: There are 3 types of members

- (a) Regular members
- (b) Ad-hoc members and
- (c) Ex-officio members

Regular Members

There may be adequate prescribed number of regular members appointed to the committee and the tenure of them in these committees may be initially for a year and subject to renewal. They must attend the meetings of the committee regularly and perform the tasks of the committee.

Ad-hoc Members

Few ad-hoc members are invited by the regular members to the meetings of the committee and they assist in the functioning of the committee. They need not attend all the meetings but as and when required. Their tenure in the committee is also for a year subject to renewal.

Ex-officio Members

Some higher officials of the department or hospital will be nominated or invited to the committee meetings and they are called as ex-officio members. They attend the meeting as and when needed and advise the committee on all important matters before the committee.

For any committee to function effectively certain documents are needed. Important among them are the Minutes book, Periodical Reports, and inter office communications. In the Minutes book, the agenda of each meeting and discussion on each topic is recorded by the secretary of the committee. It also contains the decisions taken, the resolutions passed and action taken on the previous meeting decisions. The members present put their signature at the end of the meeting below the minutes recorded. Similarly periodical reports submitted to higher authorities and inter office communications are separately maintained.

Functions and Responsibilities

The general functions of hospital committees are to frame the policies, coordinate and supervise hospital-wide activities on given area of responsibility. They may also be given some specific functions such as training and education to people concerned to achieve the goal and conducting research for the same.

In order to function effectively each committee is given certain responsibilities. The common responsibilities for all the committees are:

1. To conduct regular monthly meetings
2. To report monthly to next higher authority like Executive Committee of the Medical Board and
3. To report annually to the Medical Board.

The specific responsibilities are:

I.   Antibiotics committee

The members of this committee include chief pharmacist, nurses and physicians of clinical departments and others considered to be useful in this committee by the chairman of the committee. This committee is mainly formed to promote rational and safe use of antibiotics in the hospital. Hence the responsibilities are:

1. Review of antibiotic prescriptions dispensed.
2. Regular periodic review of antibiotic usage.
3. Detect, enquire and supervise the antibiotic resistant cases.
4. Guide and advice on the products useful in infection control.
5. Carry out research on new antibiotic formulations.

Among the above, antibiotic resistance is considered critical and needed full attention by the committee because of its danger to the society.

II.   Infection control committee

Members of this committee include epidemiologist, nurses and physicians from various clinical departments; others deemed appropriate by the chairperson of the committee can be included. The primary responsibility of the committee is to control infections spreading from the patient to the employees and others inside the hospital. The other responsibilities are:

1. To frame policies and procedures for isolation, outbreak investigation, surveillance and environment control.
2. To advise on products that has impact on infection control.
3. To frame policies and monitor their implementation concerning use of equipment, sterilization and procedures.

4. To make recommendations to control occurrence and spreading of infections.

5. To approve department wise infection control policies and procedures and

6. To evaluate significant infections occurring in hospital employees.

III. Research and ethics committee

The main responsibilities of this committee are to control and monitor the clinical trials and researches conducted in the hospital. This responsibility acquires significance in the context of many reports of unethical clinical trials and hiding the failures, errors and damages caused to the patients undergoing such trials.

The Committee looks after the following:

1. Approve new clinical trials as well as review the ongoing trials.

2. Approve the research and other experiments on the patients.

3. Promote ethical use of drugs, equipments and clinical tests on the patients by the hospital staff.

4. Help the staff involved in research by proper education, guidance and supervision.

5. Coordinate with outside agencies and organizations in research activities like post marketing surveillance of drugs etc.

IV. Pharmacy and therapeutic committee and

V. Purchase committee.

These are the other hospital committees, whose formation, function and responsibilities are discussed in separate chapters.

Role of Pharmacists in Hospital Committees

From the above discussions it is clear that hospital pharmacist has a greater role to play in all the above committees. His valuable contributions are required especially in Antibiotics committee and Research and Ethics committee.

In antibiotic committee, he can contribute significantly because he dispenses and monitor the use of antibiotics and hence in a position to detect the noncompliance by the patients which is one of the main reason for antibiotic resistance. He can detect them by patient medication interview as well as patients counselling, both of which are his primary functions as clinical pharmacist. As antibiotic misuse is wide spread, resulting in the danger of creating resistant strains of microorganism, his role in controlling such a situation is very much important. Hence, he is given the role of secretary or coordinator of this committee.

Similarly, he can contribute to research, by his knowledge of pharmacokinetics and pharmacodynamic of a drug, drug-drug interaction etc. Thus his role in research and ethics committee may be invaluable. He is an expert in evaluating a drug physically, chemically as well as pharmacologically and hence can help the hospital authorities in decision making and controlling unwanted incidences.

Thus the role of pharmacist in hospital committees is indispensable.

Questions

Short Answer Questions

1. What are hospital committees?

2. Name various committees of a hospital.

3. Discuss the role of pharmacists in hospital committees.

Long Answer Questions

4. Explain the functions and responsibilities of various hospital committees.

5. Write the functions of antibiotic committee and infection control committee of a hospital.

6. How a hospital committee is organized? Who are all its members? How its meetings are conducted and recorded?

CHAPTER 6

THERAPEUTIC GUIDELINES

Developing Therapeutic Guidelines

Introduction

Origin

We know human body, diseases and their manifestations, diagnosis and treatment; all are complex in nature and leads to different interpretations and inferences. Hence the treatment given to patients, even for a same disease, differs patient to patient, doctor to doctor and place to place. This opaque situation leads to many complications, confusions and controversies in the world of medical sciences. That is why there were many attempts by well meaning physicians and surgeons to document their observation, treatment and its results. These documents were published in medical journals and subsequently found a place in text books of Medicine, Surgery and Therapeutics. As these isolated documents were not readily available for doctors in emergency or when they are hard pressed for time, they were later organized in to reference books to guide the doctors in need.

Merck Sharp and Dohme [MSD] company of USA took lead in this and started publishing some sort of guidelines as early as 1899, in the form of a manual called 'The Merck Manual.' The manual is published after complete and thorough review of published literature and research by eminent senior doctors of developed countries. It is published in the order of diseases and disorders of organs or systems of human body. It describes Etiology, Pathogenesis, symptoms and signs, clinical procedures and lab tests for diagnosis and treatment of almost all the diseases or disorders known at the time of publishing the manual.

However by no means it can be called cent percent complete and accurate and acceptable to all. Hence after the revolution in Information Technology by way of computers and internet, attempts have been made to gather and publish more comprehensive data of all treatment procedure from the majority of medical men of the world. Thus developing therapeutic guidelines for treating diseases originated and now in 21st century, we have lot of data bases, websites and books on the subject. However the role of Merck manual as a forerunner cannot be under estimated.

Of late many countries, professional associations of specialists, hospitals and medical universities have published therapeutic guidelines to assist their members, students or employees in their practice. Mostly they are available disease or disorder wise as expected. They are very much useful not only to practicing clinicians but also to junior doctors, interns, medical, pharmacy and nursing students when they enter in to their respective professional practice. Hence they are discussed in detail below.

What are Therapeutic Guidelines?

Therapeutic guidelines are systematically developed guidelines to help the doctors to select the most appropriate line of treatment in specific clinical situations. They are otherwise known as clinical guidelines or clinical practice guidelines which are recommendations developed by health care providers to serve as a guide for diagnosis, evaluation and/ or treatment of a specific disease state as defined by Grabowski.

Why Therapeutic Guidelines are required?

As mentioned above without therapeutic guidelines, treatment and its quality differ widely hospital to hospital. In order to achieve some sort of uniformity, at least for known chronic diseases, therapeutic guidelines help. It provides an opportunity to the practitioners to assess the effectiveness of his treatment and assist him in monitoring the parameters of the patients. Without therapeutic guidelines, doctors are in dark, in the matters like what diagnostic tests to carryout and what to avoid. Because of therapeutic guidelines unnecessary tests and procedures can be omitted and he can commence the treatment earlier. This reduces the cost and duration of treatment thereby giving much wanted relief to the patient and his family.

Third party payers like insurers also welcome such a procedure for obvious reasons. Most important of all aspects of therapeutic guidelines is it gives the treating physician some international research data, which he can incorporate in his line of treatment. Moreover doctors are having limited data available with them about certain group of patients like, infants, pregnant women and ethnic minorities. In such situations therapeutic guidelines are very much useful.

Aim of Therapeutic Guidelines

From the above discussions it can be safely concluded the aim of therapeutic guidelines are,

1. To improve the effectiveness of treatment
2. To minimize the duration of treatment and
3. To reduce the cost of treatment.

To achieve these aims therapeutic guidelines should be based on widely accepted guidelines and primary resources of medical literatures. There should not be any confusion about its purpose and application.

Therapeutic Guidelines Resources

There are many data bases and websites for therapeutic guidelines. Among them 'Centers for disease control and prevention' and 'National Institute of Health of USA' are important. They are free and more comprehensive in nature. American Medical Association also has therapeutic guidelines in its website. Other websites are: Agency of Health care Research and Quality [www.ahrq.gov], University of San Francisco, [http://medicine.ucsf.edu], University of Illinois at Chicago [www.uic.edu] etc,

In India website of Cardiology Society of India and other related organizations endorsed guidelines are there for hypertension. Needless to point out WHO website has many therapeutic guidelines.

Apart from the above resources there are scores of internet sites which offer therapeutic guidelines after payment or only to members after subscription. Many institution specific resources also available to be used by the employees of the particular organization [hospital] either in the form of printable booklets or link in their website protected with passwords which shows that there is some secrecy in the line of treatment as is the case with any technical work.

One of the very popular resources is by National Guidelines Clearing House [NGC] with the website http://www.guideline.gov in which U.S Department of Health and Human Resources has published many guidelines developed by various institution of the world through Agency for Health care Research and Quality [AHRQ]. If the students browse the website through Guideline Index link in the home page, hundreds of Guidelines arranged alphabetically can be seen. The site is more informative with Expert's commentaries, Guideline Synthesis, Guideline matrix, Guideline resources and comparison of guidelines. With due acknowledgement to the site authorities, a shortened version of an example guideline is given below so that students can understand how to develop a therapeutic guideline:

Guideline Title

Clinical practice guideline on the diagnosis, treatment, and prevention of tuberculosis.

Bibliographic Source(s)

Working Group of the Clinical Practice Guideline on the Diagnosis, Treatment and Prevention [trunc]. Clinical practice guideline on the diagnosis, treatment and prevention of tuberculosis. Madrid (Spain): Agency for Health Quality and Assessment of Catalonia (AQuAS); 2010. 221 p. [321 references]

Guideline Status

This is the current release of the guideline.

Contents

Scope	Qualifying Statements
Methodology	Implementation of the Guideline
Recommendations	Institute of Medicine (IOM) National Healthcare
Evidence Supporting the Recommendations	Quality Report Categories
Benefits/Harms of Implementing the Guideline	Identifying Information and Availability
Recommendations	Disclaimer
Contraindications	

Scope

Disease/Condition(s)

Tuberculosis (pulmonary, extra pulmonary, and latent tuberculosis)
  Guideline Category
  Diagnosis
  Evaluation
  Management
  Prevention
  Risk Assessment
  Screening
  Treatment
  Clinical Speciality
  Family Practice
  Infectious Diseases
  Internal Medicine
  Obstetrics and Gynecology
  Pathology
  Pediatrics
  Pharmacology
  Preventive Medicine
  Pulmonary Medicine
  Radiology
  Intended Users
  Advanced Practice Nurses
  Allied Health Personnel
  Clinical Laboratory Personnel

Health Care Providers
Hospitals
Nurses
Patients
Pharmacists
Physician Assistants
Physicians
Public Health Departments

Guideline Objective(s)

- To establish a set of recommendations for the diagnosis, treatment and prevention of tuberculosis based on the best scientific evidence available and the consensus of experts in the field

- To reduce the burden of tuberculosis in Spain through standardised, high-quality medical practice in line with Spanish healthcare strategies for the control of tuberculosis

Target Population: Adults and children of any age with the most common clinical presentations of tuberculosis

Interventions and Practices Considered

Diagnosis/Evaluation

1. Tuberculin test
2. Interferon-gamma release assay (IGRA)
3. Chest x-ray
4. Clinical symptom assessment (persistent cough or other constitutional symptoms)
5. Computed tomography (CT) scan
6. Obtaining sputum samples for smear microscopy, sample culture, identification and sensitivity tests
7. Fibre-optic bronchoscopy
8. Molecular or bacteriophage-based diagnosis techniques
9. Obtaining suitable extra pulmonary samples through biopsy or fine-needle puncture/aspiration for microbiological and histological analysis and sensitivity testing

Treatment/Management

1. Initial 2-month phase of Isoniazid, rifampicin, pyrazinamide and ethambutol and a 4-month maintenance phase of isoniazid and rifampicin for pulmonary tuberculosis
2. Alternative treatment regimens

3. Monitoring for treatment compliance
4. Intermittent treatment during maintenance phase
5. Adjuvant corticosteroid treatment (prednisolone)
6. Monitoring for liver toxicity
7. Extended treatment regimens for certain forms of extra pulmonary tuberculosis
8. Surgery for extra pulmonary tuberculosis
9. Use of directly observed treatment in certain populations
10. Treatment of challenging groups (human immunodeficiency virus [HIV]-positive patients, patients with liver disease or kidney failure, pregnant women)
11. Treating drug-resistant cases
12. Clinical, analytical, and microbiological monitoring of patients during treatment

Prevention

1. Isolation measures
2. Contact studies
3. Screening at-risk groups for latent infection
4. Treating latent tuberculosis infection
5. Bacillus Calmette–Guérin (BCG) vaccination

Note: The following were considered but not recommended for treatment: diets rich in vitamins or oligoelements, immunotherapy or laser radiation.

Major Outcomes Considered

- Rate of Tuberculosis infection
- Relapse
- Cure
- Sensitivity and specificity of diagnostic tests
- Efficacy of treatment
- Treatment compliance
- Treatment-related complications and adverse events

Methodology

Methods Used to Collect/Select the Evidence

Searches of Electronic Databases

Description of Methods Used to Collect/Select the Evidence

A search of the literature was carried out, prioritising the identification of systematic reviews (SRs) and other documents that provided a critical synthesis of the scientific literature, such as health technology assessment reports. For this purpose, an initial phase comprised a search of other clinical practice guidelines (CPGs) on the subject, in order to ascertain which SRs they had considered as a basis for their recommendations. The main CPGs used as secondary sources are listed in Appendix 6 of the original guideline document. Additional SRs were identified subsequently, following the date on which the selected CPGs were searched. The following electronic databases were consulted in this initial stage:

- TRIP Database
- National Health Service (NHS) National Library of Guidelines
- Agency for Healthcare Research and Quality (AHRQ) National Guideline Clearinghouse
- Cochrane Database of Systematic Reviews (the Cochrane Library)
- Database of Abstracts of Reviews of Effects (DARE)
- Health Technology Assessment (HTA) Database
- NHS Economic Evaluation Database (NHS EED)
- MEDLINE (accessed via Pub Med)
- EMBASE (accessed via Ovid)

To complete this stage, the publications of a number of technology assessment agencies were also consulted. These included the National Institute for Health and Care Excellence (NICE); agencies that issue CPGs, such as the Scottish Intercollegiate Guidelines Network (SIGN); and international societies.

In the second stage, an extended search of individual studies was conducted, in order to update the relevant SRs and answer the questions of the CPG. The main aim was to identify randomised clinical trials (RCTs) and observational studies, respecting the original search strategy of the relevant SRs. When these were not available, a specific strategy was designed for each question, adding validated filters in each case to identify RCTs and observational studies. The following electronic databases were consulted in this phase: the Cochrane Central Register of Controlled Trials (CENTRAL) (the Cochrane Library), MEDLINE, EMBASE and the Cumulative Index to Nursing and Allied Health Literature (CINAHL) (accessed via Ovid).

No language restriction was established for the searches carried out, but most of the studies considered were written in Spanish, English, or French. Searches covered a period from any date (varying according to the database in question) to September 2007, although relevant studies were identified in the highest-profile biomedical journals during the entire duration of the CPG development process.

Materials detailing the methodological process used for the CPG (search strategies for each clinical question, critical reading files for the studies selected, tables summarizing the evidence and formal evaluation tables) are available in Spanish at www.guiasalud.es .

Number of Source Documents

Not stated

Methods Used to Assess the Quality and Strength of the Evidence

Weighting According to a Rating Scheme (Scheme Given)

Rating Scheme for the Strength of the Evidence

Grading of Recommendations Assessment, Development and Evaluation (GRADE) Classification of Evidence Quality

Quality of Scientific Evidence	Study Design	Quality Reduced If	Quality Increased If
High	Randomised controlled trial	Design shortcoming: Significant (-1) Very significant (-2)	Association: Scientific evidence of a strong association (relative risk [RR] >2 or <0.5 and based on observational studies with no confounding factors) (+1)
Moderate		Inconsistency (-1) Direct evidence:	Scientific evidence of very strong association
Low	Observational study	Some uncertainty (-1) Great uncertainty as to	(RR >5 or <0.2 and based on studies with no chance of bias)(+2)
Very low	Other designs	whether evidence is direct (-2) Inaccurate data (-1) Reporting bias: High probability of (-1)	Dose-response slope (+1) All the possible confounding factors may have reduced the effect observed (+1)

- Methods Used to Analyze the Evidence
- Meta-Analysis
  Review of Published Meta-Analyses
  Systematic Review with Evidence Tables
- Description of the Methods Used to Analyze the Evidence

Meta-analysis of Results

In some sections for which the only evidence available consists of several individual randomised controlled trials (RCTs), meta-analysis was performed when possible and if the availability of a joint result was judged clinically relevant. In sections for which there is a systematic review (SR) and the search of the literature provided one or more subsequent individual RCTs, the main meta-analysis of the SR was updated, providing a new joint figure if possible. This was the method following for studies (SRs or RCTs) in the treatment and prevention sections. The free-access program RevMan 5 was used when performing or updating meta-analysis.

Evaluation of Evidence Quality and Grading of Recommendations

Evaluation of evidence quality and grading of recommendations was conducted following the parameters of the GRADE (Grading of Recommendations of Assessment Development and Evaluations) system, using GRADEpro, the free-access program of the GRADE Working Group. Controversial recommendations or those with no evidence were resolved by consensus of the group that developed the Clinical Practice Guideline (CPG).

Classification of Outcome Variables' Relative Importance

In this stage, the GRADE system recommends that during the initial phase of formulating clinical questions, the group developing the CPG explicitly establishes the outcome variables that are relevant to the questions, and classifies their relative importance. Importance should be classified using the following nine-point scale:

1-3: An unimportant outcome variable. It should not be included in the table evaluating quality to the results table. These outcome variables will not play an important role in formulating recommendations.

4-6: The outcome variable is important, but not a key to decision-making.

7-9: A key outcome variable in decision-making.

The relative importance of outcome variables is established by consensus.

Evaluating the Quality of Scientific Evidence

Quality is evaluated for each selected outcome variable. This means that for a single clinical question there will probably be outcome variables with various different levels of quality. Initially, scientific evidence must be evaluated on the basis of study design and studies' suitability for answering each type of question in the guideline. RCTs are assessed as "high-quality" and observational studies as "low-quality". However, there are a number of issues that may reduce the quality of RCTs or increase that of observational studies. They are outlined below. Finally, the quality of scientific evidence will be assessed as high, moderate, low or very low (see "Rating Scheme for the Strength of the Evidence" field). The following issues many reduce the quality of RCTs:

1. *Shortcomings in design or conduct*: possible examples are failure to hide the randomisation sequence, inadequate blinding, major losses, absence of analysis by intention to treat and early study termination due to benefit.

2. *Inconsistent results*: widely differing estimates of the effect of treatment (heterogeneity or variation in results) in available studies suggest real differences between these estimates. The differences may be due to differences in the population, the intervention, the outcome variables or the quality of the studies. Heterogeneity that cannot be reasonably explained reduces quality.

3. ***Lack of direct scientific evidence***: Evidence is considered indirect if there are no direct comparisons of two treatments (comparison of each treatment with a placebo, but not of the two treatments). Also, if there is extrapolation of the results of a study with a particular drug to all other drugs in the same class in the absence of a demonstrated class effect. When there are major differences between the population to whom the recommendations will be applied and the population recruited in the studies evaluated, indirectness can also be an issue. Last but not least, aspects of the potential applicability of recommendations in one context must be assessed against other contexts, as well as the external validity of the scientific evidence.

4. ***Imprecision***: when the studies available include relatively few events and few patients, and therefore have broad confidence intervals, the scientific evidence is considered to be of poorer quality.

5. ***Reporting bias***: quality may be reduced if there is reasonable doubt as to whether the authors have included all studies (e.g., publication bias in the context of an SR) or all relevant outcome variables (reporting bias).

The following issues many increase the quality of observational studies:

1. ***Significant effect:*** when the effect observed shows a strong (relative risk [RR] >2 or< 0.5) or very strong (RR >5 or <0.2), consistent association on the basis of studies with no confounding factors. In such cases, quality may be considered moderate, or even high.

2. ***A dose-response slope***

3. ***Situations in which all possible confounding factors may have reduced the association observed:*** If patients who receive the intervention being studied have a worse prognosis than the control group and nevertheless present better outcomes, the real effect observed is likely to be greater.

Methods Used to Formulate the Recommendations

Expert Consensus

Description of Methods Used to Formulate the Recommendations

The methods used are described in detail in the *Methodology Manual for Developing Clinical Practice Guidelines* of the Spanish National Healthcare System (see the "Availability of Companion Documents" field).

The steps taken were as follows:

The group that would develop the guideline was established, consisting of primary care professionals and specialists (in preventive medicine and public health, infectious diseases, general and community medicine, pulmonology, paediatrics, microbiology and clinical parasitology, and clinical pharmacology). These professionals were contacted via the various scientific societies interested in the subject of the Clinical Practice Guideline (CPG). Various users of the healthcare system inspected materials for patients.

Clinical questions were formulated according to the PICO model: Patient, Intervention, Comparison, and Outcome.

Formulating Recommendations using the Grading of Recommendations Assessment, Development and Evaluation (GRADE) System

When recommendations are formulated, the group developing the guideline must decide to what extent it can be assumed that implementing a recommendation will result in more benefit than harm. This is not a simple decision, and it is affected by many factors, making this stage one of the most complex in guideline development.

Proposals for systems to formulate recommendations began more than twenty years ago. Even at the outset these systems distinguished between the level of scientific evidence (how suitable different study designs were for answering the various types of questions) and the strength of recommendations. Since then, the various systems have gradually developed and incorporated issues other than study design, which must be taken into account when formulating recommendations.

The methods of the GRADE working group have been followed when classifying evidence quality and grading the strength of recommendations. The GRADE working group aims to establish an explicit, transparent method to develop recommendations that is easy for teams that develop CPGs to use, in order to overcome the disadvantages of other recommendation development systems.

Grading the Strength of Recommendations

Grading the strength of recommendations is relatively simple, as only two categories are considered: *strong* recommendations and *weak* recommendations (see the "Rating Scheme for the Strength of the Recommendations" field).

With *strong* recommendations, the group compiling the Clinical Practice Guideline (CPG) are sure that the benefits of the intervention exceed its harm or, in contrast, that the harm exceeds the benefits. In the former case, the recommendation is strongly for the intervention. In the latter, it is strongly against it.

Weak recommendations can also be for or against an intervention. A recommendation is weakly in favour of an intervention if the group compiling the CPG concludes that the benefits of implementing the recommendation probably exceed the harm, although this is not absolutely certain. In contrast, a recommendation is weakly against an intervention if its harmful effects probably exceed its benefits.

A number of other factors must also be considered when grading recommendations:

1. *Risk/benefit balance:* in order to give a suitable assessment of the balance between benefits and risks, the baseline risk of the population for whom the

recommendation is intended and the effect in both relative and absolute terms must be considered.

2. *Quality of scientific evidence:* before a recommendation is implemented, the level of certainty of the estimate of the observed effect must be ascertained. If the quality of the scientific evidence is not high, confidence must decrease even if the scale is large, and therefore so must the strength with which a recommendation is made.

3. *Values and preferences:* uncertainty as to the values and preferences of the CPG's target population must also be taken into account. The values and preferences of healthcare staff, the patient population and the general public must be reflected and should affect the grading of recommendations.

4. *Cost:* costs vary much moreover time, between geographical areas, and according to various other factors than other outcome variables. This means that although a high cost reduces the probability of a recommendation being graded as strong, context will be essential to the final assessment.

Rating Scheme for the Strength of the Recommendations

Implications of the Degrees of Recommendation in the Grading of Recommendations Assessment, Development and Evaluation (GRADE) System

Implications of a strong recommendation:		
Patients	**Clinicians**	**Managers/Planners**
The vast majority of persons would agree with the recommended action, and only a small proportion would not agree.	The action recommended should be implemented for most patients.	The recommendation can be adopted as healthcare policy in the majority of situations.
Implications of a strong recommendation:		
Patients	**Clinicians**	**Managers/Planners**
Most people would agree with the action recommended but a significant number would not.	Acknowledges that different options will be appropriate for different patients, and that clinicians must help each patient choose the option most consistent with his/her values and preferences.	Significant debate and stakeholder involvement are needed.

Cost Analysis

The guideline developers reviewed published cost analyses.

Method of Guideline Validation

External Peer Review

Description of Method of Guideline Validation

External reviewers reviewed the second draft of the original guideline document (May 2009). The various scientific societies involved, which are also represented by members of the group that compiled the Clinical Practice Guideline (CPG) and external reviewers, were contacted.

Recommendations

Major Recommendations

Definitions for the quality of evidence (**High, Moderate, Low, and Very Low**) and strength of recommendations (**Weak, Strong**) are provided at the end of the "Major Recommendations" field. **Good clinical practice** recommendations are based on the clinical experience of the group that develops the guideline, in the absence of reliable clinical evidence.

Diagnosis

Diagnosing the Infection

Strong: The tuberculin test is always recommended for the diagnosis of latent tuberculosis infection.

Good clinical practice: The tuberculin test must be performed by trained staff in order to prevent errors in either performance or reading. It can be performed in children from the age of 6 months.

Weak: If the tuberculin test is positive for someone who has previously received Bacillus Calmette–Guérin (BCG) vaccination (particularly in the last 15 years) or negative for someone who is immunosuppressed or a child less than 5 years old, an interferon-gamma release assay (IGRA) must be considered as a complementary test.

Good clinical practice: Inpatients in whom it is suspected that the tuberculin test will be impossible to read, an IGRA test and chest X-ray are suggested in order to rule out active tuberculosis.

Good clinical practice: IGRA tests must be performed in laboratories with accredited quality control systems.

Diagnosing Active Pulmonary Tuberculosis

Strong: Pulmonary tuberculosis must be clinically suspected inpatients with a cough lasting more than 2 weeks, haemoptoic expectoration and fever of unknown origin.

Strong: Patients with a persistent cough lasting more than 3 weeks must undergo a chest X-ray to rule out pulmonary tuberculosis and other illnesses.

Weak: In children who have been in contact with a smear-positive patient and have a positive tuberculin test, clinical symptoms and a normal chest X-ray, computed tomography (CT) scans may be considered on a case-by-case basis. In children who have been in contact with a smear-positive patient and have a positive tuberculin test, no clinical symptoms and a doubtful chest X-ray, CT scans may be considered on a case-by-case basis.

Strong: Inpatients with clinically and radiologically suspected pulmonary tuberculosis, at least three samples of respiratory secretion (sputum) must be obtained, preferably in the mornings, and sent as soon as possible to a microbiology laboratory for smear microscopy, sample culture, identification and sensitivity tests.

Weak: If a sputum sample cannot be obtained, sputum induction or gastric aspiration should be performed to obtain a sample. Fibre-optic bronchoscopy is recommended for cases in which other methods have proved ineffective.

Good clinical practice: Clinical and radiological suspicion of pulmonary tuberculosis is sufficient grounds to begin treatment. There is no need to wait for culture results, although it is advisable that sputum samples be obtained before beginning treatment.

Weak: Sputum samples should be centrifuged and chemically homogenised.

Weak: For smear microscopy of sputum, traditional staining methods are recommended in addition to fluorescence methods of analysis.

Weak: Automated liquid-medium cultivation methods are recommended in addition to traditional methods using solid media.

Good clinical practice: Molecular or bacteriophage-based diagnosis techniques must be considered secondary to conventional techniques such as smear microscopy and cultures.

Weak: If there are major clinical grounds to suspect tuberculosis, molecular direct detection techniques must be considered for sputum samples in addition to traditional cultivation methods.

Strong: Serological diagnosis methods are not recommended for the diagnosis of pulmonary tuberculosis.

Good clinical practice: Molecular diagnosis techniques must be performed only in recognised laboratories with accredited quality control systems.

Diagnosing Extra Pulmonary Tuberculosis

Good clinical practice: A high degree of clinical suspicion is needed for not delaying diagnosis of extra pulmonary tuberculosis.

Good clinical practice: Extra pulmonary tuberculosis must always be considered if a patient presents constitutional symptoms (asthenia, anorexia, and weight loss), fever, night sweats and signs and symptoms of local organ involvement, with altered immunity or a history of pulmonary tuberculosis.

Strong: Wherever possible, a suitable sample should be taken from the affected area, if necessary via biopsy or fine-needle puncture/aspiration, for histological analysis, smear microscopy, and cultures.

Good clinical practice: The sample should be placed in a dry container and sent to the sample laboratory for processing as soon as possible. The whole sample should not be preserved in formaldehyde, as this may destroy bacilli.

Strong: The imaging test recommended to diagnose suspected extra pulmonary tuberculosis depends on the organ or system affected. A chest X-ray should always be performed in order to rule out pulmonary tuberculosis.

Strong: In addition to microbiological and histological analysis of the sample, a rapid diagnostic method should also be used if treatment needs to be started early, such as in tuberculosis meningitis or severe disseminated tuberculosis.

Diagnosing Resistance to Tuberculosis Drugs

Good clinical practice: Sensitivity tests for first-line drugs should be performed on initial isolation of all tuberculosis patients.

Weak: Sensitivity testing should initially be performed using rapid determination methods. Traditional or phenotypic methods should also be used in cases with a high risk of resistance to tuberculosis drugs, such as people from countries with high endemic rates or those undergoing repeat treatment.

Good clinical practice: Sensitivity tests for second-line drugs must be performed if microbiological resistance is detected or if clinical resistance to first-line drugs is suspected, such as when there is failure in initial response to treatment or after a relapse once treatment is completed.

Good clinical practice: Sensitivity studies must be performed in laboratories with accredited quality control systems.

Treating Tuberculosis

Treating Pulmonary Tuberculosis

Good clinical practice: Individuals diagnosed with pulmonary tuberculosis must be treated and monitored by physicians and healthcare staff with sufficient experience in handling pulmonary tuberculosis.

Strong: Most patients with pulmonary tuberculosis not previously treated should be treated using a short, 6-month regimen consisting of an initial 2-month phase of Isoniazid, rifampicin, pyrazinamide and ethambutol and a 4-month maintenance phase of Isoniazid and rifampicin.

Weak: Other treatment regimens for pulmonary tuberculosis are also recommended (see Table 1 in the original guideline document).

Weak: Treatment should be extended to 9 months inpatients with cavitary pulmonary tuberculosis who still have positive cultures at the end of the initial (2-month) phase of treatment.

Good clinical practice: Treatment compliance must be assessed if there is a positive culture at the end of the initial (2-month) phase of treatment.

Strong: For initial treatment of tuberculosis in children, the same treatment regimens (at suitable doses) are recommended as for the adult population unless there are specific contraindications.

Weak: In children and adults, intermittent treatment (three times a week) may be considered during the maintenance phase if it is directly observed and if a culture taken after 2 months of treatment is negative.

Strong: Twice-weekly intermittent treatment regimens are not recommended.

Weak: To reduce the development of drug resistance and the number of drugs taken daily, adults should be treated with fixed-dose combinations of the tuberculosis drugs currently on the market.

Weak: Rifabutin is a reasonable option if rifampicin is not tolerated or if there is a high risk of interaction with other drugs, particularly antiretrovirals.

Weak: Adjuvant corticosteroid treatment may be considered in certain cases of extensive forms of tuberculosis.

Strong: Other adjuvant treatments, such as diets rich in vitamins or oligoelements, immunotherapy or laser radiation, are not recommended for tuberculosis.

Good clinical practice: Liver toxicity must be closely monitored inpatients receiving tuberculosis treatment, particularly those with known liver disease.

Treating Extra Pulmonary Tuberculosis

Strong: Treatment regimens (drugs and duration) for patients with **pleural, lymphatic, osteal, spinal or pericardial tuberculosis** should be no different from treatment regimens for pulmonary tuberculosis.

Strong: Corticosteroid treatment is not recommended for all patients with pleural tuberculosis.

Weak: For pleural tuberculosis, corticosteroid treatment should be considered in order to improve symptoms rapidly.

Strong: Surgery should not be performed routinely in all patients with **osteal tuberculosis**.

Weak: Inpatients with **spinal tuberculosis**, corrective or orthopaedic surgery should be considered in cases with a high risk of damage to the spinal cord or spinal instability, in order to achieve mechanical stability.

Weak: A longer treatment regimen, lasting up to 9 months, may be considered for patients with **osteoarticular tuberculosis**, depending on their clinical and radiological development.

Strong: Patients with **tuberculous meningitis** must follow a longer treatment regimen, lasting up to 12 months.

Strong: Inpatients with stage II or III **tuberculous meningitis**, adjuvant corticosteroid treatment is recommended during the initial phase (prednisolone 60 mg/day for 4 weeks).

Weak: In children with **tuberculous meningitis**, adjuvant corticosteroid treatment is recommended during the initial phase (prednisolone 60 mg/day for 4 weeks).

Weak: In children with **tuberculous meningitis** and hydrocephalus, ventricular drainage should be considered.

Strong: Inpatients with **pericardial tuberculosis**, adjuvant corticosteroid treatment is recommended during the initial phase (prednisolone 60 mg/day for 4 weeks).

Strong: Routine pericardiocentesis is not recommended for patients with **tuberculous pericarditis** and any degree of pericardial effusion.

Weak: Inpatients with **tuberculous pericarditis**, evacuating pericardiocentesis can be considered for cases where there is risk of pericardial tamponade or functional compromise.

Monitoring Treatment

Good clinical practice: Responsibility for successful treatment must be shared between the healthcare professionals in charge of patients and the healthcare authorities that provide the necessary resources.

Good clinical practice: The potential level of treatment compliance must be assessed and monitored in all tuberculosis patients who begin tuberculosis treatment.

Good clinical practice: It is important to motivate patients and to highlight the importance of fully complying with treatment, both for latent infection and active tuberculosis.

Good clinical practice: The strategies available for improving compliance must be tailored to each case and agreed upon with the patient.

Strong: The generalised use of directly observed treatment for all patients receiving tuberculosis treatment is not recommended.

Strong: Directly observed treatment regimens are recommended under certain circumstances, such as for patients living in poverty, those with no fixed address, cases with significant grounds to suspect poor compliance, patients with a history of poor compliance, and children.

Strong: Various strategies are recommended for improving compliance. These include reminder letters, phone calls, education, and home visits.

Treating Challenging Groups

Good clinical practice: Tuberculosis treatment for human immunodeficiency virus (HIV)-positive individuals must be provided by a physician who specialises in both infections.

Weak: In HIV-positive adults and children with pulmonary tuberculosis that has not been treated previously, a 6-month isoniazid and rifampicin treatment regimen is recommendded, supplemented with pyrazinamide and ethambutol for the first 2 months.

Strong: In treatment regimens for HIV-positive patients with tuberculosis, rifampicin should be maintained whenever possible.

Good clinical practice: The beginning of antiretroviral treatment for a patient receiving tuberculosis treatment must be considered on an individual basis according to the patient's immune status, in order to prevent treatment interactions.

Good clinical practice: In HIV-positive patients with CD4 counts above 350, tuberculosis treatment should be given first. Antiretroviral treatment must be introduced once tuberculosis treatment is complete.

Good clinical practice: In HIV-positive patients with CD4 counts between 200 and 350, antiretroviral treatment should begin after the first 2 months of tuberculosis treatment.

Good clinical practice: In HIV-positive patients with CD4 counts below 200, antiretroviral treatment should begin after between 2 and 8 weeks of tuberculosis treatment if the latter is well tolerated.

Good clinical practice: In children, it is reasonable to begin antiretroviral treatment 2 to 8 weeks after the beginning of tuberculosis treatment. The patient's immune status and the appropriateness of combining treatments must be considered on a case-by- case basis. In severe cases, both treatments may begin simultaneously.

Weak: Replacing rifampicin with rifabutin is recommended in an 18 month tuberculosis treatment regimen if there is a high risk of interactions with antiretroviral treatment.

Good clinical practice: Patients with chronic liver disease must be treated by a specialist, particularly in advanced clinical stages.

Good clinical practice: Liver function must be tested before the beginning of tuberculosis treatment and at regular intervals, particularly inpatients with chronic alcohol consumption, those being treated with other hepatotoxic drugs, those who are HIV-positive, or those who have chronic hepatitis virus infection or known liver disease.

Good clinical practice: Streptomycin and ethambutol doses must be adjusted for patients with kidney failure.

Good clinical practice: In most cases, pregnant women should be given standard tuberculosis treatment.

General Principles for Treating Drug-Resistant Cases

Good clinical practice: Patients with multi-drug resistant tuberculosis must be treated by a specialist.

Good clinical practice: Treatment regimens for multi-drug resistant tuberculosis must consist of at least four drugs to which the patient has shown no resistance.

Strong: A directly observed treatment regimen lasting at least 18 months is recommended for patients with multi-drug resistant tuberculosis.

Good clinical practice: A patient with multi-drug resistant tuberculosis can be considered cured if he/she has completed the first year of treatment and gives at least five negative cultures (taken monthly).

Strong: A sensitivity test should be performed in cases of repeat treatment.

Good clinical practice: Inpatients whose treatment is interrupted for less than 1 month and who have been fully monitored, treatment should be resumed until the treatment regimen has been completed.

Good clinical practice: Inpatients whose treatment is interrupted for more than 1 month or who give a positive smear microscopy during the interruption, the treatment regimen should be restarted, from the beginning.

Monitoring Patients

Good clinical practice: If there are sufficient resources available, treatment, monitoring and isolation of most patients with pulmonary tuberculosis can be performed at the primary care level.

Good clinical practice: In some clinical situations, specific monitoring by specialists, and even hospitalisation, is recommended (see Figure 1 in the original guideline document).

Good clinical practice: It is important to identify the main specialised institutions in each area or region to which patients must be referred if indicated.

Good clinical practice: Monitoring of individuals who begin tuberculosis treatment must consist of clinical, analytical, and microbiological monitoring during the first 2 weeks. It then must be followed by monthly clinical monitoring, analytical and bacteriological monitoring every 2 months, and radiological and bacteriological monitoring at the end of treatment.

Good clinical practice: Clinical monitoring must be even closer if there are analytical changes or positive cultures after the second month, if complications are suspected in children.

Good clinical practice: If a patient presents liver enzyme values five times higher than normal, or signs and symptoms of cholestasis, all potentially hepatotoxic medication must be suspended. The patient must then be monitored closely to see whether treatment can be resumed or whether a treatment regimen involving non-hepatotoxic drugs must be used instead.

Preventing Tuberculosis

Home Isolation Measures

Strong: Patients with pulmonary or laryngeal tuberculosis must remain in respiratory isolation until they are no longer suspected of being infectious.

Weak: Patients may be placed in respiratory isolation at home if this is feasible, unless the disease is severe or there are complications.

Good clinical practice: All medical establishments must have a set of measures (organisational and structural) designed to reduce hospital transmission of tuberculosis.

Good clinical practice: In addition to these measures, tuberculosis patients suspected of being infectious must wear surgical masks when they are in communal areas of medical establishments.

Good clinical practice: Healthcare staff working in high-risk areas must undergo tuberculin tests when they are hired, and at regular intervals if the initial test is negative.

Conventional Contact Studies

Strong: Contact studies should begin promptly when pulmonary, pleural or laryngeal tuberculosis is diagnosed. This is particularly important in the most infectious forms, such as cavitary pulmonary forms and/or cases with positive sputum smear microscopy.

Good clinical practice: Contact studies must consist of clinical history, a tuberculin test for high- and medium-priority contacts, and a chest X-ray for those with positive tuberculin test results, to rule out active tuberculosis.

Good clinical practice: In a contact study, a tuberculin test must be considered positive if its induration is ≥5 mm, regardless of whether the person tested has received BCG vaccination.

Good clinical practice: The tuberculin test must only be repeated if the first test was negative and less than 8 weeks have elapsed since the individual's last contact with a tuberculosis patient.

Weak: An IGRA is recommended in addition to the tuberculin test if the tuberculin test is positive for someone who has previously received the BCG vaccine (particularly in the last 15 years), or negative for someone who is immunosuppressed or is less than 5 years old.

Treating Latent Tuberculosis Infection

Strong: Tuberculin tests are not recommended for populations at low risk of infection to screen for latent tuberculosis infection.

Strong: In most immunocompetent individuals with positive tuberculin tests, isoniazid should be administered for at least 6 months to prevent tuberculosis.

Strong: In individuals with positive tuberculin tests and a high risk of developing tuberculosis, isoniazid should be administered for 9 months.

Strong: 12-month treatment regimens are not recommended for the prevention of tuberculosis.

Strong: In immunocompetent individuals, rifampicin should not be used in combination with pyrazinamide due to its high toxicity.

Weak: Alternative treatment regimens such as a combination of rifampicin and isoniazid (3 months) or rifampicin alone (4 months) are also recommended for the prevention of tuberculosis.

Weak: If there is potential resistance to isoniazid in the index case, contacts should be treated with rifampicin for 4 months.

Strong: In HIV-positive individuals with positive tuberculin tests, isoniazid should be administered for at least 9 months to prevent tuberculosis.

Weak: In HIV-positive individuals with positive tuberculin tests, a combination of rifampicin and isoniazid (3 months) is also recommended for the prevention of tuberculosis.

Weak: In HIV-positive patients with positive tuberculin tests, a combination of rifampicin and pyrazinamide may be considered (2 months).

Weak: To prevent tuberculosis in children and adolescents with positive tuberculin tests, treatment with any treatment regimen routinely used in adults, at appropriate doses, is recommended.

Good clinical practice: Children born to mothers with pulmonary tuberculosis and positive smear microscopies, 6-month prophylactic treatment with isoniazid is suggested, in addition to a mask until the mother is no longer infectious, or separation of the neonate from the mother if drug resistance is suspected.

Good clinical practice: Regardless of gestational age, isoniazid and vitamin B6 supplements are suggested for pregnant women with recent positive tuberculin tests (less than 2 years ago) after contact with a smear-positive patient.

Weak: Treatment for latent infection should not be begun in contacts of patients with multi-drug resistant tuberculosis.

Good clinical practice: A proactive attitude must be taken to assess and promote compliance throughout treatment. If intermittent treatment regimens are used, direct observation of medication intake should be used.

Good clinical practice: Analytical monitoring of liver function should be performed every 2 months in individuals receiving treatment for latent tuberculosis infection, particularly those receiving isoniazid.

Weak: Primary prophylaxis with isoniazid (300 mg/day or 5 mg/kg/day) is recommended for 8-12 weeks in children less than 5 years old, HIV-positive individuals, and those with immune system alterations, if they have come into contact with infectious patients.

Vaccination

Strong: Routine BCG vaccination is not recommended in Spain.

Good clinical practice: BCG vaccination is suggested for healthcare staff and those contacts of multi-drug resistant tuberculosis, and in whom other control strategies cannot be implemented or have failed.

Good clinical practice: The BCG vaccine must not be administered to those who have already been infected.

Good clinical practice: A diagnosis of tuberculosis must not be ruled out in a vaccinated individual in whom clinical findings suggest tuberculosis.

Definitions

Grading of Recommendations Assessment, Development and Evaluation (GRADE) Classification of Evidence Quality

Quality of Scientific Evidence	Study Design	Quality Reduced If	Quality Increased If
High	Randomised controlled trial	Design shortcoming: Significant (-1)	Association: Scientific evidence of a strong association (relative risk [RR] >2 or <0.5 and based on observational studies with no confounding factors) (+1)
Moderate		Very significant (-2)	Scientific evidence of very strong association (RR >5 or <0.2 and based on studies with no chance of bias)(+2)
Low	Observational study	Inconsistency (-1)	Dose-response slope (+1)
Very low	Other designs	Direct evidence: Some uncertainty (-1) Great uncertainty as to whether evidence is direct (-2) Inaccurate data (-1 Reporting bias: High probability of (-1)	All the possible confounding factors may have reduced the effect observed (+1)

Implications of the Degrees of Recommendation in the GRADE System

Implications of a strong recommendation:		
Patients	Clinicians	Managers/Planners
The vast majority of persons would agree with the recommended action, and only a small proportion would not agree.	The action recommended should be implemented for most patients.	The recommendation can be adopted as healthcare policy in the majority of situations.

Table Contd...

Implications of a strong recommendation:		
Patients	**Clinicians**	**Managers/Planners**
Most people would agree with the action recommended but a significant number would not.	Acknowledges that different options will be appropriate for different patients, and that clinicians must help each patient choose the option most consistent with his/her values and preferences.	Significant debate and stakeholder involvement are needed.

Clinical Algorithm(s)

The following algorithms are provided in the original guideline document:

- Managing liver toxicity during treatment for active tuberculosis or latent infection
- Beginning a conventional contact study according to form of tuberculosis and confirmation of diagnosis
- Examination and treatment of high- and medium-priority contacts (immune-competent adults, children aged 5 or above)

Evidence Supporting the Recommendations

Type of Evidence Supporting the Recommendations

The type of supporting evidence is identified and graded for each recommend-dation (see the "Major Recommendations" field).

Benefits/Harms of Implementing the Guideline Recommendations

Potential Benefits

Appropriate early diagnosis, treatment availability, and follow-up, as well as actions that target vulnerable groups at high risk of infection or those with poor living conditions

Potential Harms

Side Effects of Drugs for the Treatment of Tuberculosis

- Side effects of isoniazid affect mainly the liver, and to a lesser extent the nervous system. Hepatic side effects can take the form of self-limiting increases in liver enzymes at any time during treatment, mainly during the first 4 months (10% to 20% of cases). Peripheral neuropathy is dose-related and affects mainly patients with some predisposition (malnutrition, alcoholism, diabetes, human immunodeficiency virus [HIV] infection, kidney failure) (2%). To prevent this, dosage forms are often combined with pyridoxine (vitamin B6). Individuals with slow acetylation capacity are also at greater risk. The cause of liver toxicity is the metabolite of isoniazid. Less commonly, isoniazid can cause haematological reactions (agranulocytosis, aplastic anaemia, eosinophilia), and hypersensitivity reactions (up to 20% of patients may present antinuclear antibodies), sometimes with cutaneous symptoms.

- Pruriginous skin reactions, with or without an associated rash, occur in up to 6% of cases treated with rifampicin. They are generally self-limiting, and are rarely serious hypersensitivity reactions. Gastrointestinal reactions include nausea, anorexia, and abdominal pain, occasionally severe. It can cause transient bilirubin increases; liver toxicity is more common if rifampicin is combined with isoniazid. Thrombocytopenia and pseudoinfluenza have been reported during intermittent treatment regimens. It typically causes orange discoloration of bodily fluids (sputum, urine, tears, etc.), of which patients should be warned.

- The main side effect of pyrazinamide is liver toxicity, which is dose-related. At normal doses (25 mg/kg), the rate of liver toxicity is less than 1%. It is also a frequent cause of polyarthralgia and asymptomatic hyperuricaemia, although dose adjustment and suspension of treatment are rarely necessary. Other side effects include nausea, anorexia, and skin rash.

- The main side effect of ethambutol is optic neuritis with reduced visual acuity or reduced colour perception, affecting one or both eyes. This effect is associated with daily doses above 15 mg/kg. An intermittent treatment regimen may reduce the risk of this side effect. Patients beginning a treatment regimen that includes ethambutol must undergo a visual acuity and colour perception test, which must be repeated on a monthly basis if treatment lasts more than 2 months, if it involves high doses, or if the patient has any degree of kidney failure. Occasionally, ethambutol may cause skin reactions. In children, ethambutol doses of 15 to 25 mg/kg may be administered during the first 2 months if plasma levels of ethambutol are lower. Visual evoked potential tests can be conducted in small children who do not cooperate with the examination.

- Rifabutin can cause severe neutropoenia (up to 2%), particularly at high doses, in daily treatment regimens and inpatients who are HIV-positive. When combined with macrolide antimicrobials or other drugs that can reduce the elimination of rifabutin, it can cause uveitis. Like rifampicin, rifabutin is associated with asymptomatic liver enzyme increases and, in under 1% of cases, with clinical hepatitis. It can also cause gastrointestinal side effects, skin reactions, polyarthralgia, pseudojaundice, and pseudoinfluenza, as well as orange coloration of bodily fluids.

- Streptomycin, ethambutol and many second-line drugs can cause renal toxicity. If they need to be administered due to intolerance or resistance, dosing must be adjusted according to the glomerular filtration rate. Inpatients undergoing kidney dialysis, drugs must be administered after dialysis, as dialysis eliminates them.

Appendices 12 and 13 in the original guideline document contain additional information on side effects and liver toxicity.

Drug Interactions

There is great potential for drug interactions between rifamycins (particularly rifampicin) and antiretrovirals. The Centers for Disease Control and Prevention (CDC) recently (in 2007) published a document containing summaries of the main interactions between antiretrovirals and rifampicin, and the most appropriate dosing and treatment regimen adjustments. An adapted version of this information is provided in Appendix 9 in the original guideline document.

Paradoxical Reactions

Paradoxical reactions of the immune system (immune reconstitution syndrome) have been recorded during tuberculosis treatment. They are characterised by fever, increased pulmonary infiltrate or increased pleural exudates and enlarged lymph nodes in the neck, thorax or abdomen after treatment has begun. This type of reaction, which can be serious, has been recorded in more than a third of patients receiving both antiretroviral and tuberculosis treatment. However, paradoxical reactions after the beginning of tuberculosis treatment have also been recorded in HIV-negative individuals.

Drug Resistance

The main problem in repeated treatment is drug resistance, either to isoniazid alone or to multiple drugs. Due to this risk, if a patient requires repeat treatment his/her previous treatment must be investigated and sensitivity must be diagnosed using at least traditional methods (phenotypic methods or fluid cultivation), and ideally also using rapid diagnosis methods.

Side Effects of Bacillus Calmette–Guérin (BCG) Vaccination

Between 1% and 2% of vaccinated children may experience side effects. These are generally local, benign reactions, correlated to the concentration of bacilli in the vaccine, the child's age, the strain used, and the vaccination method used. Most adverse reactions occur in the first 5 months following BCG vaccination. The most common side effects are ulcers at the site of inoculation, caused by incorrect administration (e.g., subcutaneous instead of intradermal), excessively high doses, or secondary contamination at the injection site. However, side effects to the vaccine are considered uncommon. The risk of local reaction ranges from 0.01 to 6 per thousand live births. Disseminated infection 6 to 12 months after vaccination is much rarer (between 0.19 and 1.56 per million vaccinations), but can be fatal. This effect has been observed in vaccinated children who presented congenital or acquired immunodeficiency syndrome (AIDS) and in AIDS patients. Regional suppurative lymphadenitis is a rare side effect, with an incidence of 0.1 per thousand vaccinated children. Osteitis is another side effect, occurring in up to 46 children per million vaccinated. It can appear upto 12 years after vaccination. Although no teratogenicity has been described for the vaccine, in pregnant women vaccination is usually postponed until after the birth.

Contraindications

- Streptomycin, kanamycin, prothionamide/ethionamide, amikacin and capreomycin are contraindicated during pregnancy.

- Contraindications to treatment for latent tuberculosis infection include acute hepatitis, severe chronic liver disease, and serious adverse reactions to treatment. Mild or moderate chronic liver disease, history of adverse reactions to treatment that are not serious, and pregnancy are relative contraindications to treatment for latent tuberculosis infection.

Qualifying Statements

- This clinical practice guideline (CPG) is an aid for decision-making in healthcare. Its use is not compulsory, and it does not replace the clinical judgment of healthcare staff.

- No recommendations have been made on the organisation of medical services, control programmes or aspects of epidemiology surveillance for the disease. Also excluded are recommendations for certain situations or specific locations such as boat or plane travel, customs or prisons, as these can be applied only with the cooperation of public authorities.

- In addition, complex clinical situations that require highly specialised care have not been covered in depth. These include the specific handling of concurrent human immunodeficiency virus (HIV) infection, those with other immune system changes, tuberculosis in neonates, rare forms of extra pulmonary tuberculosis, recurrent tuberculosis, and extremely resistant tuberculosis. These issues, while certainly important, are the subjects of other CPGs, both in Spain and abroad (see Appendix 6 in the original guideline document).

Implementation of the Guideline

Description of Implementation Strategy

Dissemination and Implementation

Guideline Formats, Dissemination, and Implementation

There are various different versions of clinical practice guidelines (CPGs): full, summary, information for patients, and quick-consultation tool. All these versions are available in

HTML and PDF from the GuíaSalud website (www.guiasalud.es). A hard copy of the summary version containing a CD ROM of the full version is also published.

Dissemination and implementation strategies include the following:

- Official presentation of the guideline by healthcare authorities
- Copies sent individually to professionals and potential users
- Distribution of patient guideline
- Dissemination of the guideline in electronic format on the websites of healthcare services and scientific societies involved in the project
- Presentation of the guideline at scientific events (conferences, meetings)
- Publication of the guideline in medical journals

Proposed Evaluation Indicators

Any organisation that provides medical services must establish ongoing improvement strategies. This is the basis of quality plans, which require objective evaluation indicators. Healthcare indicators are a quantitative (and sometimes qualitative) measure that allow for objective tracking of the quality of the important processes involved, in this case, healthcare. This means that indicators are not a direct measure of quality but rather tools that require ongoing use, assessment of changes in outcomes, and reading in the context of each individual organisation providing the service being evaluated. The quality of healthcare is a gradient of probability, and improvements to healthcare can improve patients' health (or that of the public).

Indicators do not measure a single component of healthcare quality. Instead, many aspects such as the accessibility, efficacy, and suitability of healthcare are interrelated and affect the final outcome. However, it is very important for indicators to have both internal validity (they must identify what is to be measured) and external validity (results must be interpretable), and to be based on up-to-date knowledge.

Defining indicators is not easy, and still less so in Spain, where various different organisations provide often complementary medical services within a single healthcare process. In addition to proposing a formula for calculation, identifying the updated theoretical basis supporting it, and identifying the sources of information from which cases will be taken, the underlying factors that explain possible variations in results must also be outlined.

The working group has considered the complexity of healthcare provided for tuberculosis and the many different situations in Spain, and has chosen to select a series of indicators already developed by the World Health Organization (WHO), which can be adapted to Spain. Appendix 7 in the original guideline document presents and explains a list of indicators; comprehensive descriptions can be found in the full WHO document.

Finally, this CPG aims to provide a tool for interested clinicians and managers, which may be useful in the specific design of healthcare evaluation.

Identifying Information and Availability

Bibliographic Source(s)

Working Group of the Clinical Practice Guideline on the Diagnosis, Treatment and Prevention [trunc]. Clinical practice guideline on the diagnosis, treatment and prevention of tuberculosis. Madrid (Spain): Agency for Health Quality and Assessment of Catalonia (AQuAS); 2010. 221 p. [321 references]

Adaptation: Not applicable: The guideline was not adapted from another source.

Date released: 2010

Guideline Developer(s)

Agency for Health Quality and Assessment of Catalonia (AQuAS) - State/Local Government Agency [Non-U.S.]
GuiaSalud - National Government Agency [Non-U.S.]
Ministry of Health (Spain) - National Government Agency [Non-U.S.]

Source(s) of Funding

This Clinical Practice Guideline (CPG) has been funded via an agreement signed by the Instituto de Salud Carlos III (Carlos III Institute of Health), an autonomous body within the Spanish Ministry of Science and Innovation, and the Agència d'Informació, Avaluació i Qualitat en Salut of Catalonia (AIAQS – Agency for Information, Evaluation, and Quality in Health), within the framework of cooperation established in the Quality Plan for the National Health System of the Spanish Ministry of Health, Social Policy and Equality.

Guideline Committee

Working Group of the Clinical Practice Guideline (CPG) on the Diagnosis, Treatment and Prevention of Tuberculosis [Names of the members listed]

Financial Disclosures/Conflicts of Interest

The authors' and reviewers' disclosure of interests was compiled using the pre-established form included in the Methodology Manual for Developing Clinical Practice Guidelines of the Spanish National Healthcare System. The authors and external reviewers involved in developing the final recommendations contained in this guideline were not influenced in any way by the views or interests of the funding body/ies, in this case the agreement signed by the Carlos III Health Institute (Spanish Ministry for Health and Consumption) and the Catalan Agency for Health Technology Assessment. The declaration of interest by all members of the Working Group, as well as by the persons who took part in expert collaboration and external revision, can be found in Appendix 5 in the original guideline document.

Guideline Status

This is the current release of the guideline.

Guideline Availability

Electronic copies: Available in English and Spanish from the GuíaSalud Web site.

Availability of Companion Documents

The following are available:

- Quick reference guides are available in several dialects from the GuíaSalud Web site .
- A summary version is available in Spanish from the GuíaSalud Web site .
- Methodology manual for developing clinical practice guidelines of the Spanish National Healthcare System. Available in Spanish from the GuíaSalud Web site .

In addition the appendices of the original guideline document contain proposed evaluation indicators and information on interactions of the main tuberculosis drugs, combined administration of rifampicin or rifabutin and antiretrovirals, respiratory isolation, reading tuberculin tests in population screening, side effects and monitoring of treatment for latent infection, overall assessment of risk of liver toxicity caused, and treatment regimens evaluated in latent tuberculosis. The Spanish version of the guideline is available via a mobile application from the GuíaSalud Web site.

Patient Resources

Appendix 2 of the original guideline document contains information for patients. Please note: This patient information is intended to provide health professionals with information to share with their patients to help them better understand their health and their diagnosed disorders. By providing access to this patient information, it is not the intention of NGC to provide specific medical advice for particular patients. Rather we urge patients and their representatives to review this material and then to consult with a licensed health professional for evaluation of treatment options suitable for them as well as for diagnosis and answers to their personal medical questions. This patient information has been derived and prepared from a guideline for health care professionals included on NGC by the authors or publishers of that original guideline. The patient information is not reviewed by NGC to establish whether or not it accurately reflects the original guideline's content.

NGC Status

This NGC summary was completed by ECRI Institute on June 25, 2014. The information was verified by the guideline developer on August 1, 2014.

Summary of Method of Preparation of Guidelines

From the above example it is clear how a therapeutic guideline is prepared and presented. For simplicity, it can be summarized as follows: First of all the disease for which the therapeutic guideline should be prepared must be identified. Then specialists of that disease and relevant others should be organized into a group. They should be given the task of review of already available literature and then the guidelines should be prepared using evidences. The preliminary guidelines thus prepared should be circulated and opinion of various stalk holders should be ascertained. These opinions and suggestions are either incorporated or rejected into the draft guidelines after debate and discussions among the guideline developers. Then it should be published suitably. After few months or so, feedbacks received should be analyzed and the guidelines are republished and updated. Though this procedure seems to be simple there are many practical problems, nevertheless, developing therapeutic guidelines is worth venturing.

Disadvantages of Therapeutic Guidelines

The advantages of therapeutic guidelines are obvious and need not be listed; however, there are few disadvantages. They are,

1. The Clinicians freedom to treat a patient as per his decision is curtailed, if he is compelled to follow the therapeutic guidelines in a hospital.
2. The junior doctors tend to rely more and more on the guidelines for their practice, rather than innovating or finding new methods of treatment.
3. A set of pre determined line of treatment, naturally goes against the principle of individualization of drug therapy. The line of treatment has to be changed if something wrong is found during Drug therapy review or Therapeutic Drug Monitoring by the Clinical Pharmacist.

Hence while following therapeutic guidelines, all these factors should be taken into account and accommodated suitably.

Factors Affecting Implementation of Guidelines

A therapeutic guideline, if followed blindly may leads to failure. The treating physician has to use his intelligence and experience while treating patients, because no two individuals are alike as far as diseases and its manifestations are concerned.

With any professional practice, there used to be some trade or professional secret which the senior professionals don't want to reveal to their juniors [at least in initial stages]. Even a roadside automobile mechanic keeps away his juniors while repairing a gear box of a vehicle! The Pharmaceutical manufacturing chemists and analysts know it very well that there are many secrets in the manufacture and stability of formulations or its correct method of analysis. Medical profession is not an exemption to this common practice.

Chief or senior doctors while treating complicated cases simply dictate a drug or test without revealing the reason for it to the juniors. He might have observed some symptom of the disease manifestation and know the reason for it because of his long experience, which the juniors could not observe. Thus all are not told while treating a patient and hence they may not find a place in therapeutic guidelines.

Thus junior doctors, Clinical pharmacists and nurses require extreme skills of observation of patient and able to find out even a minor development and reason for it. Of course these skills are acquired by experience and therapeutic guidelines cannot be a substitute for it, at best guidelines are just guidelines!

Questions

Short Answer Questions

1. Write a note on the need for Therapeutic guidelines and its resources

2. What are the disadvantages of Therapeutic guidelines?

Long Answer Questions

3. What are therapeutic guidelines? How it is prepared? Discuss its merits and demerits.

CHAPTER 7

PHARMACY PROCEDURAL MANUAL

Introduction

It is a booklet containing policies and procedures about the administration of pharmacy and serve as a guide to the hospital pharmacist for executing efficient 'pharmaceutical care' in the hospital.

'Pharmaceutical care' is defined as the responsible provision of drug therapy for the purpose of achieving definite outcomes that improves quality of life of the patient.

Thus the manual is the guide book to the pharmacist in particular and other health professionals in general.

Purpose and Use

The purpose or reasons for preparing and publishing such a manual are many and indicate the importance given to pharmacy services in hospitals by the government and other authorities. The usefulness of Pharmacy Procedural Manual (PPM) can be listed as follows:

1. They provide definite procedure for a given work; thereby doubts, wastages and errors are eliminated.
2. As a printed version, it prevents errors in conveying policies and procedures orally
3. It is very much useful as a guide to give training to new employees of pharmacy department
4. They ensure same and similar policies are followed in all similar situations, thereby avoiding problems later.
5. Even in court cases against the hospital pharmacy, it serves as a valuable defence.
6. Finally by using the manual as yardstick, we can evaluate the services, qualities and performance of pharmacists.

Preparing a Manual

The Head of the department of pharmacy services or Chief Pharmacist of a hospital should prepare the manual. He should be thorough with the policies of the hospital and in the techniques of writing or preparing the manual. In the preparation of the manual various persons are involved and various processes are to be utilized and controlled.

The organization of this administrative and professional policy material requires a great deal of thought and planning otherwise will result in a confusing presentation which may complicate rather than clarify the matter.

The manual can have the format and content as described in the following sections.

Format of a Manual

The following is a presentation of a format which may be readily adapted to a specific operation by any pharmacist. The manual can be divided into four general sections.

1. Organization
2. Personnel
3. Facilities and
4. Services

This format is adequate and is recommended to those who may wish to organize and develop a procedural manual for their hospital pharmacy. One must, however bear in mind that no two manuals or hospitals will have the same policy, and therefore in some instances even this general format will not suffice. However let us, discuss the general contents of each section in detail.

Contents of a Manual

1. Organization

    (a) Organization of hospital pharmacy

    (b) Services by the department including drug information services

    (c) Intra and inter departmental relationships and

    (d) Role of pharmacists in various hospital committees like PTC.

2. Personnel

    (a) Job descriptions including responsibilities

    (b) Leave rules including sick leave, annual leave etc

    (c) Holidays

    (d) On duty permissions and

    (e) Salary and allowances

3. Facilities

(a) General policies relating to the use, maintenance and repair of the equipments of dispensary, laboratory central sterile service department and manufacturing section, if available.

(b) Policy and procedure governing the use of pharmacy equipments by other departments

(c) Obtaining services of maintenance department of the hospital and

(d) Obtaining services of outside agencies, fee to be paid, rules etc.

4. Services

The services of the department can be classified into two. They are administrative services and professional services

(a) Administrative services

    (i) Working hours

    (ii) Purchase procedure

    (iii) Pricing policy

    (iv) Service charges

    (v) Refund policy

    (vi) Inventory control and

    (vii) Monthly, annual or periodical reports

(b) Professional services

    (i) Narcotic regulations

    (ii) Use of research drugs

    (iii) Hospital formulary

    (iv) Policy towards drugs brought by patients

    (v) Pre-packing

    (vi) Bulk compounding

    (vii) Training programmes including educational services

    (viii) Intravenous admixture and Total Parenteral Nutrition

    (ix) Drug and poison information services and

    (x) On call services.

Some Example Policies and Procedures in the Manual

The government by an order makes it mandatory for the hospital administrator and the hospital pharmacist to prepare the written policies and procedures pertaining to the hospital drug manufacture and distribution system.

The Government Order provides the guidelines regarding what must be included in the pharmacy procedural manual. Few examples are given below:

1. Drug preparation and dispensing shall be restricted to licensed registered pharmacists.
2. A pharmacist should review the prescriber's order or direct copy thereof, before initial dose of medication is dispensed.
3. The use of floor stock medications should be minimized.
4. The unit dose system is recommended
5. Written policies and procedures that are essential for patient safety and for the control, accountability and intra hospital distribution of drugs shall be reviewed annually, revised as may be necessary and enforced.
6. All drugs should be adequately labelled.
7. Discontinued and out dated drugs or containers with damaged labels should be returned to pharmacy.
8. Drug product defects, if any, may be reported to authorities concerned, like Dean, PTC, Drugs inspector etc.
9. Drugs should be administered to the patient only on a written prescription.
10. Medication errors and adverse drug reactions shall be reported immediately in accordance with written procedures.
11. Self-administration of medications by patients shall be permitted on a specific written order by treating physician.
12. Investigational drugs shall be properly labelled and stored. They should be used only under direct supervision of the authorized principal investigator.
13. Orders for drugs must contain only the approved symbols and abbreviations.
14. Drugs compounded in the hospital for administration must be administered then and there.
15. Substitution of drugs with other brands must be done only with the approval of the physician concerned.

Publishing and Distributing a Manual

The manual prepared with the content as above must be published by the hospital authorities after thorough checking by an expert committee headed by chief of pharmacy services. The printed booklet of the manual should be made available to all the departments concerned.

The manual should be reviewed periodically, updated and new edition published after additions or deletions, if any to the content.

As the government follows equal and same policies throughout the state, all government hospitals in the state can have one pharmacy procedural manual, published at state level. Since very few deviations from the procedure mentioned in the manual are required depends upon the local conditions, they can be made to the manual with the written permission from authorities concerned. Thus with the pharmacy procedural manual in place, the goal of effective and efficient 'pharmaceutical care' to the people can be achieved.

But in reality, the situation is far from satisfactory. No Indian hospital has this pharmacy procedural manual. It is neither prepared nor distributed by anybody. Reason for this state of affairs is not difficult to understand. We have only D.Pharm holders as pharmacists in our hospitals. Preparation and implementation of all procedures of pharmacy procedural manual is beyond their capacity. Hence graduate and post graduate pharmacists must be appointed in all hospitals and a full pledged department of pharmacy services should be opened. Until and unless this is done, no meaningful service to the patient can be given by the pharmacist. The starting of Pharm.D course by PCI is a step in the right direction which must be taken forward to its logical conclusion of appointing these Pharm.D holders in all government and private big hospitals.

Questions

Short Answer Questions

1. Define pharmacy procedural manual.

2. Why pharmacy procedural manual is prepared?

Long Answer Questions

3. Enumerate the content of pharmacy manual.

4. Detail the policies and procedures given in pharmacy manual.

5. Explain the administrative and professional services listed in a pharmacy manual.

CHAPTER 8

BUDGET OF HOSPITAL PHARMACY

Introduction

A young pharmacist on joining duty in a hospital pharmacy is not required to prepare the annual budget of the department, on the other hand, he is expected to learn and have knowledge about his department's important works – the budget preparation and its implementation – as it is going to determine the overall performance of hospital pharmacy for the next one year and beyond.

The budget of hospital pharmacy is important, because it is one of the departments having direct relation with the people. Hence any deficiency in its preparation and implementation will reflect on the reputation of the entire hospital. Thus it becomes all the more important that a realistic budget is prepared by taking into consideration of all factors and circumstances and also the success of previous budget or otherwise.

Definition

A budget is nothing but a plan for future operations, in terms of finance. As we know for every activity, money is needed and hospital pharmacy is no exemption. The plan is prepared, according to financial implication of all functions of hospital pharmacy. Thus budget is an instrument to review the working of any department by higher authorities, in relation to prepared plan, in a comprehensive and integrated form expressed in financial terms.

As the overall hospital budget is the combination of all its departmental budgets, it must be prepared with utmost care and devotion. Hence, a pharmacist must be aware of its aims first, then its divisions and factors affecting a budget.

Aim or Objectives of Budget

1. It sets goal to achieve and thus standards for performance
2. By comparing the actual results with the goal in the midway appraisal of the budget it helps to identify failures.

3. By analyzing the failures, it provides the way for correcting the mistakes or identifies the factors beyond control.

If a budget is not prepared, the above objectives cannot be achieved and such organizations will end up in closure.

Factors Affecting Budget

A budget has to be prepared primarily according to the needs of a department, but it is not as simple as it looks. The budget is influenced by many factors like local conditions and compulsions, management's policies and pressures, higher authorities' confidence on the department's ability and the head of the department's skill in implementation of the budget.

1. *Local conditions and compulsions*: A budget prepared without taking into consideration of local needs will face many problems during its implementation. Obviously the local community is the beneficiary of the budget and hence their needs should be given priority while preparing a budget. For example, in a place where water borne diseases are more, the drugs for those diseases should be purchased in needed quantity and budget provisions should be made for its purchase, if not interim local purchases has to be made and that make the annual budget useless. In order to prepare a useful budget, the knowledge of demographic, epidemiological and attitudinal characters of local community is essential and that is the reason for including local people's representatives like MLA or MC in the consultative or advisory committee of the hospital.

2. *Management's policy*: The budget has to be prepared in accordance with the policy and objective of the management. These policies are not always constant and changes out of pressure. Depends on it, the budget and programs of pharmacy services should be prepared. It should coincide with the overall plan of the institution. For example the management may change its policy towards charging or pricing of drugs to patients treated in the hospital. Hence drugs suitable for charging has to be procured, similarly if it has to be given free of charge; drugs at lowest or optimum price should be purchased from the manufacturer or supplier. All these changes the way budget was prepared earlier. Overall budget allocation for drugs purchase has to be either increased or decreased according to new policy.

3. *Confidence of higher authorities*: As the budget is out and out money matter, it requires the confidence of higher authorities and trust on the budget preparing and implementing department. The previous year's performance of the department will be taken into account while according sanction for the current year budget. As the budget of hospital pharmacy department is connected with supply and services to other departments of hospital, the support from those department heads will also be useful in getting sanction for proposals of pharmacy department.

4. *Ability of head of pharmacy services*: In sanctioning the budget proposal, the ability and integrity of the head of the department of pharmacy is also considered. The personal reputation of him goes long way in achieving the goals of department. As mentioned earlier, the successful completion and achievement of target of previous year budget are the deciding factors for getting sanction for the proposed budget without cuts.

Requirement/Characters of a Budget

1. First of all, the management must define the policies and objectives of the budget, taking into consideration, the growth of the hospital.

2. These policies and objectives must be clearly understood by those in managerial position, since without their active support and participation the goals cannot be achieved.

3. The aims of the budget should be reasonable and achievable.

4. There should not be any under estimate or over estimate of the capability of department and unachievable goals should not be focused. The prevailing and anticipated conditions should be estimated correctly, as far as possible.

5. At the same time, the budget should not restrict the initiatives of the staff and discourage them from attempting new ventures or practices.

Divisions of a Budget

A budget has many sections depends on the money comes in or goes out. Thus it can be classified into (a) Revenue (income) accounts (b) Expense accounts and (c) Capital accounts. Last two are dealing with money that goes out, however, there is little difference that the former involves expenses of recurring nature and the latter deals with onetime expenses or investment in assets.

(a) *Revenue accounts*: The revenue or income for the hospital pharmacy department is through sale of drugs to inpatients, outpatients and other departments. While preparing budget, the previous year revenue has to be considered and the revenue for forth coming year has to be estimated. When calculating this all risk factors like price rise, fall in demand etc should be borne in mind. Fool proof methods should be devised to generate income from the activities of the department. Another source of income for the department is from the sale of empty containers, bottles and other packing materials which are generated in huge volumes in big hospitals. This apart any professional service rendered to outside agencies by the departments can be levied a professional or service charge and credited in the revenue account. The revenue generated by pharmacy department of a charity hospital or government hospital may be minimum, whereas it is a considerable amount from private hospitals.

(b) ***Expenses accounts:*** It can be broadly classified into administrative expenses and professional expenses. Administrative expenses include salaries and wages, stationeries, telephone and electricity bill for the office etc. Professional expenses include, drugs purchase bill, raw material and other supplies, expenses involved in maintenance of professional equipments and instruments etc. These expenses are known as recurring expenses, as they are made repeatedly many times in a financial year and also year after year.

Salaries and wages are calculated for all the employees of the department, including part time and temporary employees. If new posts are to be created in the next financial year the anticipated salary also, should be added to this heading. Overtime wages, if any, to be paid to the employees should also be calculated. In these calculations, previous year experience in the working of the department, offer valuable guidance.

Supply and expenses include all purchases to the department mainly the drugs and other pharmaceuticals and raw materials. Allowance should be made for future expansion, price rise and local and emergency purchases. While calculating the expected cost of purchase for the forthcoming year, taxes, and transport expenses, insurance, loading and unloading charges etc should not be forgotten.

(c) ***Capital accounts:*** Capital expenses are not recurring expenses and as such considered as onetime expense. Construction of new buildings, purchase of new equipments etc fall under this category. Though these are all assets added to the department, in due course of time due to wear and tear these assets depreciate in value. Once it becomes unusable they have to be replaced. That might be huge expense for the institute. Hence usually a depreciation value is detected from the revenue account and separately kept aside for future purchase. The depreciation value for each year is deducted depending on the durability or life of the equipment or asset.

Deducting and setting aside depreciation value is almost irrelevant to Government hospitals whereas it is possible in private hospitals. The head of the department of the pharmacy has to fix life period in years of depreciable machinery and instruments in consultation with their manufacturers and/or suppliers, who alone can furnish or guarantee the serviceability in terms of years as this factor depends upon workmanship, quality control factors and frequency or extend of usage of the equipment under question.

Usually, for small expenses a unit cost of say Rs. 1000 may be fixed and any expense above this value is put under capital account for which the HOD should get permission from higher authorities. The sealing is deliberately kept low, in order to have better control over finances by higher authorities.

The public health sector including hospitals are considered 'white elephants' meaning thereby they incur only expenses and not generate any income to the government. Hence it is impossible for hospitals to make any huge capital expense from its internal resources or income generated by the hospital. Almost all capital expenses are made by grants from State or Central Government or the trust which manages the hospital.

Government Hospital Budgets (The Process)

The budget preparation processes are more or less same for private hospitals or Government hospital. The budget thus prepared by HOD of hospital pharmacy should be submitted to the management in the case of private hospitals, higher authorities in the case of Government hospitals. They in turn submit the consolidated budget of all sections of their organization, through proper channel, to their higher authorities, well before the beginning of the budget session of parliament or state assembly in February of every year. The budgets thus collected from all the hospitals of the district by District Medical Officer (DMO) or District Health Officer (DHO) will be submitted to the state level directorates, after corrections if any and recommendations within their budget allocations. The State Director of Medical Services [DMS] or Health Services [DHS] or Medical Education [DME] will in turn consolidate all district level budgets, include their own office's budget and submit to the health ministry in the state secretariat. They forward these budget proposals with modifications, if any, to the finance ministry for final approval and passing in the state legislature, during state budget for the forthcoming financial year.

Each and every budget proposal thus submitted will be scrutinized by financial experts and senior officers at various levels, either approved in full or with cuts and send back to the department concerned for implementation, after state assembly passes it before 31st March of every year.

Budget approval: From the above discussion, it is clear that hospital pharmacy department is required to maintain somewhat detailed and correct records to arrive at the figures for the budget. Though it is very desirable to collect and keep one's own statistical data, it is commonly observed in practice for the pharmacist to depend upon the accounts department for many basic figures.

Hence Pharmacist must develop a close liaison and support with the accounts officer of the hospital and thus he can prepare a best budget and through its correct implementation earn reputation for himself and his department.

However, he should be ready to receive his budget proposals with cuts or modifications, in the beginning of each financial year say by April and implement it with his full efficiency, so as to get approval of his next budget proposals without cuts.

Questions

Short Answer Questions

1. List the objectives of Hospital Pharmacy Budget.

2. What are the characters of a budget?

Long Answer Questions

3. How a budget for hospital pharmacy is prepared?

4. Enumerate the factors affecting the budget of a hospital pharmacy.

5. What are different sections of a budget? Explain.

CHAPTER 9

MANUFACTURING IN HOSPITALS

Introduction

The main function of hospital pharmacy is to make available to the patient the medication required for his well being, in full, without any interruption or short supply. The pharmacy may accomplish this by purchasing the drugs from pharmaceutical manufacturing companies or may undertake the manufacture within the hospital itself. However the aim is to make quality preparations available at lower cost.

To achieve this aim, manufacture of essential drugs in the hospitals is a better option as depending on outside commercial supply has inherent drawbacks and problems as detailed below.

Advantages or Need for Manufacture in Hospitals

When manufacturing of drugs are undertaken in hospitals:

1. Cost of medicines is reduced as it avoids profit margin for the manufacture, whole saler and retailer apart from promotion cost and transport cost. It is estimated that this cost is one third of retail price and half of tender or contract price at which the Government purchases drugs.
2. It assures the supply of needed drug at needed time rather than depending on outside suppliers for timely supply.
3. Production and supply of emergency drugs can be undertaken as and when required as in the case of epidemics.
4. Manufacturing in hospitals complements the operation of hospital formulary system.
5. Hospital pharmacy manufacturing units can be used for giving training to pharmacy graduates.
6. It solves the problem of sub-standard drugs being supplied to the hospitals by unscrupulous suppliers and also mixing of standard drugs with sub-standard drugs and corruption, favouritism and other malpractices in the purchase of medicines to Government hospitals.
7. It provides Job opportunities for pharmacy graduates.

Problems in Starting Manufacturing in Hospitals

Though there are so many advantages, the hospital pharmacy manufacturing units are yet to be started in Indian Hospitals due to opposition from private pharmaceutical manufacturers. It is argued that private manufacturing companies will be affected, if manufacturing is started in hospitals. It is a misplaced concern because hospitals cannot and need not manufacture all the formulations available in the market. They may manufacture a maximum of 100 formulations listed as 'essential drugs' by WHO and other agencies.

Thousands of formulations left out from this list can be manufactured by these manufacturers and with efficient marketing they need not depend on supply to Government Hospitals. In fact hundreds of manufacturers are surviving years together without getting government orders, as very few can win the contract or biddings for government supply every year.

Only few hospitals like Christian Medical College Hospital, Vellore in Tamil Nadu, Government Medical College Hospital, Thiruvananthapuram are having hospital pharmacy manufacturing units. Their success story must be an eye opener for all concerned. If these manufacturing units are started in all the district head quarters hospitals and drugs supplied to all Taluk hospitals, dispensaries and primary health centers in that particular district, health care to the people will achieve an ideal level, devoid of shortage of drugs, sub therapeutic doses and consequent resistant microorganism and so on. Hence sound policy decisions should be made by governments.

Policy

First of all Government or Management of the hospital should take a policy decision to undertake manufacturing of drugs in hospitals. Though, it was recommended by Hathi committee few decades ago it is yet to be accepted and implemented by Government of India or State Governments. Hathi committee recommended only the manufacture of IV fluids in hospitals as it is used in huge quantities in all the hospitals and it is a life saving drug. However, given the expertise available with the pharmacy graduates and post graduates, other formulations like capsules, tablets, liquid orals and ointments can also be manufactured in hospitals. Once such a policy decision is taken, the next question to be decided is what formulation or drug should be manufactured in what quantity and very importantly whether such manufacturing will be economical. The cost of production of some drugs may be more if manufactured in small quantities and such drugs should be purchased from private manufacturers. To avoid such a situation, a thorough cost analysis must be undertaken for each product the hospital intended to manufacture.

Cost Analysis

The cost of production for each drug can be calculated by adding the cost of all inputs to manufacture those products. These inputs are, labour cost (Direct and Indirect), materials cost (Direct and Indirect), conversion cost and overhead expenses.

Labour cost: It can be divided into two, one involve the labour used directly in the manufacture, the other denote to indirect labour like clerks, store keeper, watchman, driver etc. Their salary per day should be calculated and multiplied by number of days they are used for the manufacture of particular product.

Material cost: These include items used for the manufacture of the drug. It also falls under two categories, viz. direct materials and indirect materials. The direct materials are all the ingredients of the formulation including excipients colouring and flavouring agents and packing materials, indirect materials are those which do not form part and parcel of the product but those materials which helps in smooth manufacture like lubricants for the machine.

Conversion cost: To convert the raw material into the finished product machines, equipments, electricity etc are also used. They undergo depreciation and consume energy in the form of steam, petrol or electricity. The cost of these should be calculated and added to production cost.

Over head expenses [Indirect cost]: This cost is not directly attributable to any one cost or any one product or service. They are administrative expenses, interest on the capital, cost of space, facilities like phone, water, stationary, postage, printing etc.

Adding the entire above costs one can get the total production cost for a particular drug. It should be divided by the number of units manufactured and cost per unit is obtained. This cost should be lessthan the rate at which it is available from the pharmaceutical manufacturers.

The indirect cost should be compared with the direct cost for the purpose of calculating a ratio, which may be later added to the direct costs. The following example illustrates the point.

(a) Assume the ratio of indirect cost to direct cost is 100%.

(b) If 100 L of product 'A' require Rs. 2000 as material cost and Rs. 2500 direct cost of labour, then the cost per litre is calculated as follows:

Direct cost of Materials	Rs. 2000.00
Direct cost of Labour	Rs. 2500.00
Indirect cost @ 100% of direct cost	Rs. 4500.00
Total cost	Rs. 9000.00

Cost per litre = 9000/100 = Rs. 90

If the quantity to be manufactured is doubled to 200 L, only the material cost and packing material cost are doubled. The labour cost will increase little more in packing section, negligible in manufacturing section and hence cost of production will go down. However, the increased quantity manufactured should be used within a reasonable time. Otherwise it results in problems of storage, long time storing and reduced inventory turnover etc. Hence it is important to estimate the demand for each item to be manufactured.

Estimation of Demand

The following are the methods to estimate the demand for a drug in a hospital:

1. **Judgment Method:** Senior pharmacists can project the demand for a drug by their experience with the product and is usually accurate.

2. **Statistical Method:** By extra polating the past consumption pattern to forecast the demand for the future.

3. **Mathematical Method:** By regression analysis of hospital admissions, number of surgeries performed, infection rate etc.

Manufacturing

After the policy decision to manufacture a drug in the hospital is made cost analysis and estimation of demand are finalized. Then the hospital management has to decide, in consultation with the head of the department of pharmacy, what products it intends to manufacture and in what quantity. Depends on these decisions, after providing for future requirements etc, the pharmacy department should go for four 'M's:

1. Men
2. Machine
3. Material and
4. Method

1. *Men*: In order to manufacture pharmaceutical formulations the requirement of technical manpower is given in Drugs and cosmetics act and rules. Pharmacy graduates with sufficient experience in the manufacture of specific formulation should be appointed in specific section. Thus a pharmacist having experience in the tablet manufacturing section only, given endorsement by the drugs control administration to manufacture tablets. He should be assisted by trainee graduate pharmacists and D.Pharm holders.

Similarly, to certify the drugs manufactured, by analysis, analytical pharmacists with sufficient experience should be appointed in the laboratories attached to manufacturing unit. Other than this man power, sufficient number of skilled workers and unskilled workers should be appointed to run the machines and pack the drugs manufactured.

Among the staff required for manufacturing – the technocrats – the manufacturing and analytical pharmacists should be appointed first even before the erection of the plant and others can be appointed once the plant is ready for starting production.

2. *Machines and equipments*: The size and capacity of machines or manufacturing equipment required for a manufacturing unit of a hospital will vary from institution to institution. Before purchasing and erecting the machines, consideration must be given to the scope of the manufacturing program, the quantities to be produced and time required or expected to consume the product.

Depends on the above criteria, automatic, semiautomatic or manual machines have to be purchased and installed. As mentioned earlier, future requirements should also be considered and taken into account while taking decision about the capacity of the machine. Always there should be space for expansion in any manufacturing setup.

Many producers of pharmaceutical manufacturing and packaging equipment have prepared excellent descriptive brochures and catalogues which are to be consulted, before deciding the brand, model and size of the machines for the hospital pharmacy.

The technical personnel appointed for manufacturing (B.Pharm and M.Pharm) should be consulted and their experience with various types of machines must be given due weightage while deciding the brand and model. As these are the people going to operate the machines with the help of skilled labour, their requirements should not be overlooked and they must be first appointed or available for consultation.

After erecting the machines trial run or trial batches have to be taken up with the help or presence of Technicians or Engineers of the company which has supplied the machines. Thus a pucca, foolproof set of machines must be installed before commencing the production on large scale.

3. *Material*: Once the Men and Machines for the manufacturing are ready next important requirement is materials to be used in the manufacture. They are of three types viz.

1. Raw materials
2. Packing materials and
3. Ancillary materials

1. Raw materials are those going into the composition of the finished product. Only the active ingredients of the formulation are mentioned in the label, however, we may use many excipients and adjuvants like colouring agents, sweetening agents and flavouring agents.

2. Packing materials are the labels, cartons, boxes, bottles, caps, corrugated sheets, adhesive tapes, aluminium foils or blisters, batch number printing inks, gum, paste etc., which are used to pack the finished product either individually or in bulk.

3. Ancillary materials are those which are used during the manufacturing process but do not go into the composition of it. For example, filter papers, filter pads, lubricants used in machines, cleaning brushes, cloths etc, are equally important to have a trouble free manufacturing run.

For determining the quantity of each of the material to be purchased the production in charge pharmacist must have the master formula (refer below) the procedure or method of manufacture etc. Using those records he can calculate the quantity of each and every item required for manufacturing all the formulations, the hospital management has decided to manufacture. This require considerable expertise and experience as non-availability of even one material to be used in a formulation out of 30 to 40 materials used for a batch halt the entire process. Hence care should be taken to stock sufficient quantity of all the 3 types of materials listed above, before starting manufacturing process.

As the same material (like excipients or adjuvant) may be required for different formulations, a production plan with quantity required for particular periods say a month should be prepared well in advance. Co-ordination and co-operation of purchase department is very much essential for any production program to be successful. These aspects are further explained in Chapter No. 12 [Purchase and Inventory control].

4. Methods of Manufacturing

Manufacture of Sterile and Non-sterile Preparations

I.   Manufacture of Sterile Preparations

(Injections): Sterile formulations include small volume parenteral, large volume parenteral, eye drops, eye lotions, eye ointments, dry syrups etc. Among these preparations, only the large volumes parenteral like Dextrose Injection, Normal Saline Injection, Dextrose Saline Injection, and Ringer Lactate Solutions are used in huge quantities in all the hospitals. As other preparations are used in small quantities compared to large volume parenteral (LVP), they can be purchased from outside manufacturers and need not be manufactured in hospitals. That's why Jai Suklal Hathi committee constituted by central government in late 60's recommended its manufacture in hospitals. However the manufacturing principles are same for all sterile preparations, hence the manufacture of LVP is detailed below:

The specific requirements for manufacture of sterile products are given in the part 1 A of the Schedule M of Drugs and Cosmetics Act 1940, which are very elaborate and anybody requiring the details can consult the same. In part II of the same Schedule M the requirements for plant and equipments are given which are reproduced below:

The whole operation of manufacture of parenteral preparations in glass and plastic containers may be divided into the following separate areas/ rooms, namely

II. Parenteral Preparations in Glass Containers

(a) Various areas

1. Water management area: This includes water treatment and storage
2. Containers and closures preparation area: This includes washing and drying of ampoules, vials, bottles and closures
3. Solution preparation area: This includes preparation and filtration of solution
4. Filling, capping and sealing area: This includes filling and sealing of ampoules and/or filling, capping and sealing of vials and bottles
5. Sterilization area
6. Quarantine area
7. Visual inspection area
8. Packaging area

(b) Equipment

The following equipments are recommended for the above areas:

(i) Water management area

1. Deionised water treatment unit
2. Distillation unit (multi-column with heat exchangers)
3. Thermostatically controlled water storage tank
4. Transfer pumps (steel service lines for carrying water into user areas)

(ii) Containers and closures preparation area

1. Automatic rotary ampoule/vial/bottle washing machine having separate air, water, distilled water jets
2. Automatic closure washing machine
3. Storage equipment for ampoules, vials, bottles and closures.
4. Dryer/sterilizer (double ended)
5. Dust proof storage cabinets
6. Stainless steel benches/stools

(iii) Solution preparation area

1. S.S tanks for solution preparation and mixing
2. Portable stirrer
3. Filtration equipment with cartridge and membrane filters or bacteriological filter
4. Transfer pumps
5. S.S benches

(iv) Filling, capping and sealing area

1. Automatic ampoule/bottle filling, capping and sealing machine under laminar air flow work station.
2. Gas lines (nitrogen, oxygen, carbon dioxide) wherever required.
3. S.S. benches/stools

(v) Sterilization area

1. Steam sterilizer (preferably with computer control for sterilization cycle along with trolley sets for loading/unloading containers before and after sterilization)
2. Hot air sterilizer (preferably double ended)
3. Pressure leak test apparatus

(vi) Quarantine area

1. Storage cabinets
2. Raised platforms/steel racks

(vii) Visual inspection area

1. Visual inspection units (preferably conveyor belt type and complete white and black assembly supported with illumination).
2. S.S. benches/stools

(viii) Packaging area

1. Batch coding machine (preferably automatic)
2. Labelling unit (preferably conveyor belt type)
3. Benches/stools.

(c) Area

(i) A minimum area of 150 sq. meters for the basic installation and an ancillary area of 100 sq. meters for small volume injectable are recommended. For large volume parenteral, an area of 150 sq. meters each for the basic installation and for ancillary area is recommended.

Those areas shall be partitioned into suitable enclosures with air lock arrangements.

(ii) Areas for formulations meant for external use and internal use shall be separately provided to avoid mix up.

(iii) Packing materials for LVP shall have a minimum area for 100 sq. meters.

III Parenteral Preparations in Plastic Containers by form Fill Seal or Blow Fill Seal Technology

(a) Various areas

The whole operation of manufacture of LVP in plastic containers including plastic pouches by automatic (all operations in one station) form-fill-seal machine or semi automatic blow molding, filling-cum-sealing machine, may be divided into following separate areas rooms:

1. Water management area
2. Solution preparation area
3. Container molding-cum-filling and sealing area
4. Sterilization area
5. Quarantine area
6. Visual inspection area
7. Packaging area

(b) Equipment

The following equipments are recommended for above areas:

(i) Water management area

1. Deionised water treatment unit
2. Distillation unit (multicolumn with heat exchangers)
3. Thermostatically controlled water storage tank
4. Transfer pumps
5. Stainless steel service lines for carrying water into user areas.

(ii) Solution preparation area

1. Solution preparation tanks
2. Transfer pumps
3. Cartridge and membrane filters.

(iii) Container molding-cum-filling and sealing area

1. Sterile form-fill-seal machine (All operations in one station with built in Laminar Air flow work station saving integrated container output conveyor belt through box).

2. Arrangement for feeding plastic granules through feeding cum filling tank into the machine.

(iv) **Sterilization area:** Super heated steam sterilizer (with computer control for sterilization cycle along with trolley sets for loading/ unloading containers for sterilization).

(v) **Quarantine area:** Adequate number of platforms/racks with storage system.

(vi) **Visual inspection area:** Visual inspection unit (with conveyor belt and composite white and black assembly supported with illumination).

(vii) **Packaging area**

1. Pressure leak test apparatus (pressure belt or rotating disc type)
2. Batch coding machine (preferably automatic)
3. Labelling unit (preferably conveyor belt type)

(c) **Space**

1. A minimum area of 250 sq. meters for the basic installation and an ancillary area of 150 sq. meters for LVP in plastic containers by form-fill-seal technology are recommended. These areas shall be partitioned into suitable enclosure with air-lock arrangements.

2. Areas for formulations meant for external use and internal use shall be separately provided to avoid mix up.

3. Packaging materials for LVP shall have a minimum area of 100 sq. meters.

IV   Manufacture of Non-Sterile Preparations

In a hospital set-up next to large volume parenteral (LVP), non-sterile preparations like tablets, liquid orals, capsules and ointments are dispensed in large quantities in that order. Hence a hospital pharmacy decided to undertake manufacture in the hospital, should take steps to manufacture these non-sterile items also, in order to meet bulk of the dispensing requirements.

Schedule M of the Drugs and Cosmetics Rules 1947 deals with the Good Manufacturing Practices and the requirements for premises, plant and equipment. Part I deals with the former (GMP) and part II deals with the latter (plant and equipments). Hospital authorities should organize these legal requirements to undertake manufacturing in hospitals.

Tablets: Manufacture of Tablets may be considered as one of the very important function of the hospital manufacturing unit, because almost all patients visiting or staying in the hospital (OP and IP) are given either one or other type of tablet. That is to say almost all the prescriptions contain a tablet or other. Hence undertaking tablet manufacturing in hospital will satisfy up to 90% of hospital requirement for drugs.

Tablet manufacturing has the following steps:

1. Mixing
2. Granulating
3. Drying
4. Punching
5. Coating and
6. Packing.

These sections require the following machineries:

1. *Mixing*

   Any one or more of the machines depends on the need, of the following:

   (a) Ribbon blender
   (b) Planetary mixer
   (c) Double cone blender

2. *Granulating*

   (a) Oscillating granulator
   (b) Fitz mill or Pulveriser

3. *Drying*

   (a) Tray dryers (24 Tray or 48 Trays)
   (b) Fluidized bed dryer

4. *Punching*

   (a) Rotary punching machines (16 stations, 32 or 64 stations)
   (b) Single stroke multiple punch or single punch machines.

5. *Coating*

   (a) Coating pans (Stainless steel) of different sizes
   (b) Polishing pans
   (c) Film coating machines or
   (d) compression coating machines.

6. *Packing*

   (a) Blister packing machines
   (b) Strip packing machines
   (c) Tablet counting machines
   (d) Sealing machines
   (e) Labelling machines.

Using the master formula file and the procedure mentioned in it, various active ingredients are made into Tablets. They are packed according to the need and the policies of the hospital either into 1000's packing or Blisters or strips. After the mandatory quality control clearances, they are sent to the hospital stores for future dispensing.

Capsules: Compared to the manufacture of tablets, manufacture of capsules is easier, as it require just the enclosure of active ingredients and diluents into the shell of the empty capsules. The various steps involved are,

1. Mixing
2. Filling
3. Polishing and
4. Packing.

The equipments needed for the above sections are, Double cone blender, capsules filling machines, (Automatic, semi-automatic or manual), polishing equipments and Blister or strip or Bulk packing machines. Prior to mixing, the raw materials are checked for moisture content and dried using any one of the dryer, if required. Similarly depends on the flow properties of raw materials, they are made into granules, or sufficient lubricants and glidents are added or mixed with inert pre-granulated diluents.

Empty capsules of good quality and standards should be used to fill the ingredients. After polishing they are packed according to the hospital requirement and policies.

Liquid orals: Though these preparations – some liquid in a bottle – were famous and popular among the hospital patients long ago, they have lost their glory to more convenient and easy to carry formulations like Tablets and capsules. Nevertheless some drugs need to be supplied in liquid form – most important among them are cough syrups and suspensions. The important steps in the manufacture of these formulations are:

1. Washing and drying of bottles
2. Preparation of purified water
3. Preparation of vehicle like sugar syrup
4. Mixing
5. Filtering, if applicable
6. Filling
7. Sealing
8. Labelling and
9. Packing.

As these steps are self explanatory, let us straight away go to the equipments required for these sections.

1. ***Bottle washing section***: Bottle washing machines with arrangement for different sizes of brushes, detergents, water jets with purified water supply and tray dryers for drying the bottles. (New bottles are just rinsed in purified water and dried].

2. **Purified water section:** Potable water supply, deionizer or demineralizer of sufficient capacity, storage tanks.

3. **Syrup section:** Large tanks, agitators or stirrers, heating source (steam or gas or electricity), filter press or filter pump, storage tanks made up of stainless steel; weighing balance etc.

4. **Mixing:** Large stainless steel tanks of various capacity like 100, 200, 250, 500, 1000 and 2000 litres, stirrer or agitator, purified water supply etc., colloid mills for suspensions.

5. **Filtration:** Filter pump or filter press with various filter medium like, filter pads, filter cloths, transport pipelines or hoses (sterile) to filling section.

6. **Filling section:** Automatic or semiautomatic filling machines of required capacity. Arrangement for visual checking of floating particles, checking of volumes filled.

7. **Sealing section:** Bottle sealing machines (automatic semiautomatic or manual), bottle caps of different sizes.

8. **Labelling section:** Labels, batch number etc., printing machines (in small scale operations) labelling machines, gum, paste etc.

9. **Packing section:** Cartons, corrugated sheets, automatic or manual packing, card board boxes etc.

External Use Preparations (Ointment, Paste, Creams etc)

It may not be economical to manufacture these items in hospitals, as the requirements for these items may not be bulk. However some ointments or creams can be prepared in the hospital, in small quantities at a time, so as to meet the requirement for 6 months or so. The various sections are,

1. Mixing
2. Filling and sealing
3. Labelling and
4. Packing.

The equipments needed are.

1. **Mixing:** Steam jacketed stainless steel tanks (or) electrically heated S.S. tanks, agitators or stirrers.

2. **Filling and sealing:** Triple roller mill; storage tanks with heating arrangement, automatic or manual filling in collapsible tubes or bottles. Tube sealing or cramping machines with Batch No. and Mfg. Date.

3. **Labelling:** If bottles are used for packing, labelling machines can be used in small scale operations, batch number printing machines etc.

4. **Packing:** Cartons, cardboard boxes, corrugated sheets.

As it is out of place to explain the entire manufacturing process or working of machineries used in manufacturing, students are advised to refer to any standard book on Pharmaceutics for unit operations as well as Pharmaceutical Jurisprudence for premises, plant and equipments, needed as per law.

Methods of Analysis

Drugs and Cosmetics Act 1940 and rules thereunder require all the drugs produced by the manufacturer must be tested for its quality and certified by competent person – the analytical chemist. As in the case of manufacturing here also four 'M's must be arranged. The first 'M' is the qualified and approved man, the analytical chemist, who should be given free hand to establish the next three 'M's - the machine, material and methods for analytical laboratory. Though machine and materials can be purchased comparatively easily, the methods of analysis for each and every raw material and formulations proposed to manufacture in the hospital is rather a difficult job.

These methods are sometimes difficult to get and hence the laboratory must have adequate expertise and facilities to develop its own foolproof method of analysis. Good Laboratory Practices [GLP] as stipulated by regulatory agencies must be followed and thus quality of each and every batch manufactured in the hospital must be ensured. The analytical and quality control processes involve testing by chemical, biological and instrumental methods of analysis. Hence all these three sections must be established with needed equipments, chemicals and space as per statutory requirements.

Quality Control: For each batch of the product, there shall be appropriate laboratory testing to confirm the final specifications. It includes test for identity and strength of each active ingredient. Tests for sterility and tests for pyrogen are conducted as per requirements of law and till the quality control people approve the particular batch for release, the entire batch is kept in quarantine stores.

Sampling and testing procedures are described in written form that shall include the method of sampling and the number of units per batch to be tested. The accuracy, sensitivity, specificity and reproducibility of test methods employed by the hospital shall be established and documented.

Batch failing to meet established standards of specification and any other quality control criteria shall be rejected. Reprocessing may be performed and once again tested to confirm the standards. Thus after getting approval of quality control people only each batch is released for distribution.

Questions

Short Answer Questions

1. What are the advantages of manufacturing in hospitals?

2. How estimation of demand for a drug in hospital is made?

3. Explain the salient features of cost analysis for manufacturing drugs in hospitals.

Long Answer Questions

4. Explain the requirements for manufacturing drugs in hospitals.

5. Write an essay about sterile manufacturing in hospitals.

6. Write briefly about manufacture of Non-sterile preparations in hospitals.

7. Enumerate the role of analysis and quality control of drugs in hospitals.

CHAPTER 10

TOTAL PARENTERAL NUTRITION AND INTRAVENOUS ADMIXTURE

Introduction

Total Parenteral Nutrition and Intravenous admixture are essentially part of manufacturing activities and hence it is more appropriate to study them next to manufacturing in hospitals. Needless to point out the above mentioned works can be carried out better by manufacturing pharmacists in a formulation manufacturing unit than in any other set up including dispensary of the hospitals, as all the space and facilities for compounding, mixing, filtering, filling and testing are readily available in the hospital manufacturing units. Without such manufacturing facilities in hospital, the medical practitioners in the hospitals are finding it difficult to get the appropriate formulations to suit the specific needs of particular patients. They are either compelled to use available formulations or administer multiple formulations to the patient, making the treatment process much more complicated. Hence they welcome these facilities and expertise in their hospitals.

Total Parenteral Nutrition

Definition

Intravenous administration of calories, nitrogen and other nutrients in sufficient quantities to achieve tissue synthesis and anabolism is called Total Parenteral Nutrition (TPN). Long ago this was described as hyper alimentation, but now a days it is referred to as TPN, as this name is more suitable and explain the technique.

Indications

From the above definition it is clear that parenteral nutrition (PN) is the intravenous administration of a nutritionally balanced and physically and chemically stable, sterile, solution. It is indicated, if the gastro intestinal tract is inaccessible, inadequate or inappropriate to meet the patient's ongoing nutritional needs. Parenteral nutrition may meet the total nutritional requirements of the patient or supplement the enteral feed or diet.

It is given to patients who are unable to eat due to carcinoma or extensive burns or who refuse to eat like geriatric cases. It is also indicated to young patients suffering from anorexia nervosa and surgical patients who should not be given food orally.

After the patient's condition is improved, depends on his external food intake, the TPN should be gradually reduced and should not be stopped abruptly.

Composition of TPN

The objective of including various components of TPN is to provide appropriate sources and amounts of all the building blocks in a single daily admixture. Thus in addition to water, six main groups of nutrients need to be included in the TPN formulation. They are amino acids, glucose, lipid with essential fatty acids, Vitamins, Trace elements and Electrolytes.

Water: In general an adult patient requires fluids up to 20 to 40 ml/kg/day. This is regulated by homeostasis of the body in normal people and may be ineffective in patients. Hence appropriate amount of water should be administered to the patient avoiding over or under hydration. Some of the factors affecting fluid requirements are dehydration or overload, fever, acute anabolic state, high environmental temperature, or low or high humidity, abnormal GI loss, burns or open wounds, blood loss or transfusion, drug therapy and cardiac or renal failure. Taking into consideration of all these factors the fluid input is either increased or reduced.

Amino acids: 20 amino acids are required for protein synthesis and metabolism. A majority of these can be synthesized by our body. There are some 8 amino acids which are called essential amino acids because they cannot be synthesized, whereas even some of the synthesized amino acids may not be sufficient in diseased conditions. Neonates, infants and children may need some amino acids, due to ineffective or immature metabolic pathways. All these factors are taken into consideration while formulating TPN. Crystalline amino acids serve as source of nitrogen in TPN fluids. The crystalline amino acids injections contain all the essential and non-essential amino acids in the L form. For optimum use of amino acids and for promoting tissue regeneration, the nitrogen to calorie ratio should be 1:150. Amino acid solutions are hypertonic and should not be administered alone into the peripheral circulation.

Glucose: Glucose is the ideal source of carbohydrate. Glucose 5% solution is isotonic with blood, but to meet the energy requirement of 2500 calories/day, this concentration may not be sufficient as it provides only 170 calories/litre. Hence higher concentrations, say 25% is administered, but it causes phlebitis, if administered directly to peripheral veins and hence should be given by a central vein (sub-clavian vein into the super vena cava) or after diluting with compatible solutions like amino acid injections, to reduce the toxicity.

Lipid: Lipid emulsions are used as a source of energy and for providing essential fatty acids, like linoleic acid and linolenic acid. They are energy rich and directly administered into peripheral veins as they are isotonic with blood. Earlier soyabean oil was used in TPN formulations, now-a-days olive oil, fish oil and medium chain triglycerides are used. Lipid clearance should be monitored by the clinical pharmacist for diabetic and other patients with impaired renal or hepatic functions.

Vitamins: The daily requirement of both water soluble and fat soluble vitamins should be added to TPN formulation. It is usually added in the form of multivitamin infusion concentrate. Combinations of different vitamin formulations are used, as no formulation meets the guideline requirement of all vitamins.

Electrolytes: The requirement of electrolytes used to vary with individual patient and the electrolyte content in the amino acid injections also should be taken into account while deciding the TPN components. The following are the concentration range of electrolytes to be used.

Sodium	-	100-120 mEq.
Potassium	-	80-120 mEq.
Magnesium	-	8-16 mEq.
Calcium	-	5-10 mEq.
Chloride	-	100-120 mEq. and
Phosphate	-	40-60 mEq.

Trace elements: There are 10 trace elements required for the body. They are iron, copper, zinc, fluorine, manganese, iodine, cobalt, selenium, molybdenum and chromium, out of this iron can be administered separately from the PN fluids. Others are concern only in longterm cases and can be added when required. Some of the factors to be considered while deciding the requirement of micronutrients (including vitamin) are, baseline nutritional state, increased loss, increased requirement and organ function like liver or kidney impairments.

Advantages of TPN and its Handling

Parenteral nutrition was administered from a series of separate bottles earlier. Health care staff had to accurately and safely manage, different trip sets, infusion rate and infusion time. Now it is possible to administer the total requirement of patient's nutrition from a single daily bag of a pharmaceutically stable formulation.

There are many advantages of TPN. They are: It is convenient and time saving, permit optimum utilization, reduce the infection risk, reduce risk of error, reduce scope for incompatibility, easy storage and stock management and possibility of home management. There are few disadvantages like potential time delay in preparing specific TPN, potential wastage of TPN if patients need changes, also variation of physical and chemical stability need to be known for storage and infusion time.

Overload of fluid, nutrition and electrolytes can have serious consequences; hence an infusion control pump must be used along with compatible infusion set. TPN should be administered when it is at room temperature, hence it should be removed from refrigerator 3 hours before administering. Initially it should be given at a slow rate for first 24 hours, later it can be increased if the patient tolerated it. Patient should be monitored for adverse events like nausea, vomiting, sweating and flushing.

Formulation Problems

After identifying the various nutrients and their quantities required by a patient, it is necessary to formulate a physically and chemically stable sterile preparation.

These preparations, at times, contain more than 50 ingredients and hence are extremely complex. Reference books should be consulted before making a preparation. The following are the problems of a TPN formulation.

1. *Physical stability*: Precipitation and lipid destabilization are the two important problems of physical stability of TPN. Precipitation may occur due to various factors like pH, temperature, presence of amino acids, magnesium, calcium and phosphorus and mixing order. Lipid destabilization results in creaming flocculation and coalescence.

2. *Chemical stability*: It is identified by chemical degradation of the vitamins, amino acids, oxidation of vitamin C, photolysis of vitamin A, photo oxidation of vitamin E are common. They can be avoided by protecting the preparation from light and high temperatures.

3. *Microbial stability*: TPN formulation itself a high nutritious medium for microbial growth. Hence it should be sterilized properly and handled carefully so as, not to contaminate the product. As with any IV infusion TPN also must be carefully examined visually and then used.

4. *Drug stability*: PN should not be mixed with other drugs as far as possible, as it will affect the above stabilities of the PN as well the drug being mixed. It may also affect the bioavailability of the drug. Strict aseptic technique should be adopted to minimize the risk of contaminating the line while adding a drug.

   In addition to the above problems, particulate matter contamination during administration and photo-degradation during storage and transport must be taken care of by using terminal in line filters, quality trip sets and raw materials, and protection from light.

I.V. [Intravenous] Admixtures

Introduction: Mixing of intravenous solutions with additional substances is done by Nurses and House surgeons or Doctors in India even today in majority of the hospitals. It is done on the assumption that all the Injections or sterile preparations are same and can be mixed with IV fluids. Just because all they add to IV fluids are also sterile, nothing will happen to those fluids, they believe. Obviously they look only at the sterility aspect of IV fluid and added drugs and have no knowledge what so ever, about its stability solubility, pH, incompatibility etc. Now, at least a section of this health care team has realized that, the IV Admixture is a sort of Injection manufacturing process and requires the skills of manufacturing pharmacist. Still a vast majority of these peoples are unaware and has to be educated by the pharmacists and in the meanwhile, to avoid mixing of additional drugs, various devices are developed by IV trip set manufacturers with different ports (openings) for additives in the set itself (VENTPLAN) or at the point of insertion of needle into the body of the patient, thus making the admixture of drugs a rare requirement. However a pharmacist must know the task of preparing IV admixture.

Definition: When one or more sterile products are added to an IV fluid for administration, the resulting mixture is known as IV admixture.

Objectives of Preparation of IV Admixtures
1. IV admixture must be done under strict aseptic conditions.
2. Drug interactions should be avoided by correct choice of additives and mixing techniques.
3. The final product should be appropriately labelled, dispensed and stored.

Suitability of Pharmacists

As addition of any ingredient to a formulation is a manufacturing activity, only a technical hand with the knowledge of the process is suitable. Thus a pharmacist who undergoes training and education in the manufacturing process, and learn about the physical, chemical and pharmacological properties of drugs during his graduation is perfect suit for the process than anybody else.

Moreover, to maintain the characteristics of sterile products, namely, sterility, freedom from particulate matter and pyrogen, it is imperative that they be performed by pharmacist in a suitable environment using aseptic techniques.

Purpose and uses of IV Admixture Service by Pharmacists

If the IV admixture service is undertaken by the pharmacist,
  (a) It saves the nursing time,
  (b) It provides for screening of physical and chemical incompatibilities by him
  (c) It minimize the calculation errors and medication errors
  (d) It centralizes the responsibility on the pharmacist rather than on multiple workers of health care team
  (e) Specific directions on the label like rate of infusion is possible and
  (f) It provides for solutions not commercially available.

Thus IV admixture service by pharmacists has many advantages and uses.

Preparation Area

Laminar flow Hoods provide an area for aseptic handling of IV admixture. In laminar flow hoods, the air is filtered through High Efficiency Particulate Air (HEPA) filter. HEPA filters remove 99.9% of all particles larger than 0.3 μm.

Since microbes are found on particles, removal of particles results in a flow of air free from both particles and microorganisms. Regardless of the type of laminar air flow, the Hood must be maintained properly to achieve an environment suitable for IV Admixture.

It must be placed in an air-conditioned room, free from any movement in front of it and its inside work bench should be wiped with a suitable disinfectant, 30 minutes before the process. It must be remembered that laminar flow hood is not a means of sterilization, but only maintain an area for IV admixture, if prepared, maintained and used properly by operator with proper aseptic techniques.

Operation and maintenance of Laminar flow Hoods can be had from the supplier and/or manufacturer of it, which should be strictly followed to get best results.

Mixing of Additional Drugs

These drugs may be injections in ampoules or vials. If solids, they must be reconstituted with suitable diluents before adding to IV fluid. A new, sterile, disposable syringe should be used for each drug and its needle may be replaced with a sterile aspirating needle. Aspirating needles have stainless steel or nylon filter with 5 μm pores. Additional drugs are drawn from their containers using this needle and then replaced with original regular needle.

Some of the additional drugs may be light sensitive, and hence the syringe can be wrapped with aluminium foil, and added to the IV fluid. The procedure for adding a drug in an IV fluid will vary depending on the type of IV fluid container.

Usually an IV admixture is considered as a unit dose. However if intermittent administration of drugs is essential, three methods are available:

1. Direct IV injection
2. Addition of drug to pre-determined volume of IV fluid in a volume control chamber attached below the main IV bag or bottle.
3. Use of second container (mini bottle/bag) with already hanging IV fluid and joining them by using 'Y' tube at the bottom.

Parenteral Incompatibility

When one or more drugs are added to an IV fluid, they may modify the characters of the substances present resulting in parenteral incompatibility. They are classified into Physical Incompatibility, Chemical Incompatibility and Therapeutic Incompatibility.

Among these, physical incompatibility can be predicted if the chemical properties of added drug and IV fluids are known. For example, sodium salts of weak acids such a Phenytoin sodium or Phenobarbital sodium, precipitate as free acids when added to IV fluids with acidic pH. Similarly calcium salts precipitate when added to alkaline medium, and water insoluble substances such as diazepam, when added to IV fluids precipitate.

Chemical incompatibilities are occurring due to hydrolysis, oxidation, reduction or complexation and can be detected by analytical methods only. An important factor which affects IV admixture is the change in acid base environment or pH of it. As the solubility and more importantly stability of IV fluids depend on a particular pH, it should not be disturbed by added drugs. Though change in solubility is visible by the precipitation etc., stability changes cannot be viewed. Example for this is the antibiotic penicillin, which is active at pH 6.5 for 24 hours, whereas it is destroyed at pH 3.5 within a short time.

Therapeutic incompatibility is better illustrated in the example of antagonizing effect of penicillin or cortisone on heparin. Thus, though it is impossible to predict and prevent all parenteral incompatibilities, their occurrence can be minimized, if the pharmacist concerned with IV admixture consults all the available literatures from parenteral manufacturers.

Quality Control

In order to maintain standards and quality of IV admixture, each hospital should have written procedures for each and every step of preparing IV admixture. Starting from the selection of additives to final administration and monitoring of patient, it is essential to maintain high standards. Suitable training programmes and re-orientation programmes should be arranged for the staff concerned with IV admixture.

In fact, all these operations are to be considered equivalent, in no way inferior to the current Good Manufacturing Practices followed by manufacturing industries and insisted by Government through Drugs Control Department.

Questions

Short Answer Questions

1. What is total parenteral nutrition?

2. Define IV Admixture.

3. What are the purpose and uses of IV admixture service by pharmacists?

Long Answer Questions

4. Describe the composition of total parenteral nutrition. What are the problems encountered during its preparation?

5. How IV admixtures are prepared? Add a note on parenteral incompatibility.

6. Why a TPN is prepared? Describe its handling and advantage.

CHAPTER 11

PRE-PACKING AND REPACKING IN HOSPITALS

Introduction

Repacking and pre-packing of drugs are carried out in some hospitals for convenience in dispensing. By definition repacking is one of the manufacturing activities as per Drugs and Cosmetic Act and Rules; however, pre-packing requires no licence.

Drugs which are dispensed too many times in a day, in big hospitals are pre-packed, whereas, other drugs which are not dispensed many times in a day are packed and dispensed as and when required. It is economical, easy and less time consuming if the items required daily for ward supply and dispensary like tablets, capsules, syrups and ointments are pre-packed. Sometime it may require separate work force, equipment and supervision to prevent errors.

Factors to be Considered

The product and quantity to be packed is determined as per the particular hospital's requirement. While deciding those aspects the following factors should be taken into account.

1. Cost of pre-packing.
2. Impact on drug's stability.
3. Storage conditions and space required.
4. Quantity of pre-packed drug required and its period of demand whether seasonal or round the year.
5. Quantity of drug in each pre-packing 10's, 12's, 20's, 24's, 30's, etc.
6. What type of packing material or container to be used.
7. Labels required for each pre-packed unit.
8. Requirement of manpower or machines for pre-packing.

9. Availability of similar packing with supplier or manufacture of the drug and its cost.

10. Need for packing again at the time of dispensing.

1. ***Cost of pre-packing:*** Obviously pre-packing in a hospital require men, machine and material, which in turn require money. The cost of pre-packing has to be borne by the hospital, if not recovered from the patient. Since drugs are already packed by the manufacturer, the pre-packing should be less and materials used should not be costlier. Again the drugs are dispensed for immediate consumption and hence not required any sophisticated packing.

2. ***Impact on drugs stability:*** The pre-packing operations should not affect the stability of drugs dispensed. Usually drugs like vitamins and antibiotics if damaged in its original packing leads to deterioration of its quality and stability. Care should be taken while pre-packing that the drug's original packing are not disturbed, but improved.

3. ***Storage conditions and space required:*** During pre-packing the drugs are removed from its original container and there is a possibility of destruction of its quality, if not stored properly, after pre-packing. Similar conditions of storage should be maintained for pre-packed drugs also, as that of original packing. That may not be possible always, as pre-packing increases the space required for storage. For example, an original packing of 1000's or 100's tablet or capsules of antibiotics or vitamins cannot be stored in the same space, after pre-packing into 10's or 15's. This problem is acute in the case of drugs which required refrigeration.

4. ***Quantity and time of pre-packing:*** How much drug is to be pre-packed and when is the difficult question to decide. Quantity of pre-packed drug required, varies with number of patients visiting and/or prescribed the drug in question. Doctors changes the drugs prescribed depend on many factors. We cannot expect, that they will be prescribing same drugs at all times. Again, the drug may be required only at particular season and may not be required throughout the year. Some drugs may be required in large quantities on outbreak of some diseases in that area, all of a sudden. Hence pre-packing is not possible always.

5. ***Quantity of drug in each pre-packing:*** Doctors prescribe various quantities of drugs depends on many reasons like, severity of diseases, requirement of review of the patient's condition and so on. Hence the quantity in pre-packing cannot be constant. Different quantities of drugs like 10's, 12's, 15's, and 20's has to be pre-packed and consequently inventory, space, cost and complications increase proportionately.

6. ***What type of packing material or container to be used?***

    This question has to be determined before undertaking pre-packing of drugs. There cannot be any compromise on the quality or stability of the drug and hence for all the packing materials and containers, minimum standards should be there. Procuring such materials at minimum cost to the hospital, require prior planning and execution.

Some containers or packing by the original manufacturer cannot be opened and resealed and hence drugs has to be dispensed as such or in similar container or packing material has to be purchased however costly it may be. Finding equally good, alternative material or container is very difficult.

7. *Requirement of labels*: When we pre-pack drugs, labels have to be printed or prepared for each pre-packed unit. It requires careful attention of supervisory pharmacist as any mislabelling will be disastrous to the entire operations. As the label has to be proportionate to the containers used and at the same time large enough to print all the statutory information, it also requires planning.

8. *Men and machines for pre-packing*: Required number of workers should be appointed in the pre-packing section of the hospital including supervisory staffs. Proper place, work table, lightings and storage area for unpacked drugs, packed drugs and labelled drugs should be marked and order of packing must be maintained. Mix up should be avoided. Labelling machines may not be required as they are for large scale manufacturing. However Label gumming machines can be installed for speedy pasting of labels on the container. These machines help in avoiding excess or less gum on the back of the label which result in ugly exterior or peeling of labels from the container. Sometimes labels without batch number, date of manufacturing. etc., printed on it is pasted on the container; hence the workers engaged in labelling should be instructed to keep an eye on the labels while fixing it on to the container.

9. *Availability of smaller packing with manufacture*: This factor demolishes the entire above requirement, as it is always economical to purchase those packing, if they are already available in the market. For example almost all the tablets and capsules are marketed as either blisters or strips of 10's or 15's. It is easy to purchase and dispense those packing. A very small percentage of patients require different quantity and that can also be dispensed by cutting those packing and writing the needed information like batch number, date of expiry etc., on the dispensing envelope. It is the general economic theory that any small scale manufacture will be costly and hence avoided.

10. *Need for packing again at the time of dispensing*: It is not possible in all the pre-packed drugs to write the name of the patient or the dose to be taken. It required a plain writable surface on the packing. Usually it is done by putting the drug into a dispensing envelope, over which all the above information is written.

It is not possible to write on the pre-packed containers; once again the pharmacist has to pack it in a dispensing envelope. Thus it increases the cost of dispensing. From the above discussion it is clear that pre-packing is not possible and feasible with all the drugs dispensed. If the number of eligible drugs for pre-packing goes down, the entire operation becomes uneconomical and waste of resources.

Pre-packing Operations

In small hospitals pre-packing operation is usually carried out by the pharmacist with the help of assistants. This is the practical approach to the problem when the volume is not more. Hence no special area need to be set aside, and there is no need for any special counting equipment other than manual tablet counter and moderately sensitive balances for weighing. Those hospitals which are required to pre-pack large quantities, establish a separate unit for the purpose. Here, a separate team of workers under the supervision of the pharmacist works using automatic or semi automatic machines.

For pre-packing of drugs in hospitals, packaging material or container, its shape and form and labels should be considered and procured. While procuring packing material or containers, not only its quality but also its commercial availability should be ascertained. Otherwise uniformity in hospital pre-packing cannot be achieved. Similarly the shape, design and form of the packing material should be in such a way that the contents can be used or administered directly from the container, without transfer to any other container. The package should be easy to open, easy to use and easy to dispose.

Once smaller packing is required, lot of labels are needed. They should be prepared according to the Drugs and Cosmetics Act and Rules and kept ready to paste as soon as packing is made.

Advantages and Disadvantages of the Pre-packing

Advantages

1. It helps in quick dispensing.
2. Error rate (in counting, measuring or weighing) is reduced.
3. Easy to control the inventory in dispensary.
4. Patients feel it is comfortable and less confusing.
5. Patients compliance can be easily checked and
6. Prescribing quantities are rationalized.

Disadvantages

1. Cost of drugs increases.
2. If the prescription is for other than packed quantity, it is required to open the pack or to keep the stock of unpacked drugs.
3. Pre-packed items require more storage space.

Re-packing

It is the process of breaking up any drug from a bulk container into small packages and the labelling of each package with a view to its sale and distribution.

It does not include the compounding or dispensing or packing of any drug in the ordinary course of the retail business. Actually it is considered as one of the manufacturing process. Hence it requires license from drug control department. It is issued for drugs other than Schedule C and C_1 and Schedule X, subject to fulfilment of some conditions.

As re-packing in hospital is normally for the purpose of dispensing, these conditions and license are not applicable. However, a pharmacist is supposed to undertake and supervise the re-packing operations in a hospital.

Recent Trends

Pre-packing or re-packing in hospitals are very rare, now a day, because all the drugs are available in pre-packed form and supplied by the manufacturers. All unit dosage forms such as tablets and capsules are supplied in blister or strip packing and multidose formulations are supplied in small quantities required. Hospitals can order whatever the packing required for them with the manufacturers, hence there is no need for hospital pharmacists to go for pre-packing or repacking.

However in order to save the cost i.e., for economical reasons, it is the Government or management of hospitals that are ordering bulk packing like 100's, or 1000's packing or 5 L jars, necessitating pre-packing or repacking.

Ultimately it is the cost that decides the packing.

Questions

Short Answer Questions

1. What is re-packing?
2. Define re-packing.
3. What are the differences between pre-packing and repacking?
4. Discuss the advantages and disadvantages of pre-packing.

Long Answers Questions

5. Describe the factors to be considered before pre-packing of drugs.
6. Explain the pre-packing and re-packing operations of hospitals.

CHAPTER 12

PURCHASE AND INVENTORY CONTROL

Introduction

Purchase and inventory control are very important operations of a hospital pharmacy. Both these works and the procedures vary with the size of the hospital, distance from the source of supply, storage facilities and turn over and of course on cost. Usually in a hospital HOD of Hospital Pharmacy or Chief Pharmacist and few other senior pharmacists are assigned these works, as they require expertise, experience and endurance to carry out and complete it successfully. However a budding pharmacist is expected to know the theoretical aspects of it and may be required to apply it in practice or assist the seniors as and when required. Knowledge of purchase and inventory control is required even if a fresh pharmacist decide to open his own community pharmacy store.

Definitions

As the three words, 'purchase' 'inventory' and 'control' are to be used repeatedly in this chapter, it is better to define them first. According to W.E. Hassan,

'Purchase' is defined as an act of getting something by paying money or its equivalent or simply to obtain or buy something for a price.

'Inventory' is defined as an itemized list of goods with their estimated worth, specially an annual account of stock taken in any business.

'Control' is defined as an act of exercising power over something.

Purchase or Procurement

Purchasing authorities: Once we decide to purchase something for an organization, the first question asked is, who should purchase or who has the authority to purchase. Then only, other aspects like what, where, when and how to purchase arise.

There are two views on the authority to be designated for purchasing. One view is all institutional purchases should be centralized and a purchase officer should be appointed for the purpose. Other view is that drugs and other related items are specialty items which require technical skills and hence its purchase should be assigned to a pharmacist. However it all varies with the policies of the Government or management of the hospitals. For example there is only one centralized agent at the state level for the purchase of drugs and other items for all the hospitals of the state in Tamilnadu (Tamilnadu Medical Services Corporation, Chennai). Some other Governments have similar or other arrangements, as it has many advantages like better control on inventory, bulk purchase and consequent large discounts and prevention of malpractices and corruption at various levels.

However, if there are purchases at institutional level and a purchase officer is appointed for the purpose, he is expected to work in collaboration with the Chief Pharmacist or HOD of the pharmacy services, each recognizing the importance of the function of the other. In this system, pharmacist provide the specification for the drugs to be purchased and have the authority to reject any article which may be below the standard and specifications, so that, the purchase officer is guided and assisted in his function. Thus there may be either one of the above authorities available for purchasing drugs for a hospital

(a) In small hospitals the purchasing function may be looked after by officer in charge of stores or Hospital superintendent with the help of store keeper. As these officers are having this work as additional duty and perform it along with their regular duties, they minimize the work and heavily depend on the store keeper who may be a pharmacist.

The following are the functions of a purchasing authority weather he is a purchase officer or Pharmacist. First of all he must collect the purchase request form, commonly called an indent, from the pharmacy. After its approval by higher authorities, purchase order should be issued to suppliers. All the records and documents pertaining to purchase should be properly maintained; so that follow up actions in case of delayed supply or discrepancy in supply can be verified in future. In order to get drugs at cheaper or economical price, competitive bidding must be arranged by those who are responsible for purchase. Similarly quotations for the required items can be obtained from various suppliers by sending the list of requirements with specifications.

(b) Role of pharmacists are very limited in purchasing drugs in Indian hospitals as we employ only D. Pharm holders as pharmacists who are being easily dominated and a full department of pharmacy services with graduate and post graduate pharmacists are yet to be established in our hospitals. However a pharmacist is supposed to know his future role in drug procurement. There are some pre-requisite before purchasing drugs for the hospital. Obviously purchases cannot be done overnight. The role of Pharmacist begins with the preparation of list of manufacturers, wholesalers or their local representatives with their addresses and phone numbers. He should keep ready the specifications for the drugs he indent to purchase. Then only, he can prepare the purchase-request form or indent and send to the purchasing authority. After his approval, drugs can be purchased from various sources depends on quantity and management's policy. The following are the suppliers of drugs to hospitals.

1. Manufacturers of drugs
2. Wholesalers
3. Retailers (in case of emergency)
4. Tender winners and
5. Contract suppliers

The pharmacist is required to inform about these sources to the purchase officer and the choice of supplier is either made by the pharmacist or left to the discretion of purchase officer. Whatever may be the way of purchase of drugs, the pharmacist and authorities should make arrangement for testing the quality and standards of the drugs supplied to the hospital. It can be tested in hospital's own testing lab, if available, otherwise the samples can be send to the commercial testing laboratories or Government laboratory and order for purchase may be executed depends on the analytical report of the samples received. After the goods are received pharmacist should acknowledge it in proper format and if any item is returned to the supplier for whatever reason, he should prepare and submit a return goods memo and send to the purchase authority. The same procedure can be repeated, after all the drugs are supplied and tested randomly for quality and then the payment for the same is recommended to the hospital management.

In order to perform above duties especially for preparing specifications-pharmacist should use the books of standards like, IP, BP, USP, National formulary, Pharmaceutical Codex etc.

Purchase Procedure

The initiation for purchase of drugs starts from the pharmacists. After determining the drugs, their specifications, price, required quantity etc., the pharmacist should prepare a purchase request form. This form will have all the details mentioned above in addition to available balance, anticipated monthly use etc. The original copy of this form is send to the administrative officer in charge for the department and upon his approval it is forwarded to the purchase department. A duplicate copy is maintained in the pharmacy department.

On receiving the purchase request form, the purchase officer prepares purchase order in multiple copies, which will contain all the specifications, quantity etc., taken from the request form. First copy of the purchase order is send to the manufacturer or supplier or his representative. The second copy is accounts payable copy and is send to the accounts department and kept in file until goods are supplied and the received report come from initiating department. Third copy is retained by the purchase officer himself for his records and follow-up. Fourth copy is sent to the initiating department i.e., the pharmacy. On receiving this copy pharmacist should check it with his purchase request form for accuracy or modifications.

Fifth and sixth copies are sent to the goods receiving department who in turn verify the goods and sent their received report to the accounts department in the fifth copy. If the goods are to be ordered again the sixth copy can be used or ignored.

If some goods are returned to the supplier for some or other reason, a return goods memo is prepared in multiple copies and sent to initiating department, purchase officer accounts department and stores.

Immediately after the goods are received, they are promptly entered in the purchase record and stock register with all the relevant details, like, invoice number and date, name of the supplier, quantity received etc.

Whenever an item is not supplied and out of stock in the pharmacy and stores, an out of stock form should be prepared in duplicate and sent to initiating, or consuming department so that a false sense of heavy demand is not created.

Control on Purchases

Almost all the superior authorities or managements of the hospitals attempt to limit the purchase volume by placing an upper limit in rupees terms on the purchase order. This method may not serve the purpose, as it is easily circumvented by issuing multiple small orders or results in fewer items and quantities, causing, shortage of drugs in the hospitals.

A more scientific method of control on purchases is to calculate the inventory turnover and order the goods accordingly. It is calculated by dividing the cost of goods sold or issued during the financial year by the average of opening and closing inventory costs. This gives the number of times the inventory has been turned over during the period.

For example if the total cost of goods sold or issued in one year in a big hospital is Rs. 20 Lakhs and the opening inventory cost is Rs. 6 Lakhs and closing inventory cost is Rs. 4 Lakhs, then the average of them is calculated to be Rs. 5 Lakhs. On dividing the total cost Rs. 20 Lakhs by this average gives a turnover rate of 4.

Inventory turnover of 4 times a year indicates the purchase was carried out properly in the previous year. That is, goods are purchased on an average 3 months once and it is considered as a satisfactory practice in trade. This turnover rate can be up to 6, meaning thereby purchase of goods once in 2 months, if the organization is running short of finance. But if it is more than 6, it denotes pessimistic attitude of management and loosing of bulk purchase discounts. Pharmaceutical manufacturers are offering more incentives on bulk purchases, for example, if you purchase 10 bottles of cough syrup they give 1 bottle free, at the same time, if you purchase 25 bottles, 3 bottles are given free, similarly for 50, ten bottles and for 100 twenty five bottles are offered, thus decreasing your cost of purchase by 10% to 25% [or increasing your profit margin from 10% to 25%]. Moreover, repeated purchase of same item many times in a year involve cost of purchase every time and waste of time and energy in the process of purchase.

On the other hand, a low turnover rate [less than 4] indicates, duplication of stock, large purchases of slow moving items and dead stock and investment.

Thus purchases should be controlled in an efficient and reasonable manner. In order to do that the purchasing authorities must know important aspects of inventory control, hence they are discussed below:

Inventory Control

While inventory is defined as an itemized list of goods with their estimated worth or value, inventory control is defined as a process of safe guarding the company's inventory and maintain it in an optimum level.

The importance and uses of inventory control are listed below:

1. It reduces the cost of production
2. It minimise the time wastage due to shortage of raw materials
3. It minimise the wastage of goods
4. It minimise the capital investment
5. It maximise customer service
6. It helps to deliver the goods at right place and right time.
7. The value of goods on storage can be seen at any time, and
8. It improves overall handling and storing of goods.

Inventory Levels

While stocking goods, the inventory level should be optimum. Excess of stock leads to huge cost of running the organization, at the same time less stock leads to many problems in supply of required item at required time. Hence store keepers follow some levels of stock and they are,

1. *Maximum level:* A level is fixed after studying various factors; beyond which, materials should not be purchased at any time, that level is called maximum level.
2. *Minimum level:* It is a level beyond which the materials should not be allowed to fall at any time.
3. *Re-order level:* This is the level at which order should be placed to replenish the stock.

Methods

Following are the various method of inventory control:

1. *Periodic inventory control*: In this method, a physical count of inventory at the end of each accounting period (a year) is undertaken.

2. *Perpetual inventory control*: In this method, entries are made in the register as and when the sale or issue is completed. Day-to-day entries thus made keep the record updated always. This is the method of inventory control followed in all the dispensaries and medical stores of the hospital as an item or medicine going out of stock, without knowing, will create lot of trouble and problems for the hospital.

3. *Special inventory -Inventory for perishable drugs*: Important life saving drugs like biologicals, (antibiotics vaccine, serum etc.,) which undergo degradation easily and have short shelf-life should have a special care. This can be achieved by the following methods:

    (a) Maintaining separate record for these items with their name, potency and expiry date.

    (b) Replacing the items nearing expiry or expired, with new one by constantly checking the record as well as physical stock.

Control of Inventory

Hospital pharmacists must control the inventory by using various measures or parameters available for the purpose. They are EOQ (Economic Order Quantity) and RQL (Re-order Quantity Level). These measures can also be used to control the purchase volume.

RQL: The greatest dilemma for a pharmacist during his professional practice in a medical store (of hospital or outside) is when and how much of an item of medicine is to be ordered. An arbitrary decision on these aspects will definitely lead to trouble and loss; hence a scientific method is needed based on which a rational decision can be made by the pharmacist.

One of the methods to determine the time of order placing is RQL (Re-order Quantity Level). It is the level that must be reached before additional stocks are ordered. Sapp, *et al.*, has developed a table to use EOQ and RQL, according to which for determining the Re-order quantity, the average usage rate per month in units of issue should be divided by 13 weeks. Then multiply the figure by the average Vender Lead Time (VLT) plus the safety factor. The following table illustrates the point:

VLT	Safety factor
0 to 2 weeks	1.0
2 to 5 weeks	1.5
5 to 8 weeks	2.0
8 to 11 weeks	2.5
11 to 15 weeks	3.0

$$R.Q = \frac{\text{Average usage rate per month}}{13} = A$$

$$= A \times (VLT + SF)$$

Simpler Method of getting RQL is by multiplying lead time in days by average daily usage of inventory. For example, if you are selling or dispensing on an average 20 bottles of B.Complex syrup per day and it require 7 days for the supplier to deliver the goods, then you must order for it when your stock reaches 140 [20 x 7] bottles.

EOQ (Economic Order Quantity): How much of an item is to be ordered, is determined by using EOQ factor. To calculate this factor, it is important to ascertain the cost of ordering and cost of carrying the inventory or holding cost. Then the EOQ is calculated by applying the following formula:

$$EOQ = \frac{\sqrt{2 \times 12 \times \text{monthly usage} \times \text{cost of ordering}}}{\text{Unit cost} \times \text{Holding cost}}$$

It may be advantageous to order expensive items on a monthly basis and inexpensive items annually. Another method of calculating the EOQ is by mathematical approach. Here the formula used is,

$$EOQ = \sqrt{\frac{2AB}{C}}$$

Where,

A is Annual usage of inventory in units

B is Buying cost per order

C is Carrying cost per unit

Example: If A = 1600 units, B = 50 Rs and C = 1Re, then

$$EOQ = \sqrt{\frac{2 \times 1600 \times 50}{1}} = \sqrt{1600}\,00 = 400 \text{ units}$$

However, in this method there are some limitations, they are,

1. The sale per year is an assumption.
2. Time taken for supply is not considered.

3. If there is unexpected demand, this calculation is useless and

4. The EOQ calculated as above may be in fraction.

Nevertheless, instead of arbitrarily determining these quantities without any basis, it is better to use some scientific calculations. A pharmacist will learn these and other skills with his experience in the job. Majority of the times, calculations made using discretion and experience of a pharmacist will be correct and rewarding.

Questions

Short Answer Questions

1. What is inventory control?

2. What are different inventory levels?

3. What are different methods of inventory control?

4. What is inventory turn-over rate? How it is calculated?

5. What is RQL?

6. What is EOQ?

Long Answers Questions

7. Explain the drug purchase procedure of a Hospital. Enumerate the role of pharmacists in it.

8. How inventory is controlled in a hospital? Explain various methods and calculations involved.

9. How purchase is controlled in a hospital or in medical store? Discuss the effect of excess or less purchase quantities.

10. Enumerate the role of purchasing authorities in purchase of drugs for a hospital?

CHAPTER 13

ORGANIZATION AND MANAGEMENT OF DRUG STORE

Introduction

"Store is a place where physical storage of materials is made which are carried into the place in a scientific and systematic manner in order to save them from all kinds of damages and losses and exercising overall control on their movement". The act of organizing and managing a store is known as store keeping.

Almost all the organizations are having one or more stores in their premises, for example, there are raw material stores and packing material stores and finished product stores in the case of manufacturing companies, saleable goods in the case of shops, or at least records and reports in the case of organization not dealing with physical inventory. Thus store keeping has become a universal function which everybody must know, pharmacists are not an exemption.

Importance of Store Keeping or Warehousing

Materials pilferage, deterioration and careless handing leading to reduced profits or even losses for an organization. It is more serious and important in the case of drugs and pharmaceuticals where the improper storage practices lead not only to loss in terms of money but also in terms of human lives. Hence the study of drugs store keeping and management is very important for a pharmacist.

Types of Stores

There are 3 main types of stores:

1. Central stores where centralized buying and handling of drugs are undertaken.
2. Central stores with sub-stores: Here buying is through central stores, but handling will be through many sub-stores.

3. Decentralized (or) Individual stores: Here buying and handling of drugs are undertaken by the buyer and store keeper of each department.

The type of stores adopted depends upon the circumstances prevailing in a hospital. Generally the first or second type of stores is common. In the first type (central stores) there are few advantages.

1. The labour required for this storage is less compared to decentralized storage.

2. Maintenance of number of records is less in this method.

However the main disadvantage is this store may not be under the control of a qualified person. By appointing one or two, assistant store keeper with required qualification we can solve this problem to greater extend.

In the decentralized method of storage, the main advantage is that it is under the control of a qualified person (pharmacist). He can adjust the inventory based on the prescribing trends and that is another advantage of this method of storage.

Organization of Drug Store

In order to organize a drug store in a hospital the following points should be considered:

(a) Location and layout

(b) Design of stores building and

(c) Management.

(a) **Location and layout:** The normal practice is to locate the drugs store near the consuming department, that is, near the outpatient dispensary and wards. The important points to keep in mind regarding location of stores are:

- Easy movement of materials.
- Good housekeeping.
- Sufficient space for men and material handling.
- Optimum use of storage space like floor, racks, shelves etc.
- Proper preservation from rain, sunlight and animals.
- The volume and variety of goods to be handled.
- Accessibility to mode of transportation such as lorry, van etc.

(b) **Design of stores building:**

(i) *Building*: The stores building must have adequate facilities for preservation of drugs. Facilities such as cold storages, air conditioning and similar facilities may be provided. The building must be strong, spacious, high enough, well ventilated and neatly arranged. The floor must be strong to withstand the pressure of frequent movement of materials.

(ii) *Lighting*: Clear and adequate lighting is essential at the same time windows are kept to minimum. Proper generator facilities should be provided in case of power failure, both for lighting and cold storage facilities.

(iii) *Safety*: The ways inside the stores must be kept clean, free from obstructions or materials, so that movement inside the stores is not affected or results in accidents. Provision of fire fighting facilities is necessary in important places, especially where inflammable materials like chloroform, ether etc., are stored and handled. The entry of unauthorized staff and persons should be strictly prohibited and the drug store should be kept under proper lock, wherever necessary.

(c) Management: See below

Types of Materials Stored

1. Tablets
2. Capsules
3. Injections
4. Ointments, pastes and creams
5. Liquid orals, and
6. Chemicals

If not stored separately in a surgical store of the hospital the following materials are also stored in medical/drug store of hospital under the control of a pharmacist.

- Bed sheets/blankets
- Bed side tables
- Cot
- LVP stands (saline stands)
- Needles
- Medical gases
- Syringes
- Surgical gloves
- Surgical dressings like bandages, gauze, cotton etc.
- Surgical equipments and instrument like scissors, forceps etc.
- Surgical suture and ligatures
- Trallies
- Wheel chairs etc.

Store Room Arrangement

Store room can be arranged under various techniques like alphabetically, pharmacologically, supplier wise, formulation wise etc. Each of these methods has its own advantages and disadvantages. Usually in a big store like hospital store, formulation wise arrangement is followed. Thus the drugs are arranged, as follows:

1. Capsules
2. Chemicals
3. External use preparations
4. Injections
5. Liquid orals and
6. Tablets

Each one of these formulations is arranged alphabetically within their respective area of storage for easy location and issue. Moreover there should be always adequate extra space for shelves to introduce as and when required, in each of this area. Thus keeping one type of formulation - say tablets - in different places of the store can be avoided.

Category Wise Storage of Inventory

There are many ways of exercising control over the inventory. For example drugs can be stored according to their cost, supply source or utility. As mentioned above each method of storage has its merits and demerits, and hence a store keeper has to decide which method is more convenient and suitable for him and his organization. As the inventory, is analyzed for its cost, source or utility, methods are referred to as ABC analysis, GOLF analysis and VED analysis.

ABC analysis: Here the drugs are grouped in according to the cost of the material as shown below:

'A' group items: This includes costly items such as biological and antibiotics. These items may not be more than 10% of total inventory, but it consumes 70% of total inventory cost.

'B' group items: These group of items are neither costly not cheap. They usually represent 20% of total inventory and the total investment on these items also does not exceed 20%.

'C' group items: These items are less expensive items but occupy 70% of total stock and the total cost does not exceed 10%.

Disadvantages of ABC analysis: Very critical and essential item for production or distribution may be included in C category because they may not be costlier or very cheap. For example magnesium stearate or talc in the manufacture of tablets, needles or plasters in the case of surgical items, water for injections in the case of drugs, are cheaper compared to other items in these categories, but if they are not available, as a result of less attention and control being paid to the cheaper items, there may be huge problem in the manufacture, operation or treatment respectively.

GOLF analysis: Here the drugs are grouped depend upon the source of supply of drug. Thus,

   G - Government controlled items
   O - Open market items
   L - Local purchase items and
   F - Foreign items are stored according to this order

This is an arbitrary method of classifying the drugs, may not be always possible for a store keeper to classify drugs according to this category. Hence, it is not followed much.

VED analysis: Here the drugs are classified based on their utility.

   V - Vital items
   E - Essential items and
   D - Desirable items

Vital items are very important items like life saving drugs without which a hospital cannot run. Essential items are little less important than vital items, however they are available always. Desirable items are not important compared to first two categories; however, if it is available it is welcomed, at the same time; non availability does not cause big problems. Some stores are arranged according to this method.

Storage of Drugs

Management of a Drug Store

1. *Manpower*: To manage a drug store, the first requirement is manpower. Thus in order to fulfil the organization of drug stores in a hospital, first the qualified staff- the pharmacists – must be appointed in adequate number, to manage and maintain the store. In addition to pharmacists, sufficient number of clerical staffs and labourers should be appointed to maintain accounts and to physically handle the materials respectively.

2. *Orderly arrangement*: As mentioned earlier, drugs can be arranged on the shelves either alphabetically, pharmacologically or formulations wise like capsules, tablets, and injections etc. whichever method followed, the drugs should be easily traceable for issuing instantly.

   The costly items must be kept under lock and key similar to narcotic drugs. The heavy materials must be stored near the entrance or exit for obvious reasons. Vaccines, sera, suppositories and similar substances which require cold storage should be stored in refrigerators.

Markings on the Inventory

In order to locate, identify and know few details about a particular item some markings are made either on the product or on the place where it is stored. Thus there are, floor marking, shelf stripping and Goods markings for the above purposes.

Floor markings: In the wooden floor or concrete floor of the stores, the name of the item stored in the particular area is marked by paint.

Shelf stripping: Paper, card, plastic or metallic strips are used for shelf stripping in which the name of the item is written. Thus the name of the item is more clearly visible and the identification and location of them are easier.

The advantages of these types of markings are:

1. A particular area is allotted for a particular product
2. It brings orderliness and
3. It is easy to check the stock

Goods marking: In this method date of receipt of goods, cost price and supplier name are marked near or on the goods. Cost price is marked in code words, thus it is easy to determine the discount while selling. Similarly if different suppliers are there for single product, goods marking help in easy identification of source of supply.

Card system: All the stored items are entered in separate cards, with its name, manufacturer, supplier, invoice no. and date, batch number, quantity, expiry date and any other details needed to refer the particular item. Receipt and Issues are then and there entered on the card, so that up to date information is available about that item. This card must be kept near or on the item. In these days of computerized inventory this may be an outdated method of inventory control, however still many hospitals are following this system, even to serve as a double check.

Stock checking: The hospital can assign the duty of checking the stock of drugs physically to certain people and they should perform their duty with or without notice to the employees of stores. The closing balance on the stock card must tally with actual balance. Damaged or expired drugs should be disposed off after necessary sanctions from the authorities.

Records: Every store should maintain the record for its purchase, issue and stock of drugs. All these entries in their register should have the supportive documents like invoices, indents and other documents. They should be maintained up to date.

Thus a store should be managed by the pharmacist in a professional and efficient manner. The efficiency of drugs store management reflects on the following aspects:

1. It must be able to purchase quality drugs at minimum cost.
2. It should scientifically store, maintain and preserve the drugs.
3. There should not be any interruption of drugs supply.

4. Suppliers should be promptly paid and there should not be any complaint from them like delayed payment or part payment etc.

5. All facilities to prevent theft, pilferage, damage or fire accident must be available.

6. Physical verification of stocks for expiry dates and stability must be under taken as often as possible.

Storage Conditions

Storage conditions stipulated in each product must be adhered in order to maintain its safety and potency. Hence a store pharmacist must be thorough with the storage conditions of drugs. General statements like protect from sunlight, protect from moisture etc should be followed and not ignored. Some products may required to be stored at some specific conditions and the temperature and that must be followed, storing either at lower temperature or higher temperatures leads to unwanted problems. The conditions of storage, even though given in general terms, are defined in all pharmacopoeias including Indian pharmacopeia. They are

(a) *Cold*: Any temperature not exceeding 8 °C and usually between 2 °C to 8 °C

(b) *Cool*: Any temperature between 8 °C to 25 °C

(c) *Room temperature*: The temperature prevailing in a working area (25 °C to 30 °C)

(d) **Warm**: Any temperature between 30 °C to 40 °C

(e) *Excessive heat*: Any temperature above 40 °C

(f) *Protect from freezing*: Freezing results in loss of strength or change in characters of the drug, in addition to the risk of breaking the container, hence, it must be carefully followed.

(g) If no specific condition is given, it is understood as protection from light, moisture, freezing and excessive heat.

Questions

Short Answer Questions

1. List the types of stores

2. What is ABC analysis?

3. What is GOLF analysis?

4. What is VED analysis?

5. Write a note on marking on the inventory.

Long Answer Questions

6. How a drug store is organized?

7. How a drug store is managed?

8. Explain category wise storage of inventory. Discuss its advantages and disadvantages.

9. Write in detail about storage of drugs. Add a note on storage conditions of drugs.

CHAPTER 14

DRUGS DISTRIBUTION SYSTEM

Introduction

The drug distribution system in hospitals can be broadly classified into two. They are,

1. Distribution to outpatients or ambulatory patients.
2. Distribution to inpatients or institutionalized patients.

An outpatient or ambulatory patient is one who after consultation and diagnosis receives treatment which could be even for further diagnosis, without being admitted in the hospital, and does not require bed or hospitalization. On the other hand, one who is in need of hospitalization for treatment are admitted and given bed in the hospital is known as inpatient. Generally the diseases of outpatients are such a nature that they require not more than a few days treatment with some exceptions like diabetes, TB and asthma whereas the inpatient's problems are complex and serious and may require close supervision, observation and treatment for comparatively long time. Hence these categories of patients are admitted in the wards.

Distribution to Outpatients

As distribution of drugs to outpatients is not complex compared to inpatients, in almost all the type of hospitals same system is followed. After consultation and diagnosis are over patients are given a prescription (and small chits [token] in which the Patient's hospital Number, name of the medicines prescribed and the quantity is written by the doctor). Then the patients or their helpers take the prescription to the dispensary or pharmacy situated near the main entrance of the hospital, so that he can collect his medicine which is usually the final work for him in a hospital and easily moves out of the hospital.

The drugs are issued to the patients through two or more windows or counters in the pharmacy one for male patients and other for female patients. Depending on the crowd or number of outpatients coming to the hospitals, the authorities may open more counters.

At least one, if required more pharmacists, will receive prescription through these counters and dispense the medicines.

Outpatients receive their medicines on the prescritions given to them by the doctors of that particular hospital only (not by other doctors). The medicines are supplied either free of cost (as in government hospital) or on payment (as in private hospitals). Free medicine cases directly get medicines from the pharmacy. Payment cases pay the cash at cash counter of the hospital (or to the dispensing pharmacist himself), produce the receipt along with the prescription to the pharmacy and get the medicines.

Drugs are then dispensed to the patients or their helpers along with necessary instructions regarding their use storage etc., orally as well as in written form on the containers or envelops of the medicine. The prescription or the small piece of paper (token) is retained by the pharmacist. He files the retained prescription or 'token' after accounts were written for the drugs mentioned in it along with patient's hospital registration number and date. If the case sheets and prescriptions are retained they are sent back to the hospital patient registration counter, after accounting as above, from where the patients get them on their subsequent visit.

Usually, seating arrangements are made for the outpatients to sit during the waiting period to get the drugs. Similar dispensing counters are opened in varies places of the hospital depending upon the requirement or policy of the hospital. Sometimes special counters are opened to dispense to special category of patients like Non gazetted Government officers (NGGO).

Dispensing to Inpatients

There are four systems in general use for distributing or dispensing drugs to inpatients. They are,

1. Individual prescription order system.
2. Complete floor stock system.
3. Combination of above two systems and
4. Unit dose distribution system.

1. Individual prescription order system

This system is generally followed in small and private hospitals where big wards for dozens of patients are not available. As the name implies patients are given prescription individually since there may be desirability for individualized service. In these small hospitals number of small rooms form the inpatient area with 2 to 4 beds in each room. Sometimes individual rooms are also provided. Hence, here bulk stock of drugs in wards (as followed in the next type of system) is not feasible. The patients receive the drugs either from the pharmacy of the hospital if available or purchase it from outside pharmacy and keep it ready. The duty nurse administers the drug as per the direction written in the prescription or case sheet. The advantages of this system are

1. Prescription is dispensed by pharmacist.
2. As drugs are not stored in this inpatient area, there is closer control over the inventory by pharmacist.
3. Patient can interact with all the members of health care team, viz, the doctor, nurse and pharmacist.

The main disadvantage is the possible delay in getting the required drugs by the patients and increased cost.

2. Complete floor stock system

In this system, medicines are brought from main pharmacy and stored in a cupboard in each ward/floor of the hospital complex. The nurse of the ward is in charge for these medicines. They distribute the drugs to the inpatients and account it. Under this system the nursing station carries both 'charge' and 'non charge' patient medications. Rarely used expensive medicines are omitted from floor stock but are dispensed upon receipt of a prescription for any individual patients. Selection of drugs to be stored in each floor/ward is done by the PTC of the hospital. In short this is a mini pharmacy inside the ward – a ward pharmacy – but without a pharmacist. This system is used most often in government and other hospitals in which charges are not collected from the patient, or when the 'all inclusive' rate is used for charging. The following are the advantages and disadvantages of the system.

Advantages

1. Drugs are readily available in the ward.
2. There is no need to return the drugs to pharmacy or stores.
3. Pharmacy work load is reduced and
4. Consequently number of pharmacists required also reduced.

Disadvantages

1. Pharmacist's services are eliminated (since dispensing is done by nurses).
2. Work load of nurses increases.
3. There are greater chances for pilferage of drugs as they are stored in dozens of wards.
4. For the same reason more drugs need to be purchased and consequently cost to the hospital increases.
5. Medication error may increase, as there is no review of prescriptions by the pharmacists.

6. Proper storage facilities need to be provided in each ward necessitating capital expenses. If not provided, drugs may deteriorate and become dangerous to the patients.

3. Combination of system 1 and 2

In some hospitals combination of above two systems are followed. Individual prescription order system as the main means of distributing drugs to the patients and also limited use of floor stock. This combination system is probably the most commonly used system in medium and large hospitals, where there are number of small rooms for patients, known as special wards and big halls as general wards available.

4. Unit dose distribution system

"Unit dose medications are those medications, which are ordered, packed, handled, administered and charged in multiples of single dose units containing a predetermined amount of drug or supply sufficient for one regular dose, application or use". If drugs are supplied in bulk packing, unit doses were felt necessary for dispensing to the inpatients by the nurses, as otherwise they are required to make calculations, measuring, weighing and packing to administer some drugs to the inpatients,. In order to avoid such unfamiliar work load to the nurses, a unit dose system was introduced. It should not be confused with what we now call as unit dose. In the above system, medicines are not to be send to the wards in bulk containers, instead they are subdivided, prepacked for a dose and labeled. Then as per the request of ward nurses, they are sent, in required number of unit doses to the ward.

With the introduction and wide spread use of tablets and capsules, these works for the pharmacist are highly minimized. Tablets and capsules are the best ready to use, unit dose forms, available in strips or blister packing. Nevertheless, few drugs like powders and cough syrups are still supplied to the hospitals in bulk containers.

The unit dose system under discussion can be best understood by the following example: consider an inpatient is prescribed cough syrup. If only 5 L jars or 500 ml bottle packing of cough syrup is supplied to the hospital, pharmacist has no option but to send one full container to the ward. Then nurses need to measure the dose every time, and give to the patient from the bulk container and keep the balance quantity within the ward.

How to account this supply in stores or dispensary is the problem. The quantity supplied cannot be debited in one patients account, nor can it be unaccounted till all the supply is consumed. Hence there is a compulsion to go for unit dose system or smaller packing, which requires empty containers, work space, equipments for filling, sealing, labeling etc in the dispensary.

Now-a-days this problem is solved by requesting the drug supplier to the hospital or hospital manufacturing unit to supply both bulk packing (for outpatient dispensing) and unit dose or small packing (for inpatients).

However, as "distribution of drugs to the inpatients by nurses" is still followed in majority of the hospitals, unit dose system's advantages and disadvantages have to be studied.

Advantages

1. Work load for nurses reduced.

2. Wastage of drugs is reduced as unused unit doses can be returned to the pharmacy and need not be discarded as in bulk packing.

3. Maintenance of records made easy as they are maintained in multiplies of unit doses.

4. Accurate delivery of medication (in the form of unit doses) is ensured due to stringent repacking conditions and expert's (pharmacist's) handling.

5. Above all, the unit doses are supplied with proper labels indicating the name of the medicine, its strength, quantity, and expiry data etc., thereby wrong administration can be minimized.

Disadvantages

1. Cost of medicines goes up due to smaller packing or re packing.

2. Require more space for storage.

3. Capital expenses need to be made to establish repacking unit in hospital, if the drugs are not supplied in unit doses.

4. The root cause for the problem is distribution of drugs to the inpatients by nurses [not by pharmacists].

Other Systems of Dispensing to Inpatients

As discussed above, the main disadvantage of above systems is dispensing by non pharmacists. Pharmacists are deprived of their work and hence their expertise, experience and service cannot be used in dispensing, leading to many problems pointed out as disadvantages of these systems. In order to overcome this problem, some hospitals have introduced a system in which, the inpatient prescription or its copy is send to the main dispensary where the pharmacist review the prescription and dispense the medicines as follows:

1. Basket (or) envelopes method

In this method, the prescribed drugs for a particular patient is put in a basket or envelope with its methods of use and other details and sent to the ward concerned. There the nurse administer the drug to the particular patient and convey the directions of the pharmacist written on the envelope or on a paper kept inside the basket. Next day the some basket or envelope is returned to the dispensary for further dispensing of drugs written.

Thus the main disadvantage of non handling of prescription by the pharmacist is solved in this method. Pharmacist is able to find out incompatibility or drug interaction possibilities and other connected problems by handling the prescription. Thus he is able to help the doctor in selecting suitable drug / formulation for the particular patient. However, still there is one deficiency in this method, that, pharmacist - patient direct dialogue is not there and whatever pharmacist want to tell the patient is conveyed through a third party- the nurses.

Thus the basket or envelop system does not solve all the problems of inpatient dispensing.

2. Mobile dispensing system

It utilizes a specially constructed stainless steel truck in which essential and frequently used medicines are taken to the wards. A worker of the pharmacy department pushes this truck to the ward accompanied by a pharmacist. It is stopped in front of each ward or in specified places and the pharmacist does dispensing to the in patients by collecting their prescriptions individually from them. The process is similar to the distribution of food and diet to the in patients by hospital authorities, three times a day, supervised by the dieticians of the hospital. The frequency of delivery of medicines and the hours during which the mobile unit will visit the ward will be selected in cooperation with nursing service.

The main advantages of this system are, pharmacist himself does dispensing and hence, his services are available for consultation by patients, nurses and medical staff. However the disadvantage of this method is non availability of all medicines in the truck as well as space for keeping required quantity. Thus pharmacist or his assistant is compelled more often to return back to the dispensary to bring and supply non available items to the inpatients. Though two main problems of previous methods, prescription handling and conveying instructions directly to the inpatients are solved, a new problem of inadequate availability of drugs arises in this method.

3. Satellite pharmacy

These are nothing but branches of main hospital pharmacy functioning around the hospital in different block, if the hospital is spread over a vast area in several buildings or in few other floors, if it is a multi-storied building.

Main pharmacy will supply the medicines to these satellite or mini pharmacies. Patients and/or nurses in charge of ward obtain their requirements of drugs from these satellite pharmacies instead of going to the main pharmacy. Sometimes these satellite pharmacies are established to cater to the special or specified category of peoples like government officers, legislatures, patients from special clinics etc. Thus it distributes drugs to both inpatients and special outpatients. However these pharmacies will have less stock only compared to main pharmacy, which receives its supply in bulk from hospital stores.

Advantage of satellite pharmacy service is that the patients are able to get the medicine quickly, without spending much time. Moreover the large crowd gathering in front of the main pharmacy and consequent problems are avoided.

The disadvantage is increase in inventory and subsequent cost. Nevertheless, almost all the problems in dispensing to inpatients are more or less solved in this method. Hence, modern hospitals or renovated old hospitals are equipped with satellite pharmacies (e.g.) Rajiv Gandhi Government General Hospital, Chennai.

Charging of Prescribed Drug

There are many methods for collecting money from the patients for the drug supplied to them. They are,

1. Direct payment by patients as in private hospitals.
2. Payment by third party like insurance company and
3. Payment through subscription as in Employees State Insurance [ESI] scheme.

1. Direct payment

In this method, the cost of medicine is calculated either by the pharmacist or the accountant and collected by the hospital cashier. After the payment is made, the patient has to produce the receipt or bill to the pharmacist, who dispenses the medicines for which payment has been made. This method is followed in all the private hospitals and in some government hospitals for specific category of patients.

2. Payment by third party

In this method, a third party like the insurance company pays the charges for the medicines prescribed, if the patient is coming under the medical/health insurance policy. In some policies, first, the patient has to pay to the hospital and later he has to get reimbursement from the insurance company after producing the bills, prescriptions and other documents required by the insurance company. But for some patients, instead of insurance company employers may be paying for their employee as per service agreements. Thus in this method patients, need not pay for their medicines.

3. Payment through subscription

This is a method in which, a fixed amount as monthly or yearly subscription is deducted from the salaries of the employees by the employers and paid to the authorities specially arranged for giving treatment, like Employees State Insurance (ESI) Corporation.

Under this scheme, the family members and dependants of the employee are also eligible to take treatment and receive medicines from ESI hospitals without paying. However even if the employee or his dependants are not sick and not taking treatment in these hospitals they have to pay every month as subscription to the corporation. A part of the expenses for these hospitals is borne by the employers also, as on welfare measure for their employees.

Pricing Policy

In all the above methods, drugs are priced with little margin or profit by the hospitals concerned. The percentage of margin differs between various hospitals. As a rule break even point is fixed as the price i.e., no loss, no profit price is charged from the patients.

Dispensing of Narcotics or Controlled Substances

During the course of dispensing to the patients, pharmacist has to dispense narcotic drugs also. Narcotics are the drugs that produce deleterious effects such as undue depression or stimulation of human brain resulting in effects like euphoria, personality destabilizing effects, addiction etc. Hence there are certain conditions and procedures to dispense such drugs enforced by the government through drugs control department. These procedures must be known to all dispensing pharmacists and they are expected to follow those guidelines in letter and spirit. Failing which may result in prosecution by the drugs inspectors and/or police personals.

Let us first look at the general conditions for dispensing narcotics, followed by specific procedures to be followed by pharmacists while dispensing to outpatients and inpatients of a hospital.

General Conditions

1. No narcotic drug should be dispensed without a written prescription of a registered medical practitioner.
2. Narcotic drugs should not be dispensed for more than one day use unless specifically prescribed by the physician.
3. Narcotic prescriptions should be retained in the pharmacy after dispensing the drug, or returned to the patient after putting rubber stamp 'issued/dispensed' and signature (with date) of the pharmacist on the prescription. If retained the prescriptions must be kept in a separate file for inspection by drugs inspectors.

4. No prescription for narcotics may be refilled. If the procedure mentioned in 3 above is properly followed, no prescription will be coming to the pharmacy for refilling.

5. No controlled substance (narcotic) which is a drug may be dispensed other than for a medical purpose.

6. Prescription for narcotics must be written in ink and shall not bear any erasing or alteration. It must be signed by the doctor, along with his name and registration number rubber stamp.

7. Prescriptions for narcotics must be complete in all aspects, that is, it must contain full address and diagnosis of the patient, as well as doctor's hospital address and phone number.

Hospital Procedure for Dispensing Narcotics

1. Responsibility for narcotics in the hospital

In general the administrative head of the hospital is responsible for proper safe guarding and handling of narcotics within the hospital. Chief pharmacist is responsible for purchase, storage and maintenance of account and proper dispensing of narcotics in particular. Similarly head nurse of a ward is responsible for the proper storage and use of controlled substances (narcotics) in the ward.

2. Dispensing to inpatients

As the administration of narcotic drugs to the inpatients is by the nurses, and these drugs are not given directly to the patient for self administration, there is always greater control over its use, compared to outpatients.

Hence, the procedure is simple, in that a separate copy of prescription should be written for narcotics for inpatients, along with the usual prescription written on the case sheet by the treating physician. This separate prescription must be complete in all aspects as described above and sent to the dispensary. The drugs supplied are kept under lock and key by the ward nurse and administered to the patient as per the directions written on the case sheet.

A *pro re nata* (prn) (occasionally) or si opus sit (SOS) (whenever necessary) prescriptions for narcotics must be discouraged except under special circumstances. The doctor may give orders by telephone in case of necessity. Then the nurse writes the order on the doctor's prescription sheet, stating that it is a telephone order. The nurse has to write the doctor name and put her own initials. The doctor must then sign the order within 24 hours. Similarly a doctor may give verbal order for narcotic drugs in an extreme emergency, where time does not permit writing the order. The nurse must write the order on prescription sheet and the doctor should sign it within 24 hours.

The doctor should not write prescription for narcotics for his own use. Narcotics obtained for ward use should not be issued to home use by the patients on discharge. These are all the procedures followed in majority of the hospitals, but may have additional or reduced conditions in a few hospitals.

3. Dispensing to outpatients

The prescription for narcotics to outpatients must contain the following information:

(a) Patient's full name

(b) Patient's address

(c) Hospital number

(d) Date

(e) Name and strength of the drug

(f) Quantity to be dispensed

(g) Directions for use

(h) Signature of the physician

The prescription must be written in ink and must not bear any correction. Narcotics should not be dispensed for more than one day's use, unless prescribed specifically by the physician. Automatic stop order for narcotics after one day's use is enforced by many hospitals in this regard. All other general conditions for dispensing narcotics are applicable to the dispensing of narcotics to outpatients.

Questions

Short Answer Questions

1. Who is an ambulatory patient?

2. Write a note on mobile pharmacy.

3. Write briefly about satellite pharmacy.

4. Write short notes on unit dose system.

Long Answer Questions

5. Write an essay about dispensing to inpatients.

6. Explain the charging of prescribed drugs.

7. Detail the procedure to be followed for dispensing narcotics.

8. Describe the complete floor stock system and its advantages and disadvantages.

CHAPTER 15

CENTRAL STERILE SUPPLY DEPARTMENT

Introduction

Central sterile supply department (CSSD) is defined as a centralized unit, which provides professional supplies and sterile equipment to all specialized departments of a hospital. Prior to centralization of this service, sterilization of surgical instruments and equipments and other items were carriedout then and there in individual departments by nurses with the help of nursing assistants. Still this is going on in hospitals were sterilization operations are not centralized. Both these methods have advantages and disadvantages.

In decentralized or local sterilization practice, the needed items in needed quantities are sterilized and used immediately and hence there is no need for careful storage of sterile items to retain its sterility. But when the requirement volume exceeds the capacity of the individual department, either they are sterilized in batches repeatedly or on barrowed equipments like autoclaves. This leads to unwanted complications time delay and possibility of incomplete or defective sterilization. Needless to mention the cost of sterilization that goes up, if sterilization is carried out in many places (wards and operation theatres) of the hospital. Another major disadvantage of this method is non availability of surgical instruments in case of emergency operations. It is worsened if operations are to be performed on dozens of patients at a time, after some natural disaster or accident.

In the centralized sterile supply services, the problems mentioned above are solved, as it ensure adequate supply of materials, at all time. However in centralizing the service elaborate arrangements has to be made, more or less similar to sterile manufacturing process. Consequently initial capital expenses goes up, however, it is just one time expense, leads to creation of assets only.

One important prerequirement for running a central sterile department is the volume of operation of the hospital should be large enough to engage the department fully. If not, it leads to waste of resources and loss to the organization. Thus in ultimate analysis, whether to go for centralized sterile services or not, purely depends on the *size and requirements* of a particular hospital.

Once a decision is taken, to centralize the sterile services, the immediate question is who is suitable to manage the services. As mentioned earlier, this large scale operation becomes an operation similar to sterile product manufacturing process, and hence, obviously a pharmacist is suitable to manage it rather than a nurse. The following paragraphs further highlight this:

Developments in Sterile Services

Usually, syringes, needles, tubing, urine collection sets, IV administration sets, gloves and small surgical instruments are frequently sterilized in a hospital. But a CSSD, if established, may be involved in the cleaning, storage, and dispensing of specialized equipments such as suction pumps, cardiac catheters, monitoring equipments, surgical dressing carts, resuscitation carts and special kits and trays. From its beginning as an equipment wash room with autoclaving facilities, CSSD has developed itself to modern production line techniques with automatic control recording devices, to insure sterility, modern washing, drying, as well as taking an active role in developing the various gas and cold storage techniques.

Hence, as pointed out earlier, modern sterilization services are akin to manufacturing operations, involving sophisticated and electronic machineries. As the pharmacist undergoes both theoretical and practical training in many engineering and technical aspects, obviously he is better suited to manage CSSD.

However, very recent developments in sterile supplies have made his job very easy. With the advent of the age of plastics and disposable items, many surgical dressings and other items are available in presterilized, ready to use and throw form. Disposable syringes, needles, IV administration sets, gloves, tubing are the examples for the inroads made by the plastic industry into the field. However still many more items, like surgical instruments and equipments, are to be sterilized regularly and frequently, hence a CSSD is not disposable!

Objectives of CSSD

1. To supply directly to operation theatre is the major objective of a CSSD.
2. To supply other sterile items needed for wards and OPD.
3. To maintain the inventory of supplies and equipments of the hospital.
4. To maintain an accurate record of the effectiveness of the various processes of cleaning, disinfecting and sterilization and
5. To contribute educational programs within the hospital relating to infection control.

Types of Materials for Sterilization

- Syringes
- Needles
- Gloves
- Blood bags
- Tubing
- Urine collection sets
- IV sets
- Suction pumps
- Cardiac catheters
- Monitoring equipments
- Surgical dressing carts
- Resuscitation carts
- Special kits
- Trays
- Surgical instruments
- Surgical dressings
- Linen like mouth mask, apron, and head covers etc.
- Glass containers and
- Any other items needed by special departments of the hospital.

Packing of Materials Prior to Sterilization

There is no 99% sterilization. It should be always 100%. Hence, it requires full attention of those who sterilize materials in a hospital. Even, packing materials prior to sterilization need careful adherence to established practices. Then they should be correctly loaded in the sterilizer, otherwise one cannot ensure 100% sterility of all the materials loaded in it. It all starts from the selection of container or packing material for putting things to be sterilized.

There are some quality materials and containers for packing articles to be sterilized. They are,

1. Metal drums
2. Card board boxes
3. Fabric packs
4. Nylon bags and
5. Paper bags

Depends upon the material to be sterilized any one of the above should be selected and packing is done according to time-tested procedures. These methods of packing are thought to technicians or nursing assistants of the hospital during their training. If such trained peoples are not available with CSSD, someone should be trained by in charge pharmacists, in the correct method of packing and loading of the autoclave or sterilizer.

Once a suitable container or packing material is selected the next step is to pack the individual items as per procedure. These procedures or methods are given in books like "Bentley's Pharmaceutics" – Old editions. These books should be consulted for guidance.

Few examples from the book are given below:

Packing of Individual Articles for Sterilization

(a) Glass apparatus, if to be sterilized, first wash and clean it thoroughly. Flasks are to be stoppered with cotton and a piece of paper is tied over the plugged openings-other pieces of glasses are packed in brown paper.

(b) If dry powder, fat or oil is to be sterilized, it should be transferred to a container, sealed and wrapped with paper and tied over the openings – packed amount should not be greater than 10 gm in weight or 1 cm depth.

(c) Glass syringes should be cleaned with soap and warm water using bottle brush rinsed and dried. Apply silicon grease over the piston, insert into the barrel and move forward and backward many times for proper lubrication. Double pack the syringe in aluminum foil.

(d) Syringe needles are washed with warm water and clean the channel. Rinse it with alcohol and keep it separately in small test tubes taking care that the needle tip should not touch the bottom of the tube and pack the tube.

(e) All containers should be completely dried before loading. It is better if the containers are oven dried at 100 °C prior to sterilization.

(f) Materials like rubber gloves, surgical cotton / ligature and sutures to be sterilized should be packed in a material which will not create any obstacle to steam penetration and removal of air. Materials can be packed in tubes, bottles closed with cotton stoppers; flask plugged with cotton or loosely applied screw caps. Wrapping cloth or plastic or Kraft paper may be used for wrapping instruments. However it should be completely dried before removing from autoclave. Covering with stout greasy paper can minimize drenching of cotton wool stoppers in tubes and bottles.

Thus complete wrapping of article is essential as it avoids contamination by the non-sterile air, which is due to contraction of air on cooling the oven and to avoid subsequent contamination prior to use.

Methods of Packing

The following points should be remembered while packing the articles in an oven or autoclave.

1. The pack should be as small as possible.
2. The contents should be arranged loosely.
3. The space between the items and folds should be parallel.
4. Heavy, tightly woven materials like hand towels, and rubber sheets should be sterilized separately in small numbers and very loosely arranged.

Loading the Sterilizer

Drums with top and bottom vents and card board boxes are loaded with lids uppermost. Drums with side vents are placed on their sides after opening the slide doors. In all the three types the contents will then be on edge. Bags and parcels should also be positioned to give the same arrangement. In addition, packing in the bottoms of side vented drums is prevented.

Sterilization Equipments

There are many type of equipment used for sterilizing different articles used in a hospital, depending upon the method of sterilization. They are,

1. Moist heat sterilization equipments
   - Saturated steam autoclaves
   - Super heated water autoclaves
   - Air over steam autoclaves
   - Steamer
   - Electric boiling water sterilizers
2. Dry heat sterilization equipments
   - Batch sterilizers,
   - Continuous tunnel sterilizers,
   - Hot air oven.
3. Gas sterilization equipments
   - An apparatus with special gas exposure chamber and heating arrangement.
4. Radiation sterilization equipments
   - Infrared conveyer oven
   - UV Lamps
5. Filtration sterilization equipments
   - Bacteria proof membrane filters

   (Note: For details about construction, working and operation of above equipments students are advised to refer any standard book on pharmaceutics or microbiology)

Supply of Sterile Materials

As most of the materials are now available in disposable sterile packing from the manufacturers, there is little work left in a hospital to supply sterile materials. However, items of day to day use like linen and surgical instruments are to be supplied in sterile conditions to the departments and or to operation theatres.

These articles are sterilized by any one of the above methods and supplied in their original packing prior to sterilization, without opening or contaminating it. If need be, they are put in other sterile outer boxes and sent to the needed department after sealing those boxes.

Alternatively they are sterilized near the place of use, by autoclaves or boiling water heater and taken to the aseptic rooms or area with special windows and used. Laminar air flow working tables are used for some instruments and equipments, either to sterilize them by showing in hot flames or for opening and keeping prior to use.

Injections and other sterile solutions are supplied by the manufacture in a ready to use containers and they can be used directly after visually checking for any floating particles or microbial growth.

Whatever method used to supply the sterile materials, it is the duty of the pharmacist, nurses and doctors to check the container and packing prior to use, for ensuring the intactness or otherwise of the packing and materials. Any slight damage should also be noted and the material inside is discarded or resterilized if permitted.

Questions

Short Answer Questions

1. Why CSSD is necessary?
2. How pharmacist is suitable to be in charge of CSSD?
3. What are the objectives of a CSSD?
4. List the materials used for packing prior to sterilization.
5. Name the equipments used for sterilization.

Long Answer Questions

6. Explain the procedure to be followed before sterilization.
7. Describe briefly the packing or loading of sterilizers. Add a note on supply of sterilized materials.

CHAPTER 16

HOSPITAL ACCESSORIES

Surgical Instruments, Health Accessories and Medical Gases

Introduction

A Hospital Pharmacist has to be familiar with not only drugs but also other accessories used in hospital like surgical instruments, equipments, health accessories and medical gases. Though they are not sold in majority of community pharmacies, the wholesalers and dealers in those items require services of pharmacists who can handle such items. In big hospitals there are separate stores for these items in the name of surgical stores where they are procured, stored and issued to needed departments of hospital by pharmacists, similar to drugs. Hence a pharmacist must learn to identify, account and dispense them mainly to surgical wards and operation theatres. A brief description of hospital & health accessories is given below:

Surgical Instruments

There are many varieties of surgical instruments, used for different purposes, before, during and after the surgery. All these instruments are needed to perform a perfect surgery, so as not to encounter any problem either during or after the surgery. Thus a good inventory of these items must be maintained by the pharmacist for which a basic understanding and knowledge on them is essential.

The Hospital equipments are classified broadly as follows:

1. Medical equipments and
2. Surgical equipments

Medical equipments are further classified into diagnostic equipments and therapeutic equipments whereas surgical equipments and instruments are classified according to the place and use. Thus there are surgical instruments used during surgery in operation theatres and those used routinely in wards and OP departments for regular and day-to-day care.

151

Moreover there are some equipments and accessories used by the patients as life supports such as caliper, crutches etc.

I. Medical Equipments

(a) **Diagnostic Equipments:** These equipments are used for the diagnosis of diseases. Due to tremendous growth of electronics industry in the last 30-40 years lot of sophisticated electronic instruments, invaded the health care sector, necessitating the services of electronic engineers and technicians in hospital. Consequently there are new branches of engineering introduced in engineering colleges like medical engineering, medical physics, etc.

The equipments used are imaging machines like ultrasound and MRI machines, PET and CT scanners and X-Ray machines. New optical micro camera attached instruments like endoscope and laryngoscope are also introduced in the recent past.

Last mentioned instruments are two in one instruments, in that they are not only used to diagnose the internal problems of human body, but attached with suitable devices to remove problematic tissues etc, thus perform the functions of a therapeutic instrument.

(b) Other therapeutic instruments are infusion pumps, medical lasers and LASIK surgical instruments.

During therapy there is vital need to monitor various parameters of the patient, for which there are equipments like ECG, EEG, BP apparatus and auto analyzers to measure haematological parameters. Blood glucose meter and clinical thermometer are other monitors used by patients in their home.

There are many other types of equipments used as life support for the patient such as heart-lung machines, dialysis machines, anaesthetics machines and medical ventilators.

All the above equipments and instruments may be purchased once in a while in a hospital and very few are stocked in surgical stores of the hospital. However unlike above medical equipments, surgical equipments and instruments have to be purchased and stocked in sufficient quantities in order to meet emergency needs.

II. Surgical Instruments and Equipments

The following are different types of surgical instruments:

1. Clamps for Blood vessels and other organs
2. Cutters like scalpels, lancets, rasp, etc
3. Catheters to be inserted into body cavities

4. Cannula which is also used to insert into body

5. Carriers and appliers for optical electronic and mechanical devices

6. Dilators and specula to access narrow incisions or passages

7. Drills and dermatomes, electrically operated devices

8. Distracters, positioners and stereotactic devices

9. Forceps for grasping

10. Needles, tips and tubes for introducing fluids

11. Rulers and calipers for measurements

12. Retractors used to spread open skin and other tissue

13. Suction tubes and tips for removal of body fluids

14. Surgical staplers used for sealing

15. Tyndallers to 'wedge' open damaged tissues

16. Ultra sound disruptors, cryotomes and cutting laser guides

17. Bone plates to fix fractures of long bones

Few commonly used surgical instruments are explained below:

Catheter: It is a thin, flexible tube or big, solid tube, called as soft or hard catheter. It can be inserted into body cavity or blood vessel. It is thus used for administering medicines or to obtain the fluids from the body. The process of inserting a catheter is known as catheterization.

Cannula: It is a tube inserted to the body, often for administering or removing fluids. It can also be used to gather data about the body condition. These tubes have sharp front end used to create a portal into the body, not necessarily inserted into an existing channel unlike a catheter.

Forceps or forcipes: It is a hinged surgical instrument used for holding objects. It is similar to tongs, clips or clamps; we use in day to day life. It is very useful to hold small objects when hands cannot be used. Various sizes of forceps like small, medium, large and extra large are available, depends on the need they are used during surgical procedures.

Needles: It is a needle with a hole through out its length to deliver fluids into the body. It is commonly used with a syringe. It is also used to draw fluids from the body like blood from the vein. Needles are used to deliver drugs through various routes like, IM, IV, SC, ID, Intrathecal etc. Depend on its use the size of the pore and/or length of the needle vary. The diameter of this pore is referred to as gauge and measured in stubs scale. Thus it range from 7 (the largest) to 33 gauge (the smallest). Smaller the number, bigger will be the size of the pore of the needle. Usually 21 gauge needles are used. Bigger ones like

16 or 17 gauge needles are used for drawing bloods quickly from donors. Due to spreading of diseases by using needles repeatedly, now a days only disposable needles are used. The upper part of the needle is covered with plastic hub, so as to fit into a barrel of a syringe.

Scalpel: It is otherwise known as lancet. It is a very small but very sharp instrument used to cut the tissue and tendon. Disposable scalpels are also available. It is made up of steel, sometimes with bone or wood handles.

Scissors: There are many types of scissors used in surgery. They may be long or short, blunt or sharp pointed, straight or curved. All these varieties are stocked in operation theatres and few on OP departments. Long or short scissors are used depends on the body organ where the surgery is performed. Curved scissors are more convenient in that they do not obstruct the place of cutting from the sight of the surgeon. Mayo's scissors are short scissors available in straight or curved size and shape. Nelson scissors are, on the other hand, long one with short blades.

Bone Plates: It is used to fix fractured bones. Usually long bones with severe fracture are fixed by screwing these plates in required place and position. They may be removed later, if the bones grow and join or they may be left in place permanently obviously the metal used for making bone plates should be non reactive and non-ionisable.

There are many more surgical instruments, which cannot be explained in the limited scope of this chapter. Students and pharmacists are advised to learn them by seeing while undergoing hospital training or immediately after appointment in hospital.

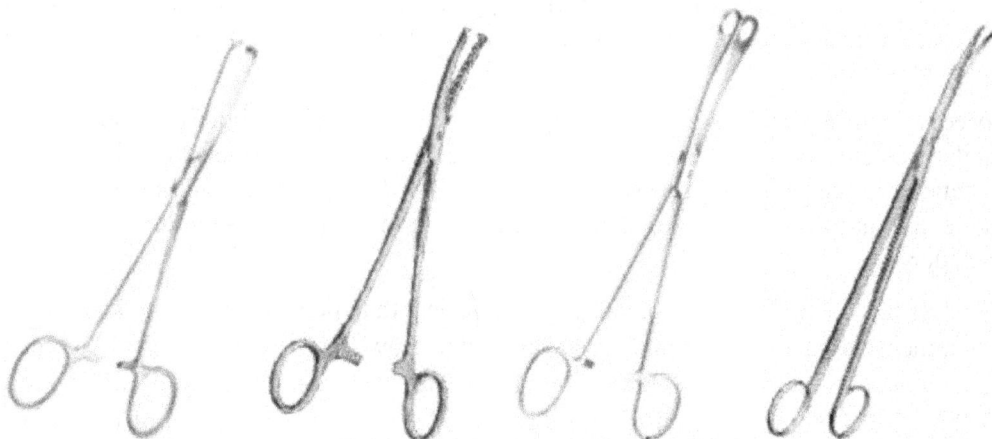

Tissue Forceps   Artery Forceps   Sponge Holding Forceps   Nelson's Scissors

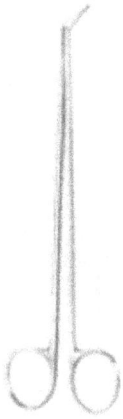

Vascular Scissors   Sharp/Blunt Scissors   Bonney Mayo's Scissors   Health's Scissors

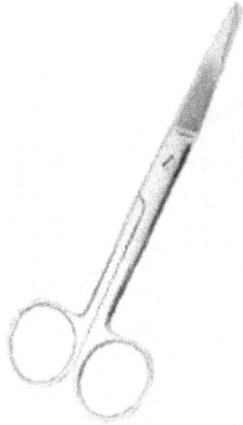

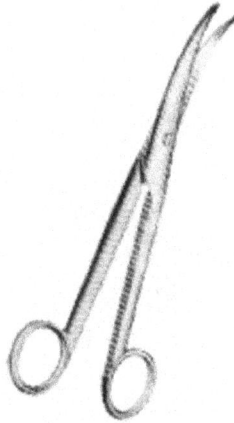

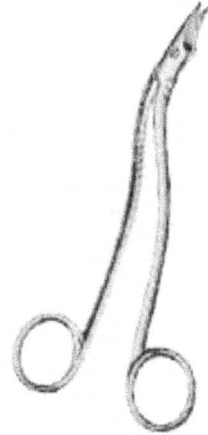

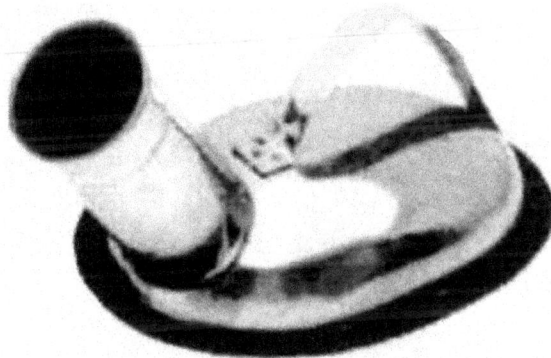

Urinal pot (male/female)

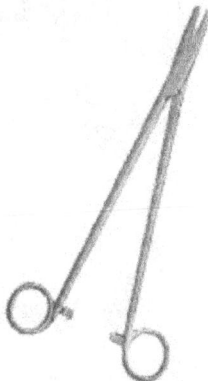

Needle Holder   Invalid Walker   Canes and Crutches

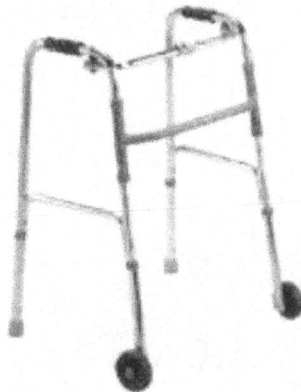

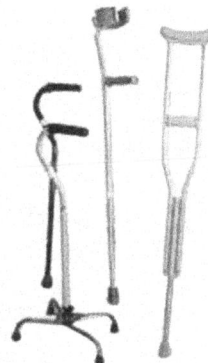

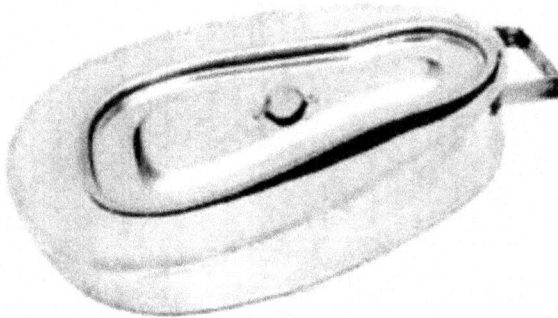

Bed pan (male/female)

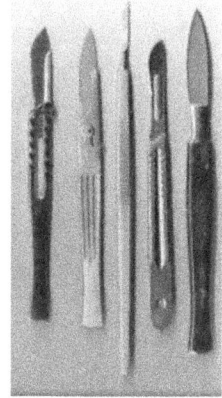

Scalpels

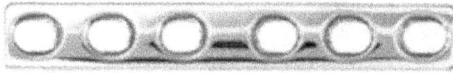

Boneplate

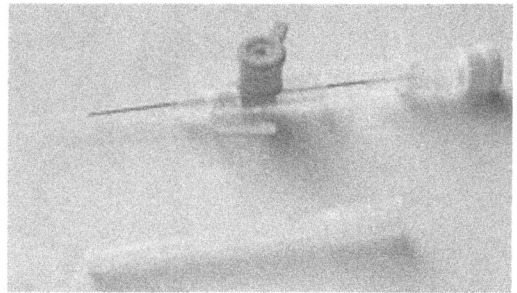

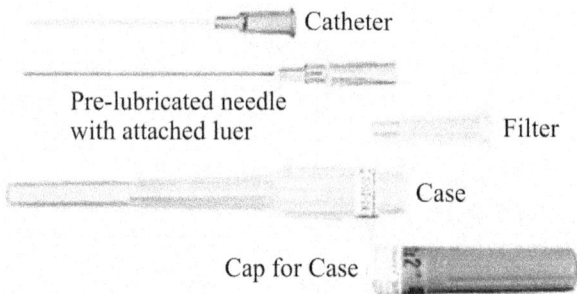

Catheter

Pre-lubricated needle
with attached luer

Filter

Case

Cap for Case

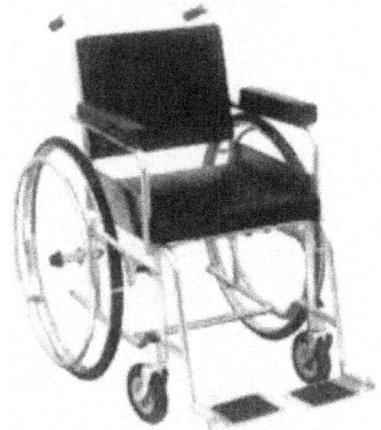

Invalid Chair (non-folding)

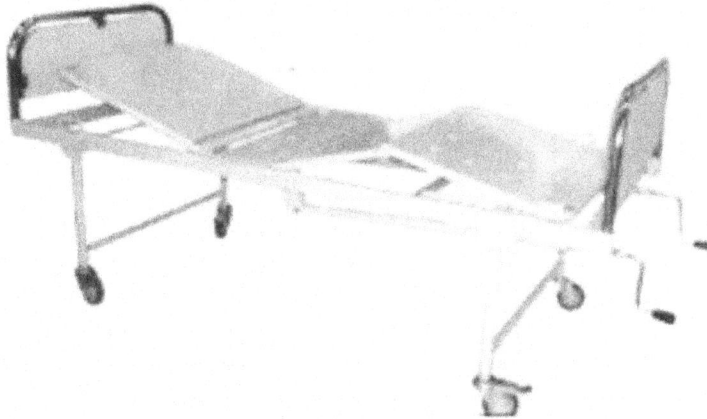

Hospital Fowler Bed

Courtesy: Wikipedia

Health Accessories

Apart from above surgical instruments many health accessories are used by a hospital. They are provided by treating physicians and surgeons to their patients depend on the need. They include hospital beds, bed pans, wheel chairs, crutches and walkers.

Hospital beds: These are not ordinary beds, but with special features to suit the need of the patient and treatment. For example the bed is divided into two equal halves in its horizontal plate, so that either the head portion or leg portion of the patient can be raised to required level. Similarly it is provided with side railings which can be screwed or unscrewed depends on the need. Saline stands and hydraulic pulley can be fixed on the sides of the bed where suitable devices are arranged. Overhead trapeze bar can also be fixed to help the patient to get up.

Bed pan: It is an object used by the patient for urinating or discharging faecal matters while in bed. This is made up of metal, glass or plastic. It is necessary for patients who are immovable due to their disease or surgery.

Wheel chair: It is a chair with wheels on both sides which can either be operated manually by the patients or his helper or by battery power. It is mainly useful for patients who are immovable due to their age, disease or surgery. Hence it is used both in hospitals and homes of the patients who are having permanent disability to walk. Wheel chairs are available with many modifications and varieties like the one with hand pedalling; hence the one which suits the patient should be used.

Canes, crutches and walkers: These are the supports used by patients who cannot walk on their own. Canes are used by patients with weak legs which cannot bear the weight of the patient. It helps to maintain balance while walking. On the other hand, crutches are lengthier and heavier which give support under the arms of the patient; hence known as arm crutches. But auxiliary crutches support both wrists and elbows. They are available with length adjustments. Walkers are 'U' shaped metal products to help the patient with disability to walk. They are available in foldable model also, so as to carry and transport them easily. They can be used by patients with strong arms and hands only.

Some patients have to be monitored continuously or very often for their clinical parameters like blood pressure, blood sugar, body temperature etc; otherwise their admission in wards is not necessary. Hence such patients are educated and trained to monitor above parameters while in their home using simple monitoring devices like dial type BP monitor, glucometer, clinical thermometer etc. Sometimes they are advised to use simple equipments like vaporizers to administer medicines by inhalation. As such all these simple equipments are available freely in the market. Though they are not accurate and dependable, they can be used at least to monitor the range of above parameters.

First aid supplies: These are usually kept ready in many places of the hospital and also in emergency, OP departments and in vehicles for transporting the patients. They are absorbent cotton, adhesive bandages, ordinary bandages, gauze, dusting powder, surgical spirit, dettol, burnol, tincture iodine, scissors, gloves and other surgical dressings like water proof self adhesive plasters, oxidized cellulose etc.

All these items should be supplied to above mentioned places by dispensary pharmacist or stores pharmacist. They are cheaper items and that should not be the reason to pay less attention towards its stock position. Sufficient quantity of all these items should be stored in any hospital to meet emergencies. Road accidents and natural disasters suddenly increase the demand for these items by manifold.

Though they are called first air supplies, these items are also regularly and daily used in all the wards and operation theatres of the hospital. Plaster of Paris, crepe bandage and Ichthammol ointment are some of the other items often required by staff treating emergency cases. Hence a hospital pharmacist must have better idea about the first aid supplies used in the hospital and a community pharmacist also keep ready these items in required quantities to supply to general public and if required, to hospitals and clinics. General public should be educated and trained in the use of first aid supplies and encourage to stock some quantity of these items in their home.

Medical Gases

These are the gases used for treatment and for producing anaesthesia, administered or inhaled as per the direction of doctors. There are many gases used for the purpose like carbon dioxide, cyclopropane, nitrous oxide, oxygen and helium.

Carbon dioxide (CO_2): Though it has no value in therapy, it is used to stimulate respiration. Along with oxygen, in 10% to 15% concentration carbon dioxide is found to be beneficial in stimulating respiration in emergencies. In case of drowning in water, poisoning by CNS depressants like morphine or carbon monoxide, it is very useful.

Cyclopropane (C_3H_6): It produces anaesthesia, the degree of which depends on its concentration. Thus small amount of it (4%) produces only analgesia, whereas 8% produces mild anaesthesia. However up to 20% in oxygen is needed to produce surgical anaesthesia. As it is explosive in nature it is not much used now-a-days.

Nitrous oxide (N_2O): It is the gas used first to produce analgesia or anaesthesia by dental and obstetric surgeons. It is otherwise known as laughing gas. A mixture of nitrous oxide and air at the percentage of 12 and 88 is usually employed. Sometimes 10 to 15% oxygen may be added to the above mixture. Nitrous oxide can also be used alone but it is not suitable for prolonged periods, in which case, addition of 10% to 15% oxygen is essential.

Oxygen (O_2): There cannot be a human life without oxygen; it is required even during anaesthetic condition. In emergency cases like Heart/lung disease, haemolytic poisons, asphyxia etc, it is absolutely essential. Usually 50% to 60% concentration of oxygen is required for normal breathing. Addition of 5% to 10%. Carbon dioxide may stimulate respiration.

Helium (He): It is a very light gas compared to other gases due to its low molecular weight; hence, useful in mechanical & pathological obstruction of respiration. Mixtures of Helium with air, oxygen or anaesthetic gases are used to make breathing without difficulties. Up to 80% helium-air mixture is used.

Cylinders and Accessories

Medical gas cylinders are made up of heavy steel and made to withstand a pressure of 200 bars. They are fitted with number of accessories to supply the content in needed quantity safely. The accessories are outlet valves, fine adjustment valves, pressure gauges, regulators, flow meters and humidifiers. Cylinders are packed with gases up to a pressure of 130 bars only and therefore there is a safety margin of 70 bars. The size of the cylinder varies from a capacity of 36 to 5112 L.

Outlet valve: There are different types of outlet valves available to release the pressurized gas from the cylinders which has to be carefully controlled. These valves are used just to open and close the gas from the cylinder, to release measured quantity and pressure. Other valves are used after this valve. Outlet valves are designed in such a way that only correct type of valve will fit into the corresponding attachments of the anesthetic apparatus, hence, administration of wrong gas is impossible. Thus a flush type (Pin Index) valve is most often used. Other valves are bull-nosed, straight type 7 and angled type 8.

Fine adjustment valves: These are simple devices to adjust the volume of gas passing through the valve. A small hand wheel is rotated clockwise or anticlockwise to move a tapered needle through a hole from which the gas comes out. Major problem with this type of valve is building up of pressure if any obstruction is there in the breathing apparatus. When the pressure inside the cylinder falls, we have to manually adjust the flow rate.

Regulators: In this accessory of the cylinder, some safety devices are incorporated so that, any pressure building up in the tube is controlled by shutting down the supply of gas from the cylinder.

Pressure gauge: Usually this accessory is engaged to measure the pressure in any apparatus for gas handling. It is a dial type meter which shows the pressure of gas passing through it. However it is not useful in cylinders with liquefied gases, as it will only show the vapour pressure inside the container which will be constant until the cylinder is empty.

Flow meters: Volume of gas administered per unit time should be measured for which flow meters are engaged. There are two types of flow meters, one is fixed orifice type, and another is variable orifice type. In the former gas is measured using dial type pressure gauge which is graduated in litre per minute, in the later type, gas is passed through a tube which is graduated on its side. A small bobbin will be floating and rotating inside this tube when gas passes through it. The height at which bobbin floats; correspond to the scale on the side. Thus the flow rate is measured.

Humidifier/nebulizer: As prolonged administration of dry gas irritates nasal mucosa, the gas is allowed to pass through water in a container. A safety valve may be attached to this container to prevent pressure being build up inside.

Colour Codes of Cylinders

As all the cylinders look similar, to avoid mix up and wrong use, medical gas cylinders are painted different colours on its outer side. The following is the chart of colour codes of cylinders.

Gas	Colour of the cylinder	
	Body	Top (valve end)
Carbon dioxide	Grey	Grey
Cyclopropane	Orange	Orange
Helium	Brown	Brown
Nitrous oxide	Blue	Blue
Oxygen	Black	White

If mixture of any of above gases is supplied, alternate bonds of colours allotted to each gas are painted on such cylinder.

Safe use and Care of Medical Gas Cylinders

1. First of all the gas to be administered to the patient is identified by the colour of the cylinder; name painted on it and also the pin index. Six possible pin positions, depends on the gas can be used which should be verified and confirmed.

2. Empty or half empty cylinders should be identified by either pressure gauge or weighing.

3. No oil or grease should be used on the valves or other parts of the cylinder, as it catches instant fire on opening the gas or due to friction.

4. Cylinders should be stored in dust free atmosphere and without dust particles adhering to the valve, otherwise, on opening the high pressure gas cylinder, fire may occur due to friction of dust particles on the valve. To avoid such a possibility, just before connecting the cylinder to the equipment, cylinder should be opened for few seconds to flow away the dust particles.

5. All joints should be checked for leaks, applying little soap water on the joint, shows bubbles of gas if there is leak. It should be immediately corrected.

6. Oxygen, cyclopropane and nitrous oxide are highly inflammable in nature; hence extra care should be taken in every stage of handling these cylinders against fire accidents.

7. Medical gas cylinders should be stored in cool, dry conditions. Cylinders should not be allowed to rust. It should be away from direct sun light falling over them.

8. Particularly in oxygen cylinders, reducing valve to control the rate of flow should be fitted. If it is of rubber bellows type, the tap of the reducer should always be opened first, before opening main oxygen tap on the cylinder, otherwise fire accident is possible.

9. All the cylinders should have the name and chemical symbol of the gas painted on it. This painting should be intact and not erased due to friction between empty cylinders while transporting.

10. A special rack should be arranged for stocking the cylinders, so that old cylinders are used first.

Questions

Short Answer Questions

1. What are diagnostic equipments? Give Examples.

2. List the surgical instruments used in hospitals.

3. Write a note on first aid supplies.

4. What are the colours used to differentiate medical gas cylinders? Explain.

Long Answer Questions

5. What are Medical Gases? Write in detail about Medical Gas cylinders and accessories used with them.

6. Write in detail about safe use and care of medical gas cylinders.

7. Explain the use of common surgical instruments. Add a note on health accessories used by patients.

CHAPTER 17

NUCLEAR PHARMACY

Need for Nuclear Pharmacy

Radio pharmaceuticals or radioactive isotope usage in hospitals is steadily increasing and hence, people concerned with its use and administrators felt the need to develop a separate wing- nuclear pharmacy. Nuclear pharmacy, if established in a hospital, will have the centralized responsibility for the dissemination of information, purchase, use, storage, disposal and monitoring of these potentially dangerous materials.

Hence, it is necessary to expose the student in hospital pharmacy to the licensing requirements of atomic energy commission, the hospital radio isotope committee and its role, which a hospital pharmacist can assume in this rapidly developing branch of the pharmacy.

Role of Atomic Energy Commission

As more and more hospitals and clinics are using radio-isotopes for diagnostic, therapeutic and research purposes, the use of these hazardous materials is subject to the control and supervision of the department of atomic energy- a government department established by an act of Indian parliament.

All the radio pharmaceuticals should be purchased from the Board of Radiation and Isotope Technology (BRIT) under Department of Atomic Energy of Government of India. A hospital pharmacist must be aware of the purchase or ordering procedure of radio pharmaceuticals. These materials are supplied to the licensed users only and the license for the same has to be obtained from the board after satisfying its terms and conditions.

Ordering Procedure

There are different forms for ordering radio pharmaceuticals. For example A1 form is for ordering radio pharmaceuticals and radio chemicals, SA4 form for standing order of radio pharmaceuticals and so on. Orders for different products and services can be placed by completing and sending the respective form. Urgent orders may also be placed by telephone or fax. However such orders should be followed by a written order in proper format clearly specifying that it is a confirmatory order.

New orders are referred to Atomic Energy Regulatory Board (AERB) for obtaining authentication and acknowledgement is sent to the customer with a key number. Orders already authorized by AERB (authorization for doctor / user / premises) are sent to respective production laboratory. Once authorization is received from AERB for new orders they are also sent to production laboratory subject to receipt of advance payment in the form of a demand draft.

Supply: The production schedule is processed at the customer service cell and a dispatch advice is sent to the customer indicating the date of dispatch. Normally a day before the dispatch, the customer support service cell prepare the packing notes and other documents like shipper's certification and sends to dispatch section and a day after dispatch the air consignment number or roadways receipt number is communicated to the customer by fax.

Conditions of Sale

This is explained in the website of Department of Atomic Energy, Government of India as given below:

1. The radioactive material supplied against the order must not be sold or transferred to any other user or otherwise disposed off except as advised by atomic energy regulatory board.

2. Facilities for the safe handling, storage and use of the material prescribed by the board from time to time must be provided.

3. Lead containers used in packing radioactive material and classified as returnable are to be returned to the board office at Mumbai.

4. Any complaint or discrepancy observed should be brought to the notice of the board within two days of the receipt of the consignment.

5. Cancellation of the orders already placed should be made at least 7 days in advance of the scheduled date of supply.

6. The order for radioactive material should be by the person who is authorized to procure radioactive material by the board and will be incharge of the use, storage and responsible for making arrangement for the safe disposal of the radioactive material.

7. He should make prompt arrangement for the collection of the consignment of radioactive material from the airways / roadways office.

8. Orders for radioactive material must be complete in all aspects. The code and the name of the product should be invariably specified. Incomplete and incorrect order forms will be returned for corrections.

9. While ordering, the pharmacist / doctor should indicate the specific activity in millicuries per gram of activated element or specify 'carrier-free' as applicable. In case of carbon 14 and Tritium labelled compounds, the specific activity in millicurie per mille mole must be indicated.

10. The board will make every effort to supply the products on the scheduled date. In exceptional cases the supply may be postponed or cancelled on account of unforeseen reactor shutdown or due to any unforeseen situation beyond their control.

Radio Isotope Committee

Hospitals which are using radioactive isotopes for diagnostic or therapeutic purposes are required to constitute a radio isotope committee. The committee should consist of a radiation physicist, a clinical radiologist, a haematologist, and a surgeon. Other members or specialists to be included in the committee and their role are usually decided by the hospital management. Usually representatives from pharmacy, nursing and administrative services are included.

The functions of the committee are as follows:

1. It considers the request for the use of particular isotope in the pharmacy and grant permission for the same. It also reviews the use of all radio isotopes in the hospital.

2. Report from the radiation protection officer is received and reviewed by the committee.

3. It strictly implements the conditions of license by Department of Atomic energy in the hospital and if somebody fails to observe protection recommendations, rules and regulations, recommend remedial actions.

4. If necessary special conditions are prescribed by the committee such as training of personnel etc. In order to educate the employees and others concerned with the use of radio isotopes, it prepares literatures and circulates among them.

Role of Pharmacist in Isotope Pharmacy

If an isotope pharmacy is established in a hospital, the pharmacist does his usual work of ordering, storing and dispensing of the radio isotopes required by the doctor licensed to use these materials.

When a physician decides to use a radio isotope, he explains his requirement to the pharmacist directly. Then the pharmacist makes necessary calculations in order to arrive at the required dosage. He places order for the same as per the procedure explained before, or if it is already available, he transfers the required quantity using a remote controlled pipette from the stock container to paper cup placed inside a lead container.

It is then safely transported to the isotope administration room. Then it is the duty of the radiation safety officer to follow the procedures for safe administration and disposal of isotopes. Thus it is a patient oriented service which requires scientific knowledge, patience and responsible behaviour by all concerned.

The role of pharmacist can be elaborated as follows:

Purchase and Storage

Unlike general drugs, radio pharmaceuticals cannot be procured from whole saler or stockist. It is under the control of Government of India and hence it has to be purchased from the Government agencies only.

Moreover, the supply cannot take long time as in the case of general drugs, as the radio isotopes are subject to decay and have half life. It should reach the potential user before it loses its activity considerably; hence, usually it is supplied by overnight delivery through airways.

While ordering it, shipping or delivery schedule, ratio activity decay etc. are to be taken into account.

Isotopes should be stored as per rules. There should be a separate room for manipulation and preparation of radio pharmaceutical dosage form and a counting area for the calibration of doses. Treatment should be given in a special room which is built and maintained as per norms.

Quality of Radio Pharmaceuticals

Like other pharmaceuticals, radio pharmaceuticals also should be tested for its quality. Many Pharmacopoeia's especially USP, specifies certain tests for radio pharmaceuticals like, radionuclide purity, radio chemical purity, chemical purity, pH, particle size, sterility, pyrogenecity and specific activity.

Radio nuclide purity is tested by γ-ray spectroscopy, half-life measurement and / or other physical methods. They help in the detection of extraneous nuclide. Thus the radio nuclide purity which is the proportion of activity present as stated nuclide is measured. For example if ^{198}Au is contaminated with ^{199}Au its radio nuclide purity is affected.

Dispensing or Handling of Radio Pharmaceuticals

Though radio pharmaceuticals are prescribed for patients they are not directly dispensed to them. Instead they are handed over to the trained health care professionals of the hospital and then administered to the patient by the authorized doctor. Therefore radio pharmaceuticals are dispensed in unit doses. While deciding the dose and other related matters, patient factors such as age, weight, surface area of body and γ camera sensitivity etc, must be considered both by the doctor and the pharmacist. Needless to mention, the decay corrections, to accommodate from when the radio pharmaceutical was prepared to the time it is actually administered to the patient should be made for each radio pharmaceutical.

If injections of radiopharmaceuticals are to be given, they are administered with lead lined special syringes supplied with the product. All the above operations should be made by using appropriate information on all products and accessories and at the place provided for it.

For example labs for radio pharmaceuticals must be provided with unidirectional flow work stations-the fuming cub-board. Drainage should be provided as per standards dictated by government agency.

Radio active isotopes are administered to patients for treatment of various conditions, e.g. radioactive iodine for hyperthyroidism, radioactive gold for malignant diffusions, and radioactive phosphorus for malignant haematological conditions. These emit β and γ rays and exposure should be reduced to the minimum by,

1. Avoiding contamination of clothing and skin from body secretions of the patient
2. Keeping the time close to the patient, as short as possible and
3. Keeping as great a distance from the patient as possible when in the unit.

Responsibility of Pharmacists and others in using Radio Isotopes

For their own safety, as well as, the safety of others, pharmacist and others whoever handling or using radio isotopes has the following responsibilities:

1. To receive instruction in radiation safety as determined appropriate by the radiation safety officer.
2. To keep exposure to radiation at the lowest level possible and specifically below the maximum permissible exposure.
3. To wear recommended radiation dosimeters for personnel, such as film badges, pockct ionization chambers and finger dosimeters.
4. To examine his hand, shoes, body and clothing for radio activity and removal of all loose contamination before leaving the laboratory.
5. To use all appropriate protective measures, such as protective clothing, respiratory protection, remote pipetting devices, ventilated and shielded glove box and hoods.
6. To prohibit smoking and eating in radio isotope laboratories.
7. To check working area daily or after each radio isotope procedure.
8. To maintain good lab practices, such as keeping working area and equipment clean and orderly.
9. To use proper labels on equipment being used with radioactive materials.

10. To place all active waste in proper containers, equipped with proper labels.

11. To report immediately the details of a 'spill' or other accident involving radioactive substances to the radiation safety officer.

12. To conduct decontamination procedures as directed by the radiation safety officer.

The above guidelines are given in radio isotope manual prepared by Peter Bent Brigham hospital, Boston. Similar manuals and booklets are issued by others also, who are involved in handling radio pharmaceuticals. As mentioned in opening paragraphs, radio isotope committee of each hospital prepares and circulates such instructions to their staff concerned.

Questions

Short Answer Questions

1. What is the need for nuclear pharmacy?

2. Write short notes on radio isotope committee.

Long Answer Questions

3. Write in detail about the role of Atomic energy commission in radio pharmaceutical sales.

4. Explain the role of pharmacist in nuclear pharmacy. Detail the responsibility of pharmacists and others in using radio isotopes.

CHAPTER 18

RECORDS AND REPORTS

Introduction

Apart from usual records of drugs stock register, indents to the stores or authorities, supply receipts etc., a pharmacist in a hospital has to maintain, some other records such as, drug profile, patient medication card, records on cases of ADR etc. Further he has to maintain the prescription given to individual patient. All these records and reports are valuable documents and very much useful in providing safe and rational drug therapy to the patients. Hence a pharmacist must be well versed with those documents.

Prescription Filing

In this era of computer revolution, anything written can be stored and retrieved easily from a computer. However the biggest problem with the use of computers is original prescription which is authenticated by the signature of the doctor, who wrote it, cannot be stored as such. Scanning, microfilming are some of the advanced methods, however, little used because of cost and other factors.

Hence, the original hand written prescription by the doctor, given to a patient is retained as hard copy, rather than the soft copy or in addition to the soft copy in a hospital. Thus prescription filing is still continuing in many hospitals. They are stored in specially made steel or wooden cup boards with inside partitions for specific number of prescriptions like 100, 1000 etc.

They may be stored in numerical order, that is, as per hospital registration number given to the patient or department wise or in chronological order (date/month wise). Whichever method followed it must be easier for the pharmacist to locate the prescription without much time or confusion or not preventing ready access to other prescriptions.

Drug Profile

Records section of the pharmacy must maintain the profile of all the drugs supplied by it, for ready reference by the pharmacist and other health care staff members. A drug profile contains all the information about that particular drug viz, category, pharmacology, pharmacokinetics, indications, dose, contraindications, adverse reactions, warning and precautions, presentation and reference. Usually leading brands available in the market and its chemical structure are also included in the profile in order to have a clear idea about the drug.

Any additional information published may be added to it, so as to have up-to-date knowledge about the drug. Drug profile can be arranged alphabetically of their generic name and also under pharmacological classification for easy reference. Such a collection of drug profile will be much useful, to doctors, nurses, pharmacists and students of these branches.

Now-a-days, all these details are available as books in the form updated monthly publications and also as data-bases to be used with computers.

Patient Medication Profile

It is otherwise known as patient medication cards. In community pharmacies, not often in hospital pharmacies, they are maintained as family prescription records, by including the drugs used by the family members of the patient. It will be a complete record, if it contains the OTC drugs used by the patient. Hence he should be educated and encouraged to reveal everything concerned with his health and treatment to the pharmacist. If not the medication profile may not be valid or worth maintaining.

The patient medication profile contains:

(a)   Name and address of the patient

(b)   Age and sex

(c)   Known allergies and adverse reactions

(d)   Present and past diseases and treatment taken

(e)   Current medications and devices used

(f)   Any other relevant information and

(g)   Pharmacist's opinion

It is better to include non prescription drugs used by the patient in the profile in the column 'F', patient's habits like smoking, alcohol use etc., should be recorded, so that patient can be warned about possible side effects or problems with certain drugs like CNS depressants.

The family system of profiling in community pharmacy has both advantages and disadvantages. It reduces number of files to be maintained by the pharmacy. It helps the pharmacist in reviewing overall health status of the family and provides him with opportunities to counsel, educate or caution the family members about impending troubles if one member of the family is affected by a disease. All these services by the pharmacist will be appreciated by the family concerned and hence a good rapport and relationship develops between pharmacy and the family.

However, if all the patient profiles are clubbed together it may present a challenge when the pharmacist attempts to monitor the therapy for each patient. Obviously the individual record makes it easier to monitor the patient and is less susceptible to errors of confusion on the part of the pharmacist.

This problem can be easily solved by using a computer by creating a folder for each family and maintaining individual files inside the folder for each member of the family.

Model Patient Medication Profile

Name of the Hospital/Pharmacy:

Allergy:

Patient's Name:

Age and Sex:

Address:

Physician Name:

Source of Admission: Home / Other Hospital / Emergency Service.

Diagnosis on Admission:

Other Pathology, if any:

Operative Procedures, if any:

Pre-operative Medication used:

Any other information:

OTC Drugs, if any:

Drugs currently used:

Date	Name of the Drugs	Dose	Route of Administration	Discontinued on	Lab tests	Pharmacists Remarks

Discharged on: *Signature of Pharmacist.*

Uses of Patient Medication Profile

(a) In Hospitals

Patient medication profile is useful

(a) To improve drug prescribing practices by the doctors of the particular hospital.

(b) To prevent drug-drug interactions.

(c) To detect and prevent drug induced laboratory test abnormalities.

(d) To select appropriate drug for the disease without over lapping or wasting precious time on non-responsive drug regimen.

(e) As patient medication history for ready reference.

(b) In Community Pharmacy

Apart from the uses mentioned above, patient medication profile, if maintained in a community pharmacy, can be useful as the basis for retrospective drug utilization report and a database to facilitate communication and consultation between the pharmacist and other health care professionals.

It is the tendency of many patients to see several physicians for the same disease; hence, there is a possibility of drug interactions or over lapping, or repetition of non responsive drug regimen. However patients used to purchase their medicines usually from the neighbourhood pharmacy, the pharmacist, has thus the chance to find out above problems, if medication profiles are maintained in that particular pharmacy.

Computer based software also provides space for pharmacists to record and document intervention important to the specific patient. Thus patient medication profile plays a major role in ensuring safe and rational use of medicines.

Records on Cases of ADR

This is an important record a pharmacist has to maintain in a hospital. If every findings, test results and medicines used by the patients are correctly recorded in the patient medication profile, it is easier to find out the untoward effect and its cause easily. Any abnormal values and other symptoms lead to the suspicion that, ADR, or drug interaction or idiosyncratic reactions have started occurring in the patient. Such cases should be monitored with drug therapy review by clinical pharmacists and findings recorded.

Once an ADR is conformed it should be reported first to the hospital authorities then to the ADR monitoring committees of the government, in the ADR reporting form, model of which is given below, available in all the wards and dispensaries.

Every case of ADR must be reported by the attending physician to the authorities or to the chairman of PTC. They, in turn, advice the physician how to proceed on the particular case and also monitor the treatment given to the patient.

Adverse drug reactions should be recorded as diagnosis wherever applicable. All these records are maintained by medical record room incharge of the hospital who is usually the pharmacist of the hospital.

Thus starting from the prescription to ADR report, the patient's entire medication history is maintained by the pharmacist and thereby he helps the hospital administration in providing best possible treatment for all the patients.

Model ADR Reporting Form
Name of the Hospital and address:
Patient's Name and Address:
Age and Sex:
Drug or Agent suspected to have caused ADR:
Source of Drug: Prescription / OTC
Full Detail of the above Drug: [Dt.of Mfg, Dt. of Exp, Batch No.]
Type of Reaction:
Therapy Given:
Progress and Result:
Date: *Signature of Attending Physician:*

Questions

Short Answer Questions

1. Write a note on prescription filing.

2. What is a drug profile?

3. What are the uses of patient medication profile?

Long Answer Questions

4. What is patient medication Profile? Explain the uses of it.

5. Explain the records used in case of ADR.

CHAPTER 19

PROFESSIONAL RELATIONS AND PRACTICES

Introduction

A pharmacist's public relation and professional relation are the important aspects of pharmacy practice. As pharmacy profession require constant touch and movement with general public, it can be promoted easily among them and earn respect and glory for the profession. Compared to other health professional like doctors, nurses and physiotherapists, pharmacists occupy a pivotal role because of his round the clock service and access to the public. He is available always among them in the community pharmacies and approachable freely in hospital pharmacies whereas a patient require prior appointment or wait for his turn in a quae to meet a doctor or physiotherapists and nurses are busy with their professional duties inside the ward and all these professional have little time to spare and share with public. Hence pharmacists are in a unique position to serve and earn the good will and appreciation from the community

Opportunities

Obviously the above professional relation and practice requires no money but time and effort on the part of a pharmacist. A pharmacist can promote his profession by the following programs:

1. By participating in teaching and information services of the hospital
2. By organizing educational services for the public
3. By participating in activities of professional associations
4. By maintaining professional relation with medical and nursing staff
5. By maintaining professional relation with research staff
6. By maintaining professional relation with medical rep and suppliers
7. By organizing rehabilitation and consultation programs

8. By providing service through various hospital committees and

9. By participating in hospital administrative works

Thus a pharmacist has great opportunities to maintain professional relations and promote pharmacy practice.

1. Participating in teaching and information services of the hospital

In order to be in constant touch with developments of health profession, all the members of health care team are required to be educated and provided with latest information. Hence big hospitals organize many programs for the purpose. Important among them are:

(a) Continuing education programs for staff

(b) Publishing pharmacy bulletins, News Letters, etc

(c) Maintaining hospital library

(d) Establish and run Drug Information Centre and

(e) Publishing Hospital Formulary.

All the above programs have only one aim-educating hospital staff. Senior pharmacists of the hospital can be utilized as resource persons for continuing education program for the juniors as well as middle level professionals of pharmacy, medical, nursing and lab services. Topics for the above programs can be decided in consultation with heads of these departments. Day-to-day developments in the respective fields, especially in pharmacy can be selected and lectures delivered to those peoples. These continuing education programs can be of 2 to 3 days duration to a fortnight. Course or study materials or synopsis of special lectures can be printed and given to the participants. Eminent speakers and technical people from outside institutions can be engaged to make the program more productive and interesting. Pharmacists can play very active role in organizing this program. Staff of other hospitals can also be invited to these programs.

As discussed elsewhere in this book Pharmacy Bulletins or News Letters serve the same purpose of educating the staff but through print media. It is more useful than the continuing education program [CEP] because these printed matters are more frequent and pass on the latest information whereas the CEP can be organized only once or twice a year.

Apart from the above programs, a hospital should maintain a well stocked library in its premises. It should have all essential reference books of medicine, pharmacy, nursing and allied health sciences. Latest editions of these books as well as journals and other periodicals should be kept in library. Needless to mention in these age of information technology, computers with internet facility should be available. A pharmacist can be given in charge of library as he by the nature of his job is an information gatherer and giver. Also he is educated and trained in establishing and running Drug Information Center which is nothing but a library for a specific purpose.

The services provided by Drug Information Center are explained in a separate chapter and need not be repeated here. Similarly publishing and updating Hospital Formulary as per the direction of Pharmacy and Therapeutic committee is discussed elsewhere.

2.   Organizing educational services for the public

Occasions may arise during the course of hospital pharmacy practice, a pharmacist has to arrange for educational programs of the community. As no treatment is complete without the use of medications, educating the public about its proper use, storage, side effects if any, has to be carried out by pharmacists. These works assume significance during epidemics or out breaks of certain diseases throughout the community.

To do this program effectively pharmacists have to prepare display boards, banners and other propaganda materials. As there are many illiterate people in rural India, these display materials should include pictorial representations which are easy to understand by those people.

Pharmacists can also arrange for audio visual presentation using slides, short films and appeal videos by popular personalities which are well received by rural people. Hand bills [pit notices] in simple language can be prepared and distributed. Short speeches delivered through mike systems fitted in vehicle, from the street corners of villages reach indented population effectively. Educational needs of people can be undertaken by respective taluk or black level hospitals.

3.   Participating in activities of professional associations

All the pharmacists must join as member of professional association of their area of practice. They must also participate in its activities with devotion otherwise it becomes useless to be a member. These associations usually carry on the work of popularizing the profession by various themes of professional day celebrations like world pharmacist's day, National Pharmacy Week etc, every year. They also arrange periodic lectures by eminent personalities from pharmacy or other professions. These lectures not only refresh the knowledge of pharmacists but also provide opportunities to discuss different point of views among the members.

Professional associations also deliberate discuss and decide about various matters concerned with profession and convey their resolution or demand to appropriate authorities in government and elsewhere for its redress. Thus they constantly try to upgrade professional dignity and status in the society. They also provide opportunity to meet friends, class and college mates and even their family members once in a year during annual day celebrations or get-togethers which is difficult for a pharmacist in today's busy city life. Only when a pharmacist participate in association activities, he can acquire up-to-date knowledge, developments in the field and also what is going on in other branches of pharmacy without much efforts. Student members can even gather job or trainee vacancy positions from members of regulatory[DI] or industry branches of pharmacy. As meeting these people individually and in person in their offices is very difficult for a student in pharmacy, he must make use of association meetings by becoming its student member.

Only by participating in professional association meetings pharmacists can correct any deficiency in its activities or inaction or direct its course of action. Simply criticizing association without participating in its meetings is of no use and leads to nowhere and that is the mistake many pharmacists are doing.

There are many professional associations in India in our pharmacy field. Among them Indian Pharmaceutical Association [IPA] and Indian Pharmacy Graduates Association [IPGA] are the major associations, where anybody in any branch of pharmacy, even if he is not a pharmacist, can become the member in the former and only pharmacy graduates in the later.

There are other associations representing particular branch of pharmacy, like Association of Pharmaceutical Teachers of India [APTI], Indian Hospital Pharmacists Association [IHPA], All India drugs control officers Confederation [AIDCOC], Organization of Pharmaceutical Producers of India [OPPI], Indian Drugs Manufacturers Association [IDMA] and numerous State Govt Pharmacists Associations. There is a separate organization for Drug traders called All India Organization of Chemists and Druggists [AIOCD] where too non-pharmacy owners of pharmacy shops are enrolled as members.

A pharmacist should enroll himself as member of any one of the above general professional associations, as well as in the association representing his branch of pharmacy and thereby serve the profession, society and him self!

4. Maintaining professional relation with medical and nursing staff

American Society of Hospital Pharmacists [ASHP] has published a guideline for collaboration of pharmacists and nurses in institutional care settings. They are relevant to hospitals of all countries and hence discussed below:

True and sincere collaboration by way of professional relation among pharmacists and nurses reflects in the quality of patient care. The complexity of drug treatment requires this collaboration between nurses and pharmacists on a regular basis. Pharmacists on their part can supply drug information to the nurses, on the other, nurses can provide valuable information on the effect of drugs on the inpatients, as they are directly involved in patient care.

The orientation programs for the students and newly appointed nurses or pharmacists can be reciprocal, in that, orientation for nurses disseminate information about various services provided by pharmacy and the program for student pharmacists can include introduction to a patient care unit [ward] and its functions by nurses. Professional collaboration should be there whenever the roles of professionals [pharmacists and nurses] overlap. For example in the area of inpatient education, monitoring ADR, ward rounds and in nursing care plans both these professionals can co-operate and exchange information and observations.

Nurses equipped with adequate drug information and knowledge of patient are in a better position to administer the drugs properly at correct time, dose and frequency and detect undesirable drug effect if any. On his part a pharmacist should provide the following drug information in adequate level and extend to the nurses:

1. Information on new drugs.
2. Information on investigational drugs used in the hospital.
3. Probable side effects and therapeutic risks of the drugs prescribed.
4. Contraindications to particular drug therapy.
5. Compatibility and stability of drugs, including I.V admixture.
6. Drug dose calculations, if any.
7. Essential pharmacokinetic data about the drugs prescribed.
8. Possible drug interactions [Drug-Drug, Drug-Food and Drug-lab tests] and
9. Effect of patient's age and disease on drug's action.

Apart from the above, pharmacist should record information that is important to the patient's medication regimen in the patient's record. Specific allergies to drugs should be highlighted on the patient's record. As discussed elsewhere in this book, nurses should be supplied with pharmacy news letters or bulletins and latest edition of hospital formulary, all prepared by hospital pharmacists.

Clinical pharmacists by participating in ward rounds with doctors and nurses can review patient medications. A fruitful exchange of information and discussions among Physicians, Pharmacists and Nurses results in better therapy, speedy recovery and discharge of the patient and that is the goal of health care team.

5. Professional relation with research staff

Though clinical research is carried out by exclusive organizations [CRO] established for the purpose of research, hospitals also play an important role in research activities. CROs have their own limitation in that they can not have human volunteers of all varieties and all diseases can not be artificially induced in them, hence big hospitals with varieties of patients and varieties of diseases are unavoidable in research activities.

Research can be undertaken for new drugs or new indication for old drugs, as well as on drugs suspected of ADR. In all these researches, pharmacist can provide needed back ground information gathered through hospital drug information center to the research staff. Extensive research literature survey is possible only through Drug Information Centre, as it has all the primary, secondary and tertiary sources of information.

If needed and requested formulations can be prepared and supplied by pharmacists using the raw materials given by research staff. Pharmacist can also organize double or triple blind study for the evaluation of research drug. Moreover pharmacist as a person in charge of stores of the hospital and procurer of raw materials for hospital drug manufacturing unit can arrange inventory of investigative materials for the research staff.

As a clinical pharmacist's work involves pharmacokinetic and pharmacodynamic study of drugs used by patients, he himself has lot of opportunities to do research on these subjects. He can co-opt physicians as co-investigators of these researches and that co-operation and professional relation will open many doors for inventions in therapeutic and pharmaceutical sciences.

6. Professional relation with medical rep and suppliers

Medical representative are the people who supply latest information about drugs and formulations newly introduced in the market. Thus they are considered as part of educational program and objectives of the hospital. Hence a pharmacist has to develop appropriate rapport with them so that hospital staff starting from pharmacist himself will benefit from his specialized knowledge.

Most of the time these representatives are considered as interruptions in busy work of pharmacists and physicians and hence not much time is allotted for his detailing and display materials. It is a wrong approach on the part of hospital staff especially for pharmacists, as pharmacists are required to gather and give drug information to the staff which is being readily supplied at his desk by the medical representatives. Thus a medical representative is helping the pharmacist in his job, so he must be provided with quality time and attention.

In order to do that properly, time must be allocated for visit by medical representative every week or fortnight as required. They must be encouraged to adhere to that time schedule and their genuine concern regarding the allotted time should be addressed. Fixing prior appointment avoid embarrassment and/or disappointment for both parties. But its success lies in adhering or honouring the appointment by both of them.

Medical representatives supply drug or product information through literatures and samples. Pharmacist should collect them and forward to the physicians and members of PTC for getting approval for future purchase. While medical representatives make a presentation or detailing pharmacist must make a note of it in product information sheet, model of which adopted from William Hassan is given below:

PRODUCT INFORMATION SHEET

NAME OF THE PRODUCT:……………………………………

MANUFACTURER………………………………………………..

GENERIC NAME…………………………………………………

ADDRESS…………………………………………………………

CHEMICAL NAME………………………………………………

SYNONYM………………………………………………………

COMPOSITION [IF IT IS A FORMULATION]   THERAPEUTIC USE OF EACH INGREDIENT

…………………………………………   ……………………………………………..

…………………………………………   ……………………………………………..

…………………………………………   ……………………………………………..

…………………………………………   ……………………………………………..

…………………………………………   ……………………………………………..

…………………………………………   ……………………………………………..

…………………………………………   ……………………………………………..

…………………………………………   ……………………………………………..

INDICATION……………………………   CONTRAINDICATION………………………..

TOXICOLOGY…………………………   ANTIDOTE……………………………………

DOSAGE & ADMINISTRATION ------- DOSAGE FORM ---------- EQUIVALENT PRODUCT

………………………………………   …………………………………

………………………………………

………………………………………   ……………...………………

………………………………………

………………………………………   …………………………………

………………………………………

PACKING AND PRICE   LITERATURE: YES/ NO

....   SAMPLES: YES/ NO

DATE: ....   PHARMACIST'S SIGNATURE:.....................

SPACE FOR PTC'S OPINION / RECOMMENTATION:

....

....

The above form is submitted to the PTC during its agenda for product approval for purchase and its inclusion in Hospital Formulary. Thus in a institutionalized modern hospital pharmacy, pharmacist's professional relation with medical representatives and drug suppliers goes long way in providing better treatment for the patient with latest drugs.

In the hospital with PTC and modern hospital pharmacy set up and control over the freedom of doctors in prescribing drugs [only those listed in hospital formulary has to be prescribed] even samples given by medical representatives has to be used only after approval by PTC. Hence these samples are supplied to the hospital stores only, not to the individual doctor in the ward or OPD. As with other drugs, physician has to order these samples through prescription to the patient and the same is dispensed by the pharmacist. Hence the list of samples available with dispensary or stores will be periodically circulated to the doctors. Thus use of drugs by a patient of the hospital is completely under the control of PTC.

7. Organizing drug rehabilitation and consultation programs

A hospital pharmacist has to organize and /or participate in drug rehabilitation and consultation program, as he is considered as expert and custodian of drugs. Hence misuse or abuse of drugs by the patients or members of public must provoke his inner consciousness. Adhering to established rules and regulations and following good pharmacy practice, reduces misuse of drugs to a great extend. However there are still minor percentages of people who misuse drugs and undergo rehabilitation program.

Pharmacists must cooperate in those programs and his advice, counseling and empathy with patients prevent relapse or failure of treatment. He must be familiar with legal and ethical issues and psychiatric approaches to the treatment of drug abuse. He must procure and stock the drugs for such detoxification and treatment program. Similarly he must be available for drug consultation by the discharged patients of the hospital. It was found in a survey that discharged patients who are in touch with the hospital, showed less deviation from the prescribed drug regimen and fewer medication problems at home than did patients who had not been provided with this service. Obviously drug consultation program promote patient safety and helps in preventing relapse of disease and consequent readmission of the patient in hospital. Most of the advice to the patients like what to do and what not to do are given at the time of discharge counseling by clinical pharmacists, however, availability of such a service through the day and year will make the patient adhere to the instructions and results in successful treatment.

8. Providing service through hospital committees

Pharmacists can play an active role in various committees of the hospital especially in PTC, Antibiotics Committee, Infection control committee etc. His role in these committees is explained in a separate chapter [No.5].

These services ensure proper and orderly functioning of the hospital and thereby the hospital earns reputation and respect among the patients and public. Hence a pharmacist must strive hard to put in his best possible service through the activities of these committees.

9. Participating in hospital administrative works

Apart from his professional duties outlined above, a pharmacist has to assist in hospital administration by few other services. For example he can serve as one of the member or even secretary of the purchase committee of the hospital. As drugs, chemicals and surgical items are the major consumable items of the hospital and pharmacists are in charge of stores and accounts of these materials, he is the natural choice to serve in purchase committee.

The major responsibility of hospital administration is to procure and distribute the above consumables without shortage and interruption. Hence pharmacist's work in this area is well received and appreciated. By the very nature of this work, pharmacist has the golden chance of establishing and maintaining cordial relationship with dozens of manufacturers, wholesalers, retailers and their representatives of these items. Thus the next important work of hospital administration also gets remarkable contribution by the pharmacists.

Many non-governmental social service organizations like, Lions Clubs, Rotary Clubs etc are in the service of their members as well as general public by arranging meetings, seminars, health camps etc. They are constantly in need of speakers in professional topics to enlighten and educate their members and people of their area. They approach hospitals for such speakers, though they prefer doctors for such speeches, doctors, unfortunately are hard pressed for time and reluctant to accept such assignments. Post graduate senior pharmacists can substitute in **accepting outside speech assignments** and many hospital managements are willing to entrust such works to pharmacists. Thus pharmacists can help hospital administration. If nobody is spared for such programs from the hospital, they cannot expect cooperation from outside organizations for its public activities. Reciprocating the gesture of outside agencies by hospital administration is one of its duties and if pharmacist can extend a helping hand to the administration in this aspect his services will be appreciated by one and all.

Questions

Short Answer Questions

1. Write a note on pharmacists and professional associations

2. Enumerate the professional relation ship between Pharmacists and Medical representatives.

Long Answer Questions

3. List the professional relations and practices of Hospital Pharmacists. Explain any two practices in detail.

4. Explain the pharmacist's professional relation with health care professionals.

PART - II

CLINICAL PHARMACY

CHAPTER 20

CLINICAL PHARMACY

Introduction

Clinical Pharmacy is a new branch of pharmacy introduced in the health care system. It is well accepted and currently practiced in USA, UK, Australia and other developed countries where the pharmacists perform the clinical pharmacy services. Though this service was introduced in those countries decades back, it is yet to be started in India. As no one can stop the forward movement of the wheels of science, it will be definitely introduced in India eventually, and hence today's pharmacy students have to be familiar with this subject.

Need / Concept of Clinical Pharmacy

What is the need for clinical pharmacy? Why suddenly a new branch of pharmacy was started? How the concept of clinical pharmacy was evolved? All these questions need to be answered for the introduction of the subject.

In order to survive and to catch the new markets, big pharmaceutical companies are spending millions of dollars in research and development of new drugs. As a result, new drugs are introduced into the market at regular intervals. Even before these drugs gets acceptance and widespread use, another drug or formulation is introduced by the competiting company, with claims of superior action etc. Thus there are hundreds of potent, new drugs, for the doctor to prescribe, with consequent risk of side effects, drug interactions etc. The competition between the drug companies are such that they flood the market not only with new drugs but also with literatures and information about those drugs with lot of claims and counter claims. Getting authentic and correct information from this junk is so difficult and hence an expert in *drug information* is needed.

Apart from this, we know that there is very little time a doctor can allot to each patient during the course of diagnosis and treatment. Also many patients are using one or other drug even before the treatment starts for the present disease or for already existing one. This predisposes the patient to ill effects during either present or future therapy. Hence *patient's medication history* is essential before starting the treatment. A suitable specialist is needed for this job. This specialist should also be able to decide the appropriateness of drug therapy, benefit to risk ratio, and alternative regimes if required.

All of us know that we all have common anatomy but not common physiology i.e., the degree of functions of our internal organs differ person to person and hence a generalized dose may not be suitable for all patients. Patient's conditions differ widely because they are with many complications like diabetes, hypertension, kidney damage, liver damage etc. Hence adjustment in dose for each patient is required, which involves many calculations based on scientific studies on the patient and his body fluids. Thus *individualization of dose and selection of drug to suit the particular individual* has to be performed by some expert. If not, the treatment cannot be claimed as fully scientific, at best it can be semi-scientific or pseudo-scientific.

However, the immediate reason for the evolution of the concept of clinical pharmacy was the THALIDOMIDE disaster of 1960-1961. The drug Thalidomide was developed in West Germany and marketed in several countries. It was given for controlling nausea and vomiting during the early stages of pregnancy and was available without the requirement of a prescription, as OTC drug.

However Thalidomide given to pregnant women produced 'PHOCOMELIA' – an arrested development of limbs of new born infants. In West Germany alone there were 10,000 birth deformities. The drug also affected thousands of infants in other countries such as England, Israel, Australia, Belgium, Brazil, Canada, East Germany, Egypt, Lebanon, Peru, Spain, Sweden and Switzerland, totaling few lakhs babies.

Thalidomide disaster has been a terrible lesson to the world, which shocked the entire health care team. On analyzing the disaster, it was found that new drugs were introduced into the market in haste without proper scientific studies after administration to human beings. Hence the process of introducing new drugs was lengthened and tightened. Also it was found that generally there is no one to monitor the effects of drugs, especially the adverse reactions of a drug on human body after administration of a drug. Hence the concept of clinical pharmacy was evolved, in which the pharmacist, is given the responsibility of doing *Therapeutic Drug Monitoring* (TDM) i.e., monitoring the drug's action after administration to the patients.

Also the concept of clinical pharmacy is helpful in assuaging the feelings of common people who were not only angry and also reluctant to go to an allopathic doctor for treatment or take allopathic drugs after Thalidomide tragedy. They started looking for alternative systems of medicine and from then onwards herbal drugs gained popularity. Hence the concept of clinical pharmacy gives the *assurance* that people's welfare after administering the drugs will be looked after by an expert, the Clinical Pharmacist, by regular monitoring and intervention if something goes wrong. Thus the old pattern of treatment "diagnosing, writing prescription, dispensing drugs and forgetting the patient" was put an end by this concept. The need for clinical pharmacy services is, thus crystal clear.

Definition

Clinical pharmacy is defined as a system concerned with rational selection and use of medicaments, at the patient level, so as to ensure the patient's maximum well being while on drug therapy.

Basis of Clinical Pharmacy

Because of the nature of his job a Clinical Pharmacist has to be in closer touch with medical profession and also the details of the treatment of the patients. Hence apart from usual pharmacy subjects he has to be familiar with Biochemistry, Clinical pathology, Pathophysiology etc. That is why these subjects were introduced into the diploma and degree syllabus of pharmacy. He must be thorough with subjects such as Biopharmaceutics, Pharmacokinetics and Pharmacodynamics which are the basis for clinical pharmacy.

While Biopharmaceutics deals with bioavailability, dosage regimen and different formulations, pharmacokinetics the significance of absorption, distribution, metabolism and excretion of drugs. Pharmacodynamics, on the other hand describes the effect of drugs on the body. These subjects thus lay the foundation for clinical pharmacy.

Needless to mention, the knowledge of chemical analysis of body fluids and other samples for drugs is very much essential to determine or adjust dose for individual patients which is considered to be a primary duty of a Clinical Pharmacist. Thus all the above subjects, hitherto neglected by pharmacists, form the basis of Clinical pharmacy.

Functions of Clinical Pharmacist

From the above discussions, it is clear that a Clinical Pharmacist has multidimensional role. Few of them are routine, few are rare and few yet need specialization. Thus, a Clinical Pharmacist has to perform the following duties routinely:

1. Getting patient's medication history
2. Offering consultation to physicians in the selection of suitable drug for the particular patient or himself selecting the drugs
3. Therapeutic drug monitoring including body fluid analysis and
4. Counselling the patients.

Apart from these regular functions, a Clinical Pharmacist may be assigned some specific duties as and when needed. For example he has to detect and confirm suspected Adverse Drug Reactions [ADR] occurred on a particular patient. Similarly he may be required to prepare Total Parenteral Nutrition (TPN) for some patients. Though these works are not required to be performed often, they are nevertheless assigned to senior Clinical Pharmacists.

In big tertiary care hospitals, complicated and referral cases may require some degree of specialization to attend. Thus, pediatric, geriatric and psychiatric cases need specialization in dealing with such cases. Also a Clinical Pharmacist's specialized services are required in difficult situations such as Narcotic withdrawal treatment, study of Clinical Toxicology and complicated pharmacokinetic studies.

Routine and General Functions

1. **Medication history interview:** Immediately after the admission of the patient in to the ward and the diagnostic tests begin, the medication history of the patient has to be obtained. Because a pharmacist is involved throughout his carrier in providing drugs to the patient both in hospital pharmacy and in outside community pharmacy, he can get a comprehensive medication history from the patient. As we are going to study in detail later in this book the art of obtaining useful medication history, it is suffice here to mention, a pharmacist is more suitable for the job than any body else in the health care team. He has to get the drug history involving, prescription drugs, and self medication and OTC drugs.

2. **Offering consultation for drug selection:** Because of stiff competition among the pharmaceutical companies to market their products and to get business, doctors are supplied with either biased information or half truth about a particular formulation, As a busy doctor has no time to verify the authenticity or correctness of those information, a Clinical Pharmacist can be of much helpful to him. He is able to give an unbiased report about the usefulness of a particular drug, on a particular patient in a particular condition. He is an expert on drugs and drug information. His main task is to ensure rational and safe use of drug, so he is in a better position to correct the deficiencies in the use of drugs, both by patients and doctors.

   Since in the ward where the Clinical Pharmacist is posted has all information available about the patient, he is able to advice on the best formulation to suit the particular patient needs. Similarly he can discourage the use of unnecessary drugs more effectively whilst on the ward than from dispensary where the relevant background information is not usually available. Alternatively, if the authorities agree he himself can select the drug and write the prescription, as practiced in USA.

3. **Therapeutic drug monitoring and analysis of body fluids:** As mentioned earlier, Clinical Pharmacist is mainly appointed, to monitor the patients after administration of drugs. To do that effectively he has to under take plasma/blood drug concentration studies. The blood samples at regular intervals are collected from the patient and analyzed. These results help the pharmacist to arrive at a suitable dose for the particular patient. Also it helps him, in assessing the value or usefulness of drug on that particular patient, so that he can suggest the doctor to either increase the dose or decrease the dose or altogether stop the drug and to go for an alternative.

Clinical Pharmacist is able to do this because he has not only the knowledge of pharmacological properties of a drug but also the knowledge of physical, chemical and pharmaceutical properties of drugs, which are not taught to doctors. Hence he is able to predict possible adverse effect that can be expected, any drug interaction possibilities and any other factor which modify drug activity. His attention is mainly drawn to the drugs which are having narrow therapeutic indices and require careful dose adjustment in the event of predisposing factors like old age, renal failure, hepatic damage and concurrent medication. Thus a Clinical Pharmacist is able to contribute significantly to direct patient care by performing TDM.

4. **Patient counselling:** Counselling is nothing but advising and convincing the patient about the drug therapy. As a result of counselling, patient compliance to the instruction improves. If a patient is made to realize via counseling his disease can be cured when he adhere to the instructions of health care team a successful treatment results. After all, every patient wants to go home early, after curing his disease, hence getting their co-operation need not be a problem. Few complaints like bitter tablets, frequent pricks, painful lab procedures they start tolerating once counseling is effectively done. They will realize whatever the health care team says and do is for his benefit and if he does not bear with it the severity of disease may increase. Counselling is done, not only during the treatment but also at the time of discharge of the patient from the hospital, about what to do, and what not to do after discharge. Thus patient counselling is considered as a major function of Clinical Pharmacist.

Specific Functions

5. **Detection of adverse drug reactions:** It is possible only through monitoring of the patient, closely and continuously. As therapeutic drug monitoring (TDM) is one of the main duties of the Clinical Pharmacist, he is in a better position to detect Adverse Drug Reactions (ADR). These are occurring infrequently or only after a prolonged administration of the drug and hence they can be detected only among inpatients of the hospital rather than on out patients, with few exceptions like chronic cases of diabetics, hypertension etc.

Since it is very unlikely to detect the ADR during pre-marketing studies, a Clinical Pharmacist's service in this area is considered important and invaluable. Once such ADR is detected it is fully investigated to ascertain its frequency and distribution. Then this information is passed on to authorities concerned (like National pharmacovigilance centers, WHO, Drugs Control Department etc) who in turn pass it on to the medical profession, pharmaceutical manufacturers and others.

6. **Total Parenteral Nutrition:** This is also a specific and particular patient oriented service, a Clinical Pharmacist can provide. He may be assigned the task of formulating and preparing Total Parenteral Nutrition (TPN) for a particular patient

who may not be in a position to take food via oral route. Clinical Pharmacist can take into account the need for particular mineral and/or vitamin as he is aware of the drug regimen and deficiencies of the particular patient. Thus he can be of much helpful to prescribers and nurses in providing better treatment to the patient.

Special Functions

Similar to medical specialties, a Clinical Pharmacist can also specialize in certain areas of his practice. For example treatment to the following patients need careful attention and monitoring and hence specialization:

(a) Pediatric cases
(b) Geriatric cases
(c) Psychiatric cases and
(d) Drug addiction cases

As the pharmacokinetics and consequently the Pharmacodynamics of the drugs administered to these categories of patients differ from normal adult patients, a careful selection of drug, its dose and monitoring are needed. For example in the case of Narcotic withdrawal treatment a correct dose need to be administered to control the episodes of violence, seizures etc. Hence a Clinical Pharmacist after some experience, need to specialize in these areas and help the medical profession in treating this risky cases. Also he may have to specialize in clinical toxicology and poison cases in order to improve the safe and rational use of drugs and save the lives.

Functions of a Clinical Pharmacist

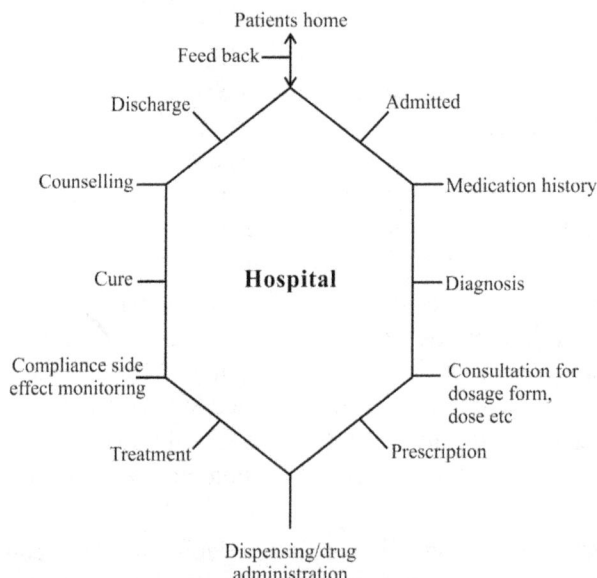

Fig. 20.1 Sides of hexagon: Existing functions of a hospital (without Clinical Pharmacist) Joints of sides of hexagon: Functions of a Clinical Pharmacist.

Skills required for a clinical pharmacist

In order to perform the functions discussed above, a Clinical Pharmacist needs to develop and acquire many skills and talents. For example to obtain a medication history useful and complete in all aspects, he needs to have good communication skills and convincing abilities. As he is going to discuss patient's personal life during medication history interview the answers may not be coming with full facts. Pharmacist must able to develop rapport with patients by making him to realize that he is working for the patient's welfare and concern with treatment outcome. Such a rapport if developed will lead to successful medication interview. He needs to have ability to put clever questions without hurting the feelings of the patient to get the correct and complete answer.

Similarly to offer consultation to the treating physician who has already a fair knowledge of drugs and formulations, its dose and uses, a Clinical Pharmacist need to know over and above what a physician has. Hence a thorough, up to date and full knowledge of drugs, therapeutics and problems with particular drugs are essential. This knowledge should be ready in mind and he should able to provide it on the spot, without referring to books and or other sources and providing it later. Thus very good subject knowledge is must for a Clinical Pharmacist.

Therapeutic Drug Monitoring (TDM) requires keen observation of the patients for the progress in treatment as well as for signs and symptoms of Adverse Drug Reactions. Once identified, he must be able to establish ADR by necessary tests and analysis. Analyzing body fluids and other samples is very difficult because the samples are collected from a living, dynamic human body. It has many variations and interferences and so, it requires sound analytical skills.

Counselling of patients again point to the need of effective communication. It also requires empathy, patience and convincing skills. All the patients' doubts must be cleared and Clinical Pharmacist must make him understand the need for adhering to instructions. Thereby compliance and consequently outcome of the treatment are highly improved.

Once these basic skills are acquired by education and experience, Clinical Pharmacist needs to specialize in his area of interest or requirement. He must able to do research in his area of specialization and acquire wide and in-depth knowledge in that field. Research papers must be published in reputed journals and conferences by him and thus a Clinical Pharmacist will become unavoidable and most wanted link in the health care team.

Questions

Short Answer Questions

1. Define clinical pharmacy.

2. What are the basics of clinical pharmacy?

3. What are the special functions of clinical pharmacy?

Long Answer Questions

4. Explain the need or concept of clinical pharmacy.

5. What are the functions of a Clinical Pharmacist?

6. Enumerate the skills required for a Clinical Pharmacist. Explain how communication skill is useful to perform his duty better?

CHAPTER 21

MEDICATION HISTORY INTERVIEW

Introduction

At the outset Clinical pharmacist must keep it in mind that this is not an interview of a candidate for some job or place in an institution. He must remember that he is going to interview a patient, who is sick, in anxiety and not in a position to oblige him, even if he wishes. Hence the interview must be planned in such a way, to get maximum information, with minimum trouble and time to the patient. Moreover the clinical pharmacist must remember that his approach must be in a manner that the patient should not feel that he is being questioned by a superior officer. At no point of time the patient should feel that he is under pressure to disclose personal information and other details.

Difference between Interview and Counselling

Clinical pharmacist has to interact with the patient, from the very beginning of patient's stay in the hospital to his discharge from the ward. He has to interact with the patient on many occasions, from the date of admission in the ward to end of treatment and beyond. During these interactions, on initial days he gathers information about the patient and at the end gave information about his post hospital routines. Generally information gathering is known as interview and information giving is counselling. However, there is no hard and fast rule that it should be like this, because it may be interchanged in many situations, so that, information may be given during interview and gathered in counselling session.

Pre-requirements for an Interview

The patient who is to be interviewed by the pharmacist might have had the same or some other disease earlier and that illness experience and the present mood bring in lot of stress on the patient. Hence out right co-operation from the patient cannot be expected. We know if some one is sick in our family, not only the patient but the entire family is worried and disturbed. All routine works of all family members gets disturbed, if it is the bread winner of the family got sick. These patients are more worried about expenses and loss of income than the disease itself. Moreover they exaggerate everything in their mind and worried about permanent disability, helplessness and even death. Hence a Clinical pharmacist must be sympathetic and helpful to the patient, so that he can cope with the situation. This is the most important pre-requisite for a medication history interview.

The success or otherwise of an interview depends on pharmacist's approach. He must start the interview with as much as information about the patient in his possession. At least he must know the patients name, age and present complaint from hospital records. Also he should know the physical condition of the patient like whether the patient is in acute pain, conscious and communicative. Usually patients are admitted in the wards after first aid and other emergency or essential clinical procedures in the out patient department (OPD). Pharmacist must verify this and hence he can safely assume that the patient may be in a position to answer his questions during interview. Similarly knowing the probable diagnosis may help in providing some idea about the severity of the disease, the possible diagnostic procedures ahead etc. Thus a thorough preparation before the interview is the pre requirement for an interview.

Structure of Patient's Case History

What is patient's medication history and its content is discussed below in detail. Let us first summarize its structure.

- Patient's name, age, sex and address
- Date of admission and patient hospital registration number
- Present complaint
- Already existing diseases like, T.B, Asthma, Diabetes etc
- Medicines currently using [Prescription and OTC drugs with dose used]
- Use of drugs of alternative systems medicine like, Siddha, Ayurveda etc
- Allergy to drug, food and others
- Problems encountered, if any, during drug use [ADR, Drug Interaction]
- Immunization [if relevant]
- Pregnancy and any problem faced [if applicable]
- Any surgery undergone and its current status
- Social drug use habits [alcohol, tobacco etc]
- Any evidence of drug abuse or misuse
- General attitude towards medicine use [compliance/ non compliance]
- Patient's opinion for present illness.

As mentioned earlier all the above information cannot be obtained in one sitting by the Clinical Pharmacist, follow up may be needed to get the left out information. For example, patient may not remember the name of the medicine he already used for his present or past illness. That has to be gathered from his old prescriptions or discharge note or bills of community pharmacies or by seeing unused balance medicines. Even a direct contact with community pharmacist where the patient used to purchase medicines through phone may be required. By all means, clinical pharmacist must try to get the full information listed above by clever questioning and efforts during medication history interview. Only a complete and comprehensive interview will serve its purpose of ensuring correct, quick and cheaper therapy for the patient and help the hospital authorities to conduct an effective Drug Utilization Evaluation [DUE] later.

How to conduct a useful Interview?

The interview should be started with polite introduction which leads to long time relationship and rapport between the pharmacist and the patient. Medication history interview is not an exemption to this. Clinical pharmacist must open the interview with self introduction after verification of patient's identity. This must be followed by defining his role as interviewer, the purpose, probable time required for the interview etc. Thus patient's mood is brought to normal and he is inclined to co-operate. Then without going for specific details, his general daily routines, hobbies and his social history like neighborhood environment etc. can be enquired.

Once this preliminary part of the interview is over, pharmacist should use his communication skills to get full and correct information about his medication history. He should get details about the prescription and non-prescription medicines currently taken by the patient. He should also gather information about previous diseases or chronic diseases under treatment at present, allergies or problems with adverse effects and possible drug misuse. All these information will not be coming out straight away, hence pharmacist has to put clever questions, some may be open questions and some may be closed questions.

Open questions are the one, for which patient can give lengthy, descriptive answers and the closed questions are required to be answered with 'yes' or 'no'. Obviously closed questions offer no option to the patient to avoid or circumvent the answer and hence should be used judiously without offending the feelings of the patient. If offended, further interview will be a waste and ends in failure as patient's co-operation ends with his wounded personality.

Careful questioning will not lead to such unpleasant end. Hence pharmacist must be attuned to the types of questions asked, the manner in which questions are asked and avoid repetitions. As far as possible technical terms should be avoided, if absolutely necessary its meaning should be explained.

Patients are always in a mental setup that once a person is willing to listen, they open up and exhaust all their problems and feelings. Pharmacist must make use of this mentality of patients to gather needed information. He should cleverly make the patient to speak about his real body problems without much interruption.

This apart, a successful interview requires use of correct body language by the interviewer. Body language helps in conducting a useful interview rather than using mere spoken words.

Role of Body Language

In order to communicate with others body language plays an important role. Not only the words but also the body communicates lot of messages to others. Communication through sign language by deaf and dumb persons is the example for this. When a message is delivered with facial expressions, hand gestures and other body movements and postures as in cinema and drama, it reaches the receiver quickly. Pharmacist also uses it instead of sitting idle with blank looks in front of the patient.

Looking at the eyes of the patients while he speaks, head nod and inclining towards the patient are some of the signs of the body which indicate, the pharmacist is actively listening to the patient. Similarly even the voice of the pharmacist while speaking to the patient has a significant role. The tone and tempo of voice conveys the message that one is sympathetic towards other or not. A voice filled with concern for the patient will definitely influence him. Thus a sweet empathetic voice is of great help to the pharmacist to achieve what he wants.

Role of Prompts

Irrespective of pharmacist's sympathetic behavior and good body language, all the needed information from the patient cannot be obtained due to various reasons. Few among them are patient's forgetfulness or lack of concentration or ignorance about what medicine they are taking and what for. It is more acute in the case of illiterate and semi-literate patients. They may not be able to answer pharmacist's questions accurately, as such, the medication history interview may not be useful.

In such situations, interviewing pharmacist has to adopt few techniques like prompting or getting help from the family members of the patient. Prompting is nothing but stimulating or leading a person to start and sustain something. Pharmacist can ask prompting questions, so that the patient starts recollecting the answer for the questions. Prompting help trigger the patient's memory. For example pharmacist can ask do you take medicines for your hypertension. Or do you apply anything externally for any skin infection? Such questions make the patient to recollect even treatments given to him long time back. Thus prompting questions asked by pharmacist results in fruitful interview. If correct answer is not forthcoming even after prompting, pharmacist has to rely on patients family members or care givers.

Interview Questions

Apart from above pharmacists can ask questions about new medicines given by doctor, medicines stopped or changed by him, etc. In order to get full information pharmacist can ask number of questions on the use of OTC drugs mentioning the symptoms and diseases usually treated by OTC drugs. Invariably many chronic patients go to doctors of alternative systems of medicine, out of their anxiety to get cure for their long time diseases. They try to hide such treatments and medicines from the health care team out of guilty consciousness. They also hide their visits to many doctors of modern medicine at the same time. Only by winning the patient's faith and confidence pharmacist can bring out such truths. While questioning patients pharmacists should ask non-biased questions and avoid leading questions like, 'you don't smoke, do you?' Leading questions prompt the patient with a particular answer.

Even pharmacists forget to ask some important questions during the interview. In order to avoid such lapses, pharmacist can follow some pattern of asking questions such as 24 hours survey and review of systems of human body. In the 24 hours survey pattern, questions can start from the patient's life of getting up from the bed in the morning to going to bed at night. Similarly if questions are asked body system wise diseases or treatment a complete interview is possible.

Sometimes even after so much preplanning and organization, important, needed information on medicines previously and currently used by the patient cannot be obtained due to the single factor that, patient don't remember anything worth about his medicines. In such cases the patient or his care givers should be asked to bring all medicines–even the empty containers–used by the patient as early as possible to complete the interview. Patients should be educated to carry the list of current medication–both prescription and OTC medicines and also they should be encouraged to purchase from the same pharmacy always by explaining its benefits.

However information about patient's non-compliance with instructions of doctors, pharmacists and other health care team members is difficult to get. Nobody admits their mistake easily. Hence clever probing questions like the following should be asked to find out non-compliance:

1. Do you carry medicines to your work place?
2. Do you forget some doses?
3. What will you do if you forget to refill the prescription?
4. If the medicine is inconvenient to you in any way what will you do?
5. Do you use costly medicines as and when needed or as per doctor's instruction?
6. Have you ever increased or decreased the dose of a drug?

From the answers to these and similar questions, non-compliance, drug misuse and abuse can be guessed and such findings should be promptly intimated to the treating physician through the final report after medication history interview.

Essential Skills for Medication History Interview

Candace W Burnett, et al, has listed in American Journal of Pharmaceutical Education [vol. 66, 2002] some 14 skills which are needed for conducting a good medication history interview. They are given below:

1. Formal form of addressing the patient. [Good Morning Mr. X!]
2. Rapport with patient. [self introduction, purpose, time required]
3. Active listening, empathetic responding.
4. Open ended questions
5. Closed ended questions
6. Transition from one subject to another.[mention it for mental preparation]
7. Verbal involvement/ repeating patient's own words.
8. Avoidance of leading questions
9. Avoidance of 'why' questions
10. Timing [giving time to adopt to series of questions]
11. Clarifying conflicting information
12. Silence [allowing patient to show emotion, digest information etc]
13. Answering questions by the patient and
14. Mentioning previous answer and question [to link current question]

If clinical pharmacist develops the skills suggested above, a useful medication interview can be obtained. Thus the quality of the information obtained from the patient and/ or their care givers depends on the quality of the pharmacist's interviewing and reviewing techniques, knowledge and skills.

Closing an Interview

To close the interview pharmacist must highlight a part or entire interview to the patient, which permits the patient or the interviewer to correct any error, clear any confusion, confirm information already given or add new information.

At the end of the interview, pharmacist can ask for additional information which the patient think might be useful. Also he can ask patient's opinion or reasons for the present problem. One more opportunity can also be given to the patient to make corrections if any. All these points should be noted in a short form, then and there, during the interview itself and elaborately written immediately after the interview as a report for the reference of treating physician and health care team.

Use of Patient's Case History in Evaluation of Drug Therapy

Evaluation of drug therapy or Drug Utilization Evaluation [DUE] is actually a quality improvement program by the hospital. As described in a separate chapter, patient medication history, medication profile and lab test profile are the three important documents used to carry out DUE. Among the three, medication history play an important role in that it is used as the starting point to commence the treatment. Hence other members of health care team like, doctor, nurse and lab technologist also ask the patient few questions to get his medication history. They too record it in the document they prepare. There may be discrepancies or conflict of information in the histories noted by pharmacist and others. Those things should be discussed with the staff concerned and needed corrections have to be carried out, if necessary by clarifying with the patient.

As all this information is to be evaluated and compared during DUE, importance must be given to present a correct and reliable data to the DUE committee. These data help the DUE committee to identify

1. Medication error either during present or earlier therapy

2. Untreated indications or undetected illness

3. Correctness of present therapy and

4. Improvement anything required in present drug's use etc.

Above all, the DUE team appreciates the usefulness of medication history in DUE.

Thus patient medication history not only helps to commence the treatment but also to conclude it with DUE.

Conclusion

If an interview is conducted properly and all the relevant information is obtained from the patient, it helps the medical fraternity enormously. The advantages are numerous and beneficial to all the persons involved in the health care of the patient, including the patient himself. It helps in speedy and correct diagnosis. It avoids unnecessary repetitions of earlier ineffective treatment; it saves the patient from unpleasant exposure to drugs allergic to him; it prevent patient from ADR, drug interaction etc.

It also gives an idea about patient's habits, weakness and dependence or requirement. Hence clinical pharmacist can effectively monitor the drug therapy later or modify the drug therapy to suit the need or condition of the patient. Without prior medication history of the patient on hand, these things are not possible and it may be too late to have such data at a later stage.

To summarize the advantages, the interview open the possibility for best treatment and consequent reduction in time, energy and money involved in the treatment.

Questions

Short Answer Questions

1. Explain briefly the difference between patient medication interview and counselling.

2. How to prepare for conducting a medication history interview?

3. Write a note on structure of patient's case history

4. How patient's case history is useful in DUE?

5. List the skills required for conducting Medication History Interview

6. What are the advantages of Medication History Interview?

Long Answer Questions

7. How to conduct a medication history interview?

8. Explain the role of body language while conducting medication history interview.

9. List different types of questions with examples and discuss their importance.

10. Conduct a mock medication history interview using one of your classmates as patient and submit a report.

CHAPTER 22

MEDICAL ABBREVIATIONS AND TERMINOLOGIES

Introduction

A pharmacist in clinical settings needs to understand the medical abbreviations and terms used by clinicians, nurses and other health care professionals. Hence he must have a fair knowledge of those words and thereby able to understand whatever discussed during ward rounds, DUE and other occasions. He has to use, interpret and apply these words while performing his duties. This knowledge can be acquired fast only in practical settings and hence he should spend more time in wards and OPDs rather than in Drug Information centers or Medicine Stores or Dispensaries.

Though pharmacists have some basic understanding of medical terms through the subjects they have studied like, Anatomy, Physiology, Biochemistry and Pharmacology, they are not sufficient in a hospital arena where a team of health care professionals are practicing. Hence he must try to learn these terms as much as possible. It may not be possible to list all the medical abbreviations and terms here as it is very large and require hundreds of pages. Hence only very important terms with their meanings which are often used are given here. Students are advised to have a standard pocket medical dictionary in their coat pocket while undergoing training and refer it then and there to understand the language spoken by their trainers or until they gain experience. They should learn to speak quickly in professional language with the members of health care team.

These terms are available in scores of websites of internet, like popular Wikipedia, medicine plus, quizlet, medlexicon etc and hence what is required is initiative and willingness to learn. To understand the medical terms which are in Greek or Latin language the root wards must be learned first. These root wards are used as prefixes or suffixes of medical terms. If its meaning is understood and remembered, it is easier to decipher the medical terms. Hence they are given here before the medical terms.

Medical Root Words – Prefixes and Suffixes

1. PREFIXES

a, an	–	without
ab	–	away from
ad	–	near, toward
ante	–	before, forward
brady	–	slow
carpo	–	wrist
cephalo	–	head
de	–	remove, take away
dys	–	difficult
gyne	–	women
hemi	–	one side
hemo	–	blood
heap/ hepato	–	liver
hystrep	–	uterus
lip	–	fat
masto	–	breast
metro	–	uterus
myo	–	muscle
myringo	–	ear drum
nephro	–	kidney
oophoro	–	ovary
orchido	–	testicle
osteo	–	bone
oto	–	ear
podo	–	foot
pro	–	coming, preceding
procto	–	rectum, anus
reno	–	kidney
rhino	–	nose
sacro	–	sacrum
spindylo	–	vertebra

stetho	–	chest
stomato	–	mouth
tachy	–	fast
vaso	–	vessel
veno	–	vein

II. SUFFIXES

- algia	–	pain
- cele	–	swelling
- ectasis or ectasia	–	stretching [dilating]
- ectomy	–	removal of
- itis	–	inflammation of
- malacia	–	softening
- ocentesis	–	puncture
- ogram	–	picture/recording
- ography	–	procedure [diagnostic]
- ograph	–	equipment
- oid	–	similar to
- olysis, olytic	–	separate, destroy
- oma	–	tumor
- ometer	–	instrument that count or measure
- opexy	–	surgical fixation
- oplasty	–	plastic surgery on
- orrhagia	–	excessive bleeding
- orrhea	–	flow or discharge
- osis	–	condition of
- ostomy	–	new permanent opening
- otomy	–	incision into
- otripsy	–	crushing
- plasia	–	growth
- plegia	–	paralysis
- trophy	–	development

MEDICAL ABBREVIATIONS

ABC	–	AIRWAYS, BREATING, CIRCULATION
ABG	–	ARTERIAL BLOOD GASES
ACL	–	ANTERIOR CRUCIATE LIGAMENT
ADHD	–	ATTENTION DEFICIT HYPERACTIVITY DISORDER
AFIB	–	ARTERIAL FIBRILLATION
ALP	–	ALKALINE PHOSPHATASE
ALT	–	ALANINE AMINO TRANSFERASE
AMI	–	ACUTE MYOCARDIAL INFARCTION
AST	–	ASPARTATE AMINO TRANSFERASE
AVM	–	ARTERIO VENOUS MALFORMATION
BMI	–	BODY MASS INDEX
BPH	–	BENIGN PROSTATIC HYPERTROPHY
BUN	–	BLOOD UREA NITROGEN
CABG	–	CORONARY ARTERY BYPASS GRAFT
CAD	–	CORONARY ARTERY DISEASE
CAT	–	COMPUTERIZED AXIAL TOMOGRAPHY
CBC	–	COMPLETE BLOOD COUNT
CHD	–	CONGENITAL HEART DISEASE
CHF	–	CONGESTIVE HEART FAILURE
CMV	–	CYTO MEGALO VIRUS
COPD	–	CHRONIC OBSTRUCTIVE PULMONARY DISEASE
CPK	–	CREATININE PHOSPHO KINASE
CPR	–	CARDIO PULMONARY RESUSCITATION
CRF	–	CHRONIC RENAL FAILURE
D & C	–	DILATATION AND CURETTAGE
DJD	–	DEGENERATIVE JOINT DISEASE
DM	–	DIABETES MELLITUS
DTP	–	DIPHTHERIA, TETANUS, PERTUSSIS
DVT	–	DEEP VEIN THROMBOSIS

ECG/ EKG	–	ELECTROCARDIOGRAM
ECHO	–	ECHOCARDIOGRAM
EEG	–	ELECTROENCEPHALOGRAM
EMG	–	ELECTROMYOGRAPHY
ERCP	–	ENDOSCOPIC RETROGRADE CHOLANGIO PANCREATOGRAPHY
ESR	–	ERYTHROCYTE SEDIMENTATION RATE
ESRD	–	END STAGE RENAL DISEASE
FSH	–	FOLLICLE STIMULATING HORMONE
GERD	–	GASTRO ESOPHAGEAL REFLUX DISEASE
GFR	–	GLOMERULAR FILTRATIO RATE
GU	–	GENETO URINARY
HAV	–	HEPATITIS A VIRUS
HBV	–	HEPATITIS B VIRUS
HCV	–	HEPATITIS C VIRUS
HDL	–	HIGH DENSITY LIPOPROTEIN
HCB	–	HEMOGLOBIN
HIV	–	HUMAN IMMUNO DEFICENCY VIRUS
HPV	–	HUMAN PAPILLOMA VIRUS
HRT	–	HORMONE REPLACEMENT THERAPY
HTN	–	HYPERTENSION
IBD	–	INFLAMMATORY BOWEL DISEASE
IBS	–	IRRITABLE BOWEL SYNDROME
ICD	–	IMPLANTABLE CARDIOVERTER DEFIBRILLATOR
IDDM	–	INSULIN DEPENDENT DIABETES MELLITUS
IUD	–	INTRA UTERINE DEVICE
IVP	–	INTRAVENOUS PYELOGRAM
LDL	–	LOW DENSITY LIPOPROTEIN
LFT	–	LIVER FUNCTION TEST
MI	–	MYOCARDIAL INFARCTION

MMR	–	MEASLES, MUMPS, RUBELLA [VACCINE]
MRI	–	MAGNETIC RESONANCE IMAGING
MRSA	–	METHICILLIN RESISTANCE STAPHYLOCOCCUS AUREUS
NG	–	NASOGASTRIC
NIDDM	–	NON INSULINE DEPENDENT DIABETES MELLITUS
NKDA	–	NO KNOWN DRUG ALLERGY
NSAID	–	NON STEROIDAL ANTIINFLAMMATORY DRUG
OCD	–	OBSESSIVE COMPULSIVE DISORDER [ANXIETY DISORDER]
PAD	–	PERIPHERAL ARTERIAL DISEASE
PAP	–	PAPANICOLAN [SMEAR TEST TO DETECT CERVICAL CANCER]
PAT	–	PAROXMAL ATRIAL TACHYCARDIA
PET	–	POSITRON EMMISSION TOMOGRAPHY
PFT	–	PULMONARY FUNCTION TEST
PID	–	PELVIC INFLAMMATORY DISEASE
PMS	–	PREMENSTRUAL SYNDROME
PPD	–	PURIFIED PROTEIN DERIVATIVE
PT	–	PROTHROMBIN TIME
PTH	–	PARATHYROID HORMONE
PTSD	–	POST TRAUMATIC STRESS SYNDROME
PUD	–	PEPTIC ULCER DISEASE
PVC	–	PREMATURE VENTRICULAR CONTRACTION
RA	–	RHUMATOID ARTHRITIS
RSV	–	RESPIRATORY SYNCYTIAL VIRUS
SOB	–	SHORTNESS OF BREATH
STD	–	SEXUALLY TRANSMITTED DISEASE
TAH	–	TOTAL ABDOMINAL HYSTERECTOMY [REMOVAL OF UTERUS]
TIA	–	TRANSIENT ISCHEMIC ATTACK

TSH	–	THYROID STIMULATING HORMONE
URI	–	UPPER RESPIRATORY INFECTION
UTI	–	URINARY TRACT INFECTION
XRT	–	RADIOTHERAPY

III. MEDICAL TERMS

ABSCESS	–	SWELLING DUE TO COLLECTION OF PUS
ACUTE	–	SEVERE, SUDDEN
ACROPACHY	–	CLUBBING OF FINGERS AND TOES
ACUTE MYOCARDIAL INFARCTION	–	HEART ATTACK
AFEBRILE	–	WITHOUT FEVER
AMBULANT	–	ABLE TO WALK
AMENORRHOEA	–	ABSENCE OF MENSES
ANGINA	–	CARDIAC PAIN DUE TO POOR BLOOD SUPPLY TO HEART
ANOREXIA	–	LOSS OF APPETITE
ANOXIA	–	WITHOUT OXYGEN
APNOEA	–	CESSATION OF BREATHING
ARTHRITIS	–	INFLAMMATION OF JOINT
ARTERIOSCLEROSIS	–	THICKENING OF LUMEN OF ARTERIES
ARRHYTHMIA	–	ABNORMAL CARDIAC RHYTHM
ATAXIA	–	AN UNSTEADINESS OF BODY/MUSCLES
AURA	–	A VISUAL DISTRUBANCE BEFORE EPILEPTIC FIT
AZOOSPERMIA	–	ABSENCE SPERM IN SEMEN
BACTERIURIA	–	PRESENCE OF BACTERIA IN URINE
BRANCHITIS	–	INFLAMMATION/INFECTION OF LUNGS
BRADYCARDI	–	SLOW HEART RATE
CARCINOMA	–	A MALIGNANT NEW GROWTH
CHOLECYSTECTOMY	–	REMOVAL OF GALL BLADDER
CIRRHOSIS	–	LIVER DAMAGE [SHRUNKEN AND HARDENED]

COLIC	–	ACUTE ABDOMINAL PAIN OR PERTAINING TO COLON
CONCUSSION	–	LOSS OF CONCIOUSNESS DUE TO SEVERE HEADINJURY
CRYTOGENIC	–	OBSCURE OR DOUBTFUL ORIGIN
CRYSTALLURIA	–	EXCRETION OF CRYSTALS IN URINE
DECUBITUS	–	LYING DOWN
DEMENTIA	–	MENTAL DETERIORATION OF FUNCTIONS
DELIRIUM	–	MENTAL DISTRUBANCE MARKED BY HALLUCINATIONS
DERMATITIS	–	INFLAMMATION OF SKIN
DIMORPHIC	–	APPEAR IN TWO FORMS
DISTAL	–	AWAY FROM CENTER
DYSCHEZIA	–	DIFFICULT OR PAINFUL EVACUATION OF FAECES
DYSPAREUNIA	–	DIFFICULT OR PAINFUL INTERCOURSE
DYSURIA	–	DIFFICULT OR PAINFUL URINATION
DYSPNOEA	–	DIFFICULTY IN BREATHING
DYSPHAGIA	–	DIFFICULTY IN SWALLOWING
ENURESIS	–	INVOLUNTARY DISCHARGE OF URINE
EMPHYSEMA	–	A LUNG DISEASE WITH LOSS OF LUNG TISSUE [IN SMOKERS]
ENCEPHALOPATHY	–	ANY DEGENERATIVE DISEASE OF BRAIN
EPITAXIS	–	BLEEDING OF NOSE
FEBRILE	–	PRESENCE OF FEVER
FISSURE	–	ANY CLEFT OR GROOVE
GASTRITIS	–	INFLAMMATION OF LINING OF STOMACH WITH PAIN
GASTRO ENTERITIS	–	INFLAMMATION OF STOMACH AND INTESTINE [WITH VOMITING]
GLAUCOMA	–	INCREASE IN INTRAOCULAR [EYE] PRESSURE

GLOSSITIS	–	INFLAMMATION OF TONGUE
GLCOSURIA	–	LARGE AMOUNT OF SUGAR IN URINE
GONORRHOEA	–	A CONTAGEOUS INFECTION OF GENITAL ORGAN
HAEMOTEMESIS	–	VOMITING OF PURE BLOOD OR WITH STOMACH CONTENT
HAEMOTOMA	–	WELL DEMARCATED BRUISE
HAEMATURIA	–	BLOOD IN URINE
HAEMOPTYSIS	–	COUGHING UP OF BLOOD
HAEMORRHAGE	–	BLEEDING [INTERNALLY OR EXTERNALLY]
HEMIPLEGIA	–	PARALYSIS OF ONE SIDE OF THE BODY
HEPATITIS	–	INFLAMMATION OF LIVER
HYPERGLYCAEMIA	–	HIGH LEVEL OF SUGAR IN BLOOD
HYPOGLYCAEMIA	–	LOW LEVEL OF SUGAR IN BLOOD
HYPOTHERMIA	–	LOW BODY TEMPERATURE
INCONTINENCE	–	LOSS OF CONTROL OF URINARY BLOODER OR BOWEL
INTUBATION	–	INSERTION OF TUBE
ISCHAEMIA	–	LACK OF BLOOD SUPPLY TO HEART
KERATITIS	–	INFLAMMATION OF CORNEA
KETONURIA	–	EXCESS OF KETONE BODIES IN URINE
LEUKAEMIA	–	BLOOD CANCER
LIBIDO	–	SEXUAL DESIRE
LUMBAGO	–	PAIN IN LUMBAR REGION
MANIA	–	AN ELATED OVER ACTIVE STATE OF MIND AND BODY
MENORRHAGIA	–	EXCESS AND PROLONG BLEEDING AT REGULAR NTERVALS OF MENSUS
MENINGITIS	–	INFLAMMATION OF MENINGES [MEMBRANE ARROUND BRAIN]

MYALGIA	–	PAIN IN MUSCLES
MYOPATHY	–	UNEXPLAINED MUSCLE WEAKNESS OR SORENESS
NAUESIA	–	FEELING OF VOMITING
NEURITIS	–	INFLAMMATION OF NEURAL TISSUE
NECROSIS	–	DEATH OF TISSUE
NEUROSIS	–	A MENTAL CONDITION WITH ANXIETY etc,
NOCTURIA	–	WAKING AT NIGHT TO PASS URINE
OEDEMA	–	FLUID COLLECTION IN TISSUES [SWELLING]
OTOTOXIC	–	TOXIC ACTION ON EAR
OSTEOARTHRITIS	–	DEGENERATION OF CARTILAGE OF BONE JOINTS
OSTEOMALACIA	–	DECALCIFICATION OF BONES [DUE TO LESS VITAMIN D]
OOPHORECTOMY	–	REMOVAL OF OVARY
PALLIATIVE CARE	–	CARE TO MINIMISE PAIN NOT CURE
PALPITATIONS	–	A RAPID AND IRREGULAR HEART BEAT
PARAPLEGIA	–	PARALYSIS OF LEG OR LOWER PART OF BODY
PROXIMAL	–	NEAREST TO CENTER
PANCREATITIS	–	INFLAMMATION OF PANCREAS
PARKINSONISM	–	IMPAIRMENT OF MOVEMENT, REGIDITY AND TREMOR
PARONOIA	–	A PSYCHOLOGICAL DISORDER OF DELUSIONS
PEDICULOSIS	–	INFESTATION OF SKIN [SCABIES]
PHLEBITIS	–	INFLAMMATION OF VEIN
PHOBIA	–	AN IRRATIONAL FEAR
POLYDYPSIA	–	EXCESSIVE THIRST PERSISTING FOR LONG TIME

PNEUMONIA	–	INFECTION OF LUNGS
POST PARTURM	–	AFTER CHILD BIRTH
PROGNOSIS	–	LIKELY MEDICAL OUTCOME OF DISEASE
PSYCHOSIS	–	AN EXTERME DERANGEMENT OF MIND
PSYCHOSOMATIC	–	NERVOUS COMPLAINT WITH BODILY SYMPTOMS
PULMONARY EMBOLUS	–	MOBILE BLOOD CLOT IN LONG TISSUE
RHINITIS [ALLERGIC]	–	NASAL CONGESTION, DISCHARGE & SNEEZING
RHEMATISM	–	INFLMMATION AND PAIN IN JOINTS
RETINOPATHY	–	ANY NON INFLAMMATORY DISEASE OF RETINA
SCHIZOPHRENIA	–	A NERVOUS DISORDER DISTRUBING NORMAL THOUGHT PROCESS
SYNDROME	–	A GROUP OF SIGNS & SYMPTOMS DUE TO DISEASE
SENILE	–	RELATING TO CHARACTERISTIC OF OLD AGE
SEPTICAEMIA	–	PRESENCE OF BACTERIAL TOXINS IN BLOOD
SPASM	–	CONVULSIVE, INVOLUNTARY MUSCULAR CONTRACTION
TACHYCARDIA	–	INCREASE IN HEARTRATE ABOVE 100/MINUTE
THROMBOCYTOPENIA	–	DECREASE IN NUMBER OF PLATELETS
URICOSURIC	–	TENDANCY TO INCREASE THE EXCRETION OF URIC ACID
VARIOLAMINOR	–	A MILD SMALL POX
XEROPHTHALMIA	–	LACK OF TEARS, DRYNESS OF EYE DUE TO VIT.A DEFICIENCY
XEROSIS	–	DRY SKIN

CHAPTER 23

WARD ROUND PARTICIPATION

Introduction

A medical practitioner going round the ward of the hospital where his patients are admitted for review or follow up of the treatment given to each patient either alone or along with his junior doctors and other members of health care team is known as ward round. This is undertaken either daily or at fixed time interval depends on the need and rules of the hospital.

Usually only chief or senior doctors goes on a ward round with his assistant doctors, house surgeons or interns and medical students. Assistant doctors who are actually involved in treating the patients get advice and suggestions from the senior or chief doctor regarding the treatment and make many visits to the ward on a single day with or without somebody accompanying him.

Thus chief doctor's visit to the ward acquires significance when the entire health care team is available for taking instructions and/ or for consultation.

Ward Rounds and Pharmacists

Till recently or even to day in many countries including India, pharmacists are not included in ward rounds, after 1970s in western countries especially in USA and UK, clinical pharmacists were asked to participate in ward rounds as the value of his services were understood and accepted by then. Doctors were provided with valuable information on different formulations, their strength, availability, side effects, suitability for the particular patient, alternative or substitute drugs etc, on the spot by clinical pharmacists during ward rounds. That is to say, those information are given when it is needed most, that is at the time of prescription writing for the in-patients. Thus he helps the medical practitioner to ensure safe and rational use of drugs and thereby improved patient care at less cost and time is achieved.

Types of Ward Rounds

There are many types of ward rounds depends on it purpose or person. Though chief doctor of the ward undertake authoritative, decision making ward rounds, prior to that, other members of health care team too make ward rounds for definite purposes. For example house surgeons or P.G Medical students go on a preliminary ward round to prepare and get ready for chief doctors round. They collect needed information about each patient and outcome of previous round's decisions. For instance they collect lab results for tests prescribed for the patient on previous round and keep ready the summary of it for chief doctor's attention. Clinical pharmacist can also undertake such preliminary round and be ready with drug related information.

The second type of ward round is by Resident Medical Officer [RMO] who is in-charge for overall activities of the hospital. Most of the time his round will be of administrative in nature and he usually don't involve in actual treatment of the patient. Nevertheless he enquires the patient or his attendants or nurses about patient's grievances or discomfort, if any, for the purpose of rectifying the same. He is accompanied by assistant doctors, Internees and nurses. These visits are not undertaken daily but few times in a month.

The third type of important ward round is by chief doctor of the ward or department. He review previous round's decisions and their results and give instructions about further course of treatment to the patient and his team make a note of it. Most of the time chief doctor explains the clinical aspects including diagnosis, symptoms, disease manifestations, treatment and its outcome during this visit to house surgeons and medical students who takes note of all these things while on the bedside of the patient. Clinical pharmacist can also use these briefings to further improve their clinical knowledge.

The fourth type of ward round is by academic staff of teaching hospitals. The associate or assistant professors of the medical or surgical or other departments of Medical colleges visit for the purpose of teaching their students about relevant cases admitted in the wards. After a brief lecture demonstration of the cases, follow up classes on the particular topic or disease will be held in class rooms available in the hospital itself or in their colleges. This ensures students to acquire practical knowledge of the subject. Most of the time clinical pharmacists have no role in this round.

Preparation for Ward Round by Clinical Pharmacist

A clinical pharmacist needs to get ready before the ward round by chief doctor of the ward. He may have to advice or suggest or offer consultation regarding the medicines prescribed for the in-patients of the ward. For which he has to prepare and keep ready the following:

1. Medication profile of each patient
2. Summary of medication history of each patient

3. Summary of Drug Utilization review

4. Recommendation he indent to make based on above documents and

5. Supportive documents and references for the above.

In spite of best care by entire health care team, there is still possibility for drug interaction, adverse drug reaction and medication error. Drug- Diet interaction Drug-Diagnostic test interaction, Drug- Disease interaction are the three DDs, a clinical pharmacist need to watch, as other type of reactions are mostly avoided by the treating team by careful planning and monitoring.

A model form of Patient Medication Profile is given on a chapter 'Records and Reports'. With slight variations they are maintained in all the hospitals where clinical pharmacy services are available. A clinical pharmacist has to keep it up dated and ready for ward rounds.

During the discussion for selection of drugs for the patient, his medication history is very much useful. Hence at least its summary, if not the full history must be available for reference by the treating clinician. The history is not only useful while prescribing immediately after diagnosis, but also during the course of treatment depends on the patient's response or otherwise for the drugs administered. This factor makes it an important document till patient's discharge.

If Drug Utilization Evaluation [DUE] has been undertaken on the particular patient by DUE team and its report is communicated to the treating team, a copy of it must be ready with clinical pharmacist. It helps to go for course correction in the light of recommendations made by DUE team.

Finally, a clinical pharmacist should prepare before hand, if he indent to make any recommendation or suggestion to change a drug or its dose or addition of another drug etc. He should able to site relevant references for his recommendations, so that, the treating clinical practitioner accept it with out any hesitation or doubt.

All the above home work by clinical pharmacist ensures better treatment for the patient and appreciation for his services.

Pharmacist Interventions

There are many contributions and few interventions a clinical pharmacist has to make during ward rounds. Clinical pharmacist has his own limitations, that, he is an authority only on drugs and related matters. Hence as far as possible he should not and need not interfere with diagnosis, pathology and etiology of diseases. However that does not mean he should not raise his doubts or toxic effect manifestations of the drug on the patient. He should be ever vigilant while watching for ADR or Drug interactions and report his observations to the treating clinician.

In many hospitals where clinical pharmacy services are fully established he is empowered to order investigative lab tests to confirm drug's toxicity. If the results of these tests confirm his suspicion, he can boldly intervene in the treatment process, equipped with test results from the lab. Thus a clinical pharmacist's intervention should be, as far as possible, based on solid evidence. Subsequently such interventions are welcomed and appreciated by health care team. After gaining confidence of chief doctor and his team in this way, his future doubts and observations will be given due attention in future even before lab results.

Pharmacist's Contribution during Ward Rounds

Most of the time a clinical pharmacist's contribution during ward rounds will be on matters relating to drugs. Doctors, nurses and medical students may require the following information on the spot; with out they resort to referring books or websites:

1. Formulations [Dosage forms],
2. Dose
3. Indications and Contraindications
4. Drugs availability and its supply source
5. Economy [price]
6. Substitute [if the above is not available]
7. Time required for getting the supply
8. Legal and administrative issues and
9. Special storage conditions, if any.

If the clinical pharmacist is able to give this information immediately, without referring any book or source of information, his value and respect among the team peaks and a fruitful team spirit develops. This results in better name for the hospital.

Limitations of Ward Rounds

A chief doctor is always hard pressed for time to undertake elaborate ward rounds. His services are required elsewhere in situations like emergency cases, on sudden complications developed in existing cases and in administrative matters. Hence he tries to make ward rounds short and useful. Clinical pharmacist needs to understand this and present his recommendations and suggestions short and precise to the point. If it is evident that less time is available for ward round, he should intervene in cases which are most important and require immediate attention. Other cases can wait till next ward round.

If there is no fixed time for ward rounds in a hospital or ward, he should make arrangement to get prior intimation about time of ward round. In some hospitals clinical pharmacist has to look after more than one ward at the same time. Suppose simultaneous ward rounds are going on these wards, clinical pharmacist has to prioritize patients in need of his intervention most and attend the ward round where the particular patient is present. For the patients in other ward he can make annotations in medication chart, if the hospital pharmacy permits it.

Drug therapy review requires medication chart endorsement by clinical pharmacist in order to ensure that prescriptions are unambiguous, clear and legible without any cause for doubt. Hence clinical pharmacists are permitted to make annotations in prescriptions in hospitals where clinical pharmacy services are fully organized. However face to face discussions among the health care team members ensure better co-ordination in the treatment process. But it may not be always possible due to various reasons. Some suggestions may not be acceptable to one or other member of the team and hence needs elaborate discussions even debate. That can not be done by standing by the side of the patient; hence the team may meet in the cabin of ward doctor or elsewhere. After thorough discussions, correct decisions are made by reviewing material facts and implemented. If the situation requires no immediate decision the team can call for additional information or evidence, till its availability, decision can be postponed. Thus ward round has its own limitations and pharmacist should learn to perform his duties within these limitations.

Skills Needed for Ward Round Participation

It is obvious that in order to communicate with multidisciplinary team of the ward round, clinical pharmacist need to acquire two important skills, the clinical knowledge and communication talent. To develop clinical knowledge pharmacists first need to understand and use the clinical terms, hence they are given in a separate chapter. Depends upon the ward where he or she is posted clinical pharmacist must learn additional clinical terms and abbreviations used in those wards. He should be able to convey his views and observations about the team clearly with out mincing words. Thus communication skills become an important pre requisite for ward rounds. Needless to point out better communication is possible, only when the person has comment over the language – English is the language usually used to communicate in a hospital among the health care team. However knowledge of local language is also required to communicate with patients and their care takers. Thus at least a working knowledge in the local language has to be acquired wherever clinical pharmacist is appointed.

While communicating with doctors and other team members, pharmacist should use polite, low pitch and firm words so as not to disturb the patients of the ward. Also he must be careful, while discussing side effects observed, alternate drugs suggested or doubt about drugs given, so that they do not make the patient to loose faith in his treatment. That will make the patient upset and depressed. Similarly he should use the words carefully so as not to hurt the feelings of team members or their services. He must always remember only a faithful co ordination among the team results in success.

Occasions may arise, when clinical pharmacists are required to give information or suggestion on a particular topic which he is not familiar with and have little knowledge about it. He must honestly admit the fact to the team and promise to get the information as and when ward round is completed. There is no need for bluffing or guessing the information. As promised he must deliver the information as quick as possible after the ward round.

Completion of Ward Round

Having discussed what to do before and during the ward round, let us discuss what to do after the ward round. During the preparation for the ward round clinical pharmacist update and keep ready the medication profile of the patient and related documents like medication history, DUE and DUR the documents and other documents. After the ward round is completed he has to update these documents with additional information discussed and decided during the latest ward round. This information are noted briefly in a hand held case diary during ward rounds and elaborately written in the registers of clinical pharmacy department.

Before attending to this work, clinical pharmacist must give priority to the information if he has promised to give his team members. They may be urgently required by the team members to complete their record or to commence the follow up treatment decided during the ward round. If no such work is there he can attend to the updating work as discussed above. Thus documentation is the one of the major work after ward rounds.

Next he can communicate the decisions to other departments concerned, if relevant and necessary. He may have to communicate with hospital administration, Head of Nursing services, Head of Pharmacy services, Head of Lab services and Head of dietary services. This information may be send via E-mails or in writing or through phone, as the case may be. Acknowledgements if required can be collected from them through messengers and filed.

Finally clinical pharmacist has to communicate some of the decisions like change in therapy, drug or procedure to the patient or his care givers. This has to be done carefully while counseling the patient. Thus patients are encouraged and their co-operation ensured to continue the treatment. Some part or entire work of this nature is assigned to nurses also. In that case clinical pharmacist has to brief the nurse concerned about matters related to clinical pharmacy services before such patient counseling sessions.

Conclusion

As discussed above, day-to-day, on the spot decisions are taken depends on the disease manifestations, drug's effect etc. This is done in a best possible way by the multidisciplinary team that ensure better treatment and achievement of its goal for which the entire team has put in its efforts. To chip in more contribution clinical pharmacists should also specialize like medical professionals. After Pharm.D or M.Pharm pharmacy practice Clinical pharmacists can specialize in Pediatrics Pharmacy, Geriatric Pharmacy,

Antibiotic therapy, Drug withdrawal treatment, psychiatric pharmacy etc, courses for which are conducted in countries like USA. If acquired these qualification will take the clinical pharmacy services to next higher level and bring respect and glory to the profession of pharmacy.

Questions

Short Answer Questions

1. Write a note on preparation for ward round by pharmacist.

2. What are the skills needed for ward round participation?

3. Explain the contribution of Clinical pharmacists in ward rounds.

Long Answer Questions

4. Write an essay about pharmacist's wards round participation.

CHAPTER 24

RATIONAL DRUG THERAPY

Safe and Rational use of Drugs

"Rational use of drugs means that patients receive medication appropriate to their clinical needs, in doses that meet their own individual requirements for an adequate period of time and the lowest cost to them and their community".

Rational Drug Therapy is possible only when the process of prescribing is appropriately followed.

Prescribing Appropriately

In order to write an appropriate prescription, certain procedures have to be followed by the physicians. First of all there should be proper diagnosis i.e., the patient's problem must be suitably defined by following the correct steps. Then the treatment process (with drugs and non-drugs) should be determined, followed by selection of appropriate drugs, dosage and duration.

Adequate information about drugs and treatment must be given to the patient in the beginning of the treatment process and the treatment response should be then evaluated.

Thus appropriate indications and appropriate drugs to appropriate patient who has been provided with appropriate information and monitoring, will ensure rational drug therapy.

Irrational Prescribing

Having seen what is appropriate prescribing, let us see, what is 'inappropriate' or 'irrational' prescribing is:

If the above mentioned criteria are not followed in writing a prescription, irrational prescription, results. The examples for irrational prescriptions are:

1. Antibiotics are prescribed for viral upper respiratory tract infections, when no drug therapy is indicated.

221

2. Wrong drugs are prescribed for a specific condition requiring a different drug. For example Tetracycline is prescribed in childhood diarrhea when ORS is enough. Similarly drugs with doubtful or unproven efficacy like antimotility drugs are used in acute diarrhoea.

3. Sometimes correct drugs are used but through wrong route of administration. For instance, Metronidazole is given IV, when oral or suppository formulations would be appropriate.

4. Unnecessary and expensive drugs are prescribed like third generation broad spectrum antibiotics, when a first line, narrow spectrum agent is sufficient.

5. Multiple drugs (polypharmacy) are prescribed even when one or two drugs are adequate.

Reasons or Factors behind Irrational use of Drugs

There are many factors or reasons behind the inappropriate use of drugs, which needs to be taken care of while prescribing or dispensing. They are:

(a) **Crowded hospitals and environment:** They bring pressure on a physician to prescribe 'something'. Even though the physician wants to prescribe after thorough investigation lack of adequate lab capacity force him to forgo the same. Insufficient staff in crowded out patient departments (OPD) is also a big handicap on rational drug use.

(b) **Patient's drug misinformation:** Due to misleading beliefs and expectations by the patients, physicians are compelled to write some drugs. Few patients even demand some particular drug like injections though unwanted for the present condition.

(c) **Prescribers lack of education and training:** Some prescribers have inappropriate role models for their practice of the profession and prescribe irrationally. Due to insufficient training and other reasons they have little drug information and they tend to generalize their limited experience for prescribing. Misleading beliefs about a particular drug's efficiency is also one of the reasons for irrational prescription.

(d) **Drug supply and promotion:** Unreliable drug supply system leads to drugs shortages in hospital which results in availability of non-essential drugs and limited supply of essential one. Hence physician has no other chance but to write whatever available in the hospital. Lack of enforcement of regulation also leads to such a bad situation.

This apart unethical promotion of drugs by pharmaceutical manufacturers, with misleading claims, offers, gifts, etc., also leads to irrational prescribing and use of drugs.

Results of Irrational use of Drugs

Irrational use of drugs results in:

(a) Sub standard therapy and thereby chances of increase in morbidity and mortality.

(b) Resources being wasted in unwanted drugs and results in availability of inadequate quantities of vital drugs in hospital.

(c) Cost of treatment goes up.

(d) Increased risk of adverse drug reactions and drug resistance and

(e) 'A pill for every ill' concept gets into the mind of patients, resulting in unnecessary demand for drugs.

Remedy for the Problem

By and large problem of irrational prescribing can be solved by proper selection of drugs before writing the prescription. Here a clinical pharmacist can be of much useful to the physician.

The following points must be remembered while selecting a drug

1. Relevance to the disease: The drug must be indicated in the treatment of the disease after proper diagnosis.

2. The efficacy, safety and quality of the drug must have been previously verified.

3. The cost of the medicine must be reasonable. The cost means, not for a unit cost but for the entire course of treatment.

4. If highly powerful and potent drugs are to be prescribed the level of expertise required to prescribe, administer and monitor safety and adverse effects of such drug or drugs must be considered.

5. Factors affecting the pharmacokinetic and Pharmacodynamics of the drug like concomitant disease, drug, body conditions like liver disease and malnutrition must be considered.

6. If many drugs are available for the particular disease or condition, the drug with most favourable risk/benefit ratio must be selected.

7. When two or more drugs are therapeutically equivalent preference should be given to;

   (a) the drug most thoroughly investigated and therefore best understood.

   (b) the drug which is suitable for more than one disease.

   (c) the drug with good pharmacokinetic properties, so as to improve the compliance and to minimize risk.

   (d) the drug that is easy to dispense as well as easy to administer.

   (e) the drugs that is easy to take by the patient and therefore having more acceptability.

   (f) the drug which are suitable for and stable in local storage conditions.

   (g) the drugs for which local, reliable manufacturing facilities available thereby avoiding import supplies.

8. Prescribe as minimum as possible, avoid multiple drug regimen.

9. New drugs should be written with great caution, only when there are definite advantages over old drugs.

10. Generic names of the drugs as far as possible should be used to write the prescription.

In order to ensure safe and rational use of drugs, apart from the measures outlined above, more precautions are devised. Thus the concept of "Pharmacotherapy" is evolved, where Clinical Pharmacist is given more roles in the treatment of patients. Similarly, for giving safe treatment to risky categories of patients like infants, old peoples and pregnant and lactating mothers, special attention has to be paid. As therapy to these groups of people acquires significance, it is dealt in the following separate chapters.

Questions

Short Answer Questions

1. What is rational use of drugs?

2. Give examples for irrational prescriptions.

3. List the reasons for irrational use of drugs.

4. What are results of irrational use of drugs?

Long Answer Questions

5. How the problem of irrational use of drugs can be solved?

CHAPTER 25

PHARMACOTHERAPY

Definition

According to American Pharmacists Association Pharmacotherapy is defined as "an area of pharmacy practice that is responsible for ensuring the safe, appropriate and economical use of drugs in patient care." "The pharmacotherapy specialist has responsibility for direct patient care, often functions as a member of a multidisciplinary team and is frequently the primary source of drug information for other health care professionals."

Putting it simply, pharmacotherapy is nothing but treatment of diseases with appropriate drugs. Of course all the diseases are treated with drugs at one stage or other, the major difference between those treatments and pharmacotherapy is, the design, execution and monitoring of therapy is carried out mainly by pharmacists in the case of pharmacotherapy.

Hence, pharmacist has to specialize in these aspects and should have extensive training and experience in therapeutics. Such trainings with specialization in pharmacotherapy are offered in developed countries, especially, there are many universities and other institutions conducting pharmacotherapy specialization in USA.

Basic Concepts

As mentioned above in pharmacotherapy, pharmacist is responsible for designing therapy and hence the first and foremost duty for him is patient specific works. Next work is the survey and collection of literature regarding pharmacotherapy and interpreting, disseminating that knowledge to the advantage of patients and health care professionals. Finally he has to gather information about Adverse Drug Reactions [ADR] and other health related problems and take initiatives to solve such problems. Thus the basic concepts of pharmacotherapy are:

1. To provide safe and patient specific treatment.
2. Documenting knowledge of pharmacotherapy to the advantage of health care team.

3. Collecting health related problems like ADR, medication error, etc and finding ways to solve them to help the society at large.

Patient Specific Pharmacotherapy

In order to give patient specific therapy the pharmacist should have all the information about the patient. Hence he should start with medication history interview of the patient. During this interview, he should collect as much information as possible about patients past and present illness, concurrent medications, OTC drugs, allergy and the reasons for his present illness. All data pertinent to patient should be interpreted in such a way that, pharmacist should able to determine treatment goals. Then he should select suitable drugs and design therapeutic regimen for the particular patient.

Any potential for drug-drug, drug-food and drug-lab test interactions should be identified and then therapeutic plan is implemented. All the plans implemented are documented. Wherever necessary pharmacist should order and perform laboratory tests and ensure the collaboration of other health care team members.

During the course of treatment, it is necessary to educate the patient and/or his attendants by devising suitable education plan. How far they understood the given information should also be assessed.

The next important step is drug therapy monitoring which gives relevant information about the successful implementation of therapeutic plan. If need be this plan should be modified and continued. Thus individualized therapy for the patient is provided by a pharmacotherapy specialist.

Pharmacotherapy Education

Successful pharmacotherapy is possible only with sustained gathering of knowledge from various sources. Such information should be interpreted, evaluated and disseminated to the members of health care team. Thus, not only health care professionals but also students, patients and even general public are educated by the pharmacist. He can also carryout research on pharmacotherapy and generate new knowledge on the subject.

Pharmacotherapy and Public

As the pharmacist himself designing and implementing the therapeutic regimen, he is in a better position to identify drug related events. By his pharmacokinetic and pharmacodynamic knowledge of the drug, he is in a position to anticipate drug's action on the patient. Any unusual event like ADR, Drug interaction, Medication errors and defects of drug or devices can be collected and reported by the pharmacist.

Similarly public health problems regarding those of drugs and its impact on health system projects can also be identified and reported by pharmacists. He can initiate remedial actions and implement them. He should monitor the results of such plans.

Thus pharmacotherapy by pharmacists not only ensures safe and rational use of drugs but also help the society to have healthy and disease free life. In order to achieve that goal pharmacist should have a sound knowledge of drugs marketed under different names and forms.

Generic and Branded Drugs

A. Generic Drugs

Definition: Generic drugs are drug products that are marketed in its general (pharmacological or chemical) name and not given any brand (special or proprietary) name by the manufacturer. They are comparable or equivalent to the branded products in its strength, dosage form and route of administration, activity and use.

The formulations with single or multiple ingredients mentioned in any pharmacopoeia, if manufactured, according to the procedure given in it, can also be referred to as generic drugs. Here, the name of the pharmacopoeia – viz – IP, BP, USP- is suffixed after the generic name indicating that it meets the standards prescribed in the monograph of that particular pharmacopoeia. e.g.: Paracetamol Tablet IP, Piperazine Citrate syrup IP.

Recent Trend: Recently generic drugs are marketed as a substitute for branded drugs whose patent has expired. As a result of it generic drugs are available at very low price, often one tenth of the branded drug concerned. However in order to maintain standards and efficiency of these generic drugs almost all countries have brought stringent conditions to manufacture and market generic drugs. Foremost among them is the condition that stipulates generic drugs must have bioequivalency to branded drugs. That is they should have acceptable range of pharmacokinetic and pharmacodynamic properties as that of original branded formulation. Hence, worldwide research and development laboratories are established to produce and market generic drugs on the day of patent expiry itself.

Economy: Generic drugs are available at very low price than branded equivalents. It is possible because generic drug manufacturer has to bear only the cost of manufacture of the particular formulation and he need not spent money on research and development, creating market, advertising etc. If a new drug or formulation is invented after considerate spending on research and marketed by a company, it is given exclusive marketing right for the product for a period of 15 to 20 years. In the name of recovering the cost of research, pharmaceutical companies charge extra ordinarily high prices to maximize their profitability. Hence when generic drugs are marketed at cost of production with little profit margins their prices are very less. Moreover, in order to make the drugs available at affordable price to the public, Government of India is giving many concessions like, not charging excise duty, etc, on the manufacture of these drugs. Hence there is economy in the use of generic drugs.

Prescriptions: In order to encourage the use of these generic drugs, doctors are requested to prescribe in generic names. If a drug is prescribed in generic name, a pharmacist can dispense any one of this generic drug, from any one of its manufactures. Anyhow, due to competitions among many manufacturers of the same formulation the price will be controlled and within the reach of general public.

Bioequivalence: The only objection for prescribing drugs in its generic name, by the doctors is their doubt on the efficacy or equivalence of generic drugs to branded drugs. To remove such apprehensions only, Governments has brought in the condition of bio equivalence of generic drugs to branded drugs. Bioequivalence of a drug is defined as the condition in which a generic drug when administered to the same individual in the same dosage (form and quantity) of branded drug results in equivalent concentration of drug in blood and tissues. To achieve this condition of bioequivalence generic drug manufacturers also do some technical works, like changes in manufacturing processes, or using different additives or pharmaceutical aids or even using pharmaceutical alternatives for the main ingredient such as its salt or ester. Thus the generic drug may be slightly chemically different but biologically equivalent to that of branded drug that is what prescribers insist.

B. Branded Drugs

Drugs manufactured and marketed by a particular manufacturer, give a name of his choice to the product and register them with Trade mark authorities. Such names are called brand names or Trade names or proprietary names. For example Paracetamol Tablet is available under different brand names such as Calpol, Tylenol, Crocin, Metacin, Panadol etc.

These names are given for 3 important reasons, viz.

1. Identity
2. Easy Marketing and
3. Promotion

1. *Identity:* Manufacturers name their product to distinguish them as being produced and marketed exclusively by a particular manufacturer. This gives them a 'brand value', depending on the company's long trouble free reputation.

2. *Easy Marketing:* Using the brand value they create, it is easy for them to market their product. Moreover, a pharmacological or chemical name (generic name) is

sometimes lengthy, complicated, confusing and difficult to remember by the doctor to prescribe. A brand name on the other hand is easy to recollect, pronounce and recorded in the minds of both doctor and the patient. Thus more sales can be achieved by these companies.

3. *Promotion:* When all companies are marketing their product in the same (generic) name, there is no need or point to promote the product among the doctors. On the other hand if specific and special name is given for the drug, companies can promote them with many propaganda techniques, like literatures, samples and small gifts with drugs name inscribed on it. Thus they can increase their sales volume and profit.

Disadvantages of Brand Name

However, this marketing and promotion cost are included in the sales price of the drug and hence the patient has to pay more price for the same quality of the drug. Thus brand names are advantageous, only to the manufacturers and aggressive marketing, affordable to only big companies, result in unequal and unethical competitions and kill the small scale industries.

A drug marketed by several companies may have several trade names. Thus there are thousands of brands available in the market. For example there are thousands of cough syrups, pain relievers, Vitamin tonic and other drugs in Indian market. A conservative estimate put it at around 75,000 brand names in India alone, out of which only about 4000 to 5000 names can be remembered by a busy practicing doctor or a pharmacist. Thus brand names create unnecessary confusions in the market.

However, as long as brand names exist in the market a pharmacist must try to remember as much as he could. At least he must memorize the names of important formulations and aware of similar sounding trade names to avoid wrong dispensing and problems to the patients.

Hence, a brief list of proprietary products available in the market belonging to some important categories like, antibiotics, antihistamines, NSAIDs, expectorants and vitamins are given below.

But the students should keep it in their mind that the list is no way exhaustive in nature and only the popular, and fast selling drugs and formulations are given here. There are many books like CIMS, MIMS etc available, which a student can keep it for ready reference. Moreover only Trade names are given here, for other details like, strength, dosage form, packing and price the above mentioned books should be referred.

Proprietary products are by their very nature, the properties of its proprietors and hence may be changed, altered or stopped at any time. Hence a constant updating of this knowledge is essential for a practicing pharmacist.

Category	Generic Name	Proprietary Name (or) Trade Name
I. Antibiotics	Ampicillin	Roscillin, Eskaycillin, Zycilin.
	Amoxicillin	Genmox, Mox, Novamox, Lupimox
	Cefalexin	Cephodex, Keeplex, Sporidex, Betaspore
	Gentamicin	Genticyn, Tamiacin.
	Tobramycin	Tobamist
	Azithromycin	ATM, Azithral, Azro.AM,
	Erythromycin	Althrocin, Erycin, Erythrocin
	Ciprofloxacin	Cifran, Ciplox, Ciprolet
	Doxycycline	Doxt, Lenteclin, Tetradox
	Oxytetracycline	Oxytetra, Terramycin
	Sulphamethoxazole + Trimethaprim	Bactrim, Septran, Ciplin
	Metronidazole	Flagyl, Metrogyl
	Rifampicin	Coxid, R-cin, Rimpacin
	Fluconazole	Fungal F, Glenflu, Zocon
	Griseofulvin	Grisovin, Walavin
	Ketoconazole	Fungicide, Ketozole
	Clotrimazole	Candid, Mycoderm.C
	Miconazole	Zole, Fungitop
II. Antihistamines	Astemizole	Acemiz, Stemiz
	Cetirizine HCl	Citrine, Cetririz, Alerrid
	Chlorpheniramine	Cadistin, Piriton
	Pheniramine	Avil, Phenal
	Promethazine	Avomine, Phenergan
III. Analgesics	Dextropropoxyphene	Proxy tab, Neurovon
	Ethyl Morphine HCl	Dionindon
	Tramadol	Trambax, Trump, Nobligan
	Analgin (Dipyrone)	Novalgin, Ultragin
IV. Anti-inflammatory (NSAIDs)	Aceclofenac	Dolavin, Valdone, Aceclo,
	Diclofenac	Voveran, Volint, Emflam
	Ibuprofen	Brufen, Ibugesic, Ibugin
	Indomethacin	Indocid, Microcid, Articid
	Mefnamic acid	Ponstan, Meftal
	Piroxicam	Dolonex, Pirox
V. Antacids	Aluminum hydroxide	Mucaine, Aludrox, Simeco
	Cimetidine	Cimet, Lock 2,
	Omeprazole	Omez, Ocid, Romesic
	Ranitidine	Aciloc, Histac, Zinetac
VI. Antispasmodic	Hyoscine	Buscopan, Belloid
	Propantheline	Propanthine

Table *Contd...*

Category	Generic Name	Proprietary Name (or) Trade Name
VII. Expectorants	Combination of Antihistamine, mucolytic etc	Benadryl, Corex, Chericof, Ephedrex, Zeet
VIII. Preparations for cold	Phenyl propanalamine	Coldact, Contac, Eskold
IX. Antidiabetics	Glibenclamide	Daonil, Glinil, Glucosafe
	Glipizide	Dibizide, Glide, Glipy
	Metformin	Bigomet, Exermet, Glumet
	Pioglitazone	G. Tase, Diavista, P. Glitz
	Tolbutamide	Rastinon
X. Vitamins	Vitamin E	Evion, EVIT, E-CAP
	Vitamin A	Arovit
	Vitamin D	Calcirol
	Vitamin A and D	Seacod. E. cod
	Nicotinic acid	Nicocin
	Pyridoxine	Pyridox
	Vitamin C	Celin, Redoxon, Cecon
	Folic acid	Foliden, Folvite,
	B.Complex	Becadex, Becosule, Beplex
	Multivitamin preparations	Dexavita, Fesovit, Revital, A to Z, Surbex T, Supradyn, Zincovit.

Questions

Short Answer Questions

1. What is Pharmacotherapy?
2. How Pharmacotherapy differs from other therapy?
3. What are the basic concepts of Pharmacotherapy?
4. Define generic drugs.
5. Define branded drugs.

Long Answer Questions

6. Explain the salient futures of Pharmacotherapy.
7. Enumerate the reasons and disadvantages of Brand names.

CHAPTER 26

PEDIATRIC PHARMACY

Introduction

For most of the drugs the pediatric dose is not indicated on the label and its calculation is left to the treating physician. Traditionally pediatric doses are calculated using the following formulae:

1. CLARK's Rule $= \dfrac{(weight\ in\ pounds)\ \times\ (Adult\ dose)}{50}$

   (This formula is common for infants and children)

2. FRIED's Rule $= \dfrac{(Age\ in\ months)\ \times\ (Adult\ dose)}{150}$

   (This formula mainly used to calculate the dose for infants and children up to 2 years.)

3. YOUNG's Rule $= \dfrac{(Age\ in\ years)\ \times\ (Adult\ dose)}{Age\ +\ 12}$

   (This rule is applicable for children of 1 to 12 years)

None of the above formulae is completely satisfactory, as they take only the age of the child into account, not any other parameter like body surface area, body weight etc. We consider children as small adults and accordingly the drugs, its dose and the entire treatment are given to them. Non-availability of specific pediatric formulations for most of the drugs marketed by drug companies is also a reason for this. In fact, during the introduction of new drugs, no clinical trial is conducted on children as it is very difficult and risky to enrol them for clinical trials. Thus there are lot of corrections to be made and precautions to be taken while using drugs in pediatric cases. Hence let us first look into the factors affecting or influencing the safe and rational use of drugs in pediatric patients.

Factors affecting use of Drugs in Children

Childhood is unique in that it ranges from one day old baby to 18 years adolescent. As it is the period of growth, the entire body and its functional ability of the child changes continuously and hence it is difficult to select a drug and its dose, to administer to such a dynamic entity.

The organs of the body, the amount of drug metabolizing enzymes and hence the drugs dose, effect of drugs and even adverse reactions vary throughout this period. As mentioned above, limited availability of specific drug's dosage forms for children make the situation more complex. Hence various factors influencing treatment of children should be thoroughly studied. They are:

1. Absorption of drugs
2. Distribution of drugs
3. Metabolism of drugs
4. Elimination of drugs
5. Monitoring the therapy
6. Non-compliance and
7. Medication errors and ADR.

Pharmacokinetics in Pediatrics

Pharmacokinetics is the study of what the body does to the drug. After the administration or application of drugs on a human body, it is absorbed, distributed, metabolized and finally excreted from the body. Each of this is influenced by many factors as described elsewhere in this book. [Chapter 34, Individualization of Dose and Pharmacist Intervention]. All these Pharmacokinetic studies were carried out on adult patients and hence very little information is available on these parameters in children. However the need for optimizing use of drugs in children has been realized in the recent past.

Absorption of Drugs

It depends on the route of administration and the dosage form to a large extent. Even in the case of IV injections, the bioavailability of drugs depends on accurate delivery of the drug, speed with which it is administered, volume of injection left out in injection port or in the infusion set tubing. This acquires more importance as the dose to be given to child is small and often in milligrams even a small loss in volume of injection has huge effect on its bioavailability. Due to less muscle mass in children, absorption from IM injection vary and should be monitored in critical cases, IM injection is also painful to children especially for certain drug like Ceftriaxone. As far as possible this route should be avoided to administer drugs to children, if other routes are available.

Rectal administration of drugs can be followed if indicated as in cases of continuous vomiting or mouth injury etc. For some drugs rectal absorption may be erratic, nevertheless it can be used for other drugs because of rapid onset of action. For example rectal diazepam solution helps to end seizures in epilepsy quickly and can be used in emergency.

Now-a-days needle free subcutaneous jet injections are available, which give comparable results of conventional SC injections with the advantage of less painful administration in children. Wherever possible topical application of drugs should be followed as there are numerous formulations like patches, plasters, creams and gels available in the market.

Out of all routes of administrations, oral route is considered to be the best as it is possible to administer the drugs, easily without the help of experts (like Nurses or Doctors) and devices (like syringe, needle etc). However oral administration has its own limitations. First and foremost is the drug must be palatable to children; otherwise, they refuse to take the medicine or vomit or spit the medicines after administration. Moreover some drugs may not be suitable for infants as their gastric emptying time reaches to the level of adults only by 6 months of age and gastric juice secretion increases slowly and reaches optimum level by 2 years of age. Thus rate of absorption differs depending on the age or growth stage of the child. For example in one clinical study delay in absorption of Ampicillin in children is noticed.

Distribution of Drugs

It is expressed in apparent volume of distribution and that depends on protein binding to a larger extent. Total body water and body mass also have significant role in determining the distribution of drugs. Obviously for drugs like amino glycoside antibiotics, which are highly distributed in ECF and tissues and hence there is larger volume of distribution, the initial loading dose should be more to reach a minimum effective concentration. These drugs are distributed in extracellular fluids which are more in neonates (50% of body weight) compared to 25% in children of 1 year age and 19% in adults. Similarly total body fat increases as the age advances from neonate to adolescent. At the age of 17 it is reduced in boys and almost double in girls!

Distribution of drugs depends on availability of protein which in turn determines the extent of binding and free drug concentration. As the later is responsible for pharmacological action, serious consideration must be given to plasma proteins and other binding sites. Usually serum albumin level reaches near adult value only at the end of a year after birth and hence decreased level in neonates is a reality, we must remember. Similarly bilirubin is also increased in neonates due to limited capacity of liver to conjugate it. While administering drugs like Phenytoin and Theophylline to pediatric cases, these factors should be taken into account.

Metabolism of Drugs

Drugs are metabolized before elimination from the body. Metabolism depends on various factors, the important among them are, amount of enzymes and the hepatic blood flow. In the neonates the enzymes for metabolism are either absent or very less compared to adults. Hence, while treating infants this should be considered. At the same time, metabolism is dramatically improved in the children of 1 to 9 years old. Phenytoin and Theophylline are metabolized greater than adults in these groups of children. Sometimes different metabolic routes are used by the children's body to metabolize some drugs, like Paracetamol and Theophylline as the later is converted to caffeine.

Oxidation, reduction, hydrolysis, hydroxylation and conjugation are the different reactions by which drugs are metabolized by the liver. Each of this reaction is carried out by corresponding enzymes and these enzymes are either less, equal or excess of adult values at different stages of growth of children.

Elimination of Drugs

Most drugs are eliminated through kidney. Hence its development and normal function are essential to excrete them from the body. Obviously due to under development of kidney in neonates excretion is limited, however they develop faster and the functions reaches adult level after few months of birth.

Renal functional abilities should be ascertained before prescribing drugs with narrow therapeutic index. Usually it is checked by calculating Creatinine clearance or serum Creatinine. However these values have their own limitations like incomplete filtration of Creatinine by the glomeruli, muscle mass etc. Methods and formulae used to calculate Creatinine clearance in adults cannot be used for calculating it in pediatric patients. New formulae have been developed taking into account, the age, weight, body surface area, and sex of the child.

Thus there are three formulae. They are:

1. Trauf and Johnson formula:

$$\text{Creatinine Clearance} = \frac{42 \times height\ in\ cm}{serum\ creatinine\ (\mu\ mol/L)}$$

2. Caunhahan formula:

$$\text{Creatinine Clearance} = \frac{38 \times height\ (cm)}{serum\ creatinine\ (\mu\ mol/L)}$$

3. Schwarz formula:

$$\text{Creatinine Clearance} = \frac{k \times height\ (cm)}{serum\ creatinine\ (\mu\ mol/L)}$$

Where k varies according to the age of the patient as follows:

In New Born (0 to 18 months) = 40

In Girls (2 to 16 years) and Boys (2 to 13 years) = 49

In Boys 13 to 16 years = 60

Any one of the above formulae can be used, but various factors affecting creatinine clearance in pediatric cases as well as in adults, like rapid change in renal function, accurate creatinine assay methods, creatinine metabolism etc should be considered.

Dosage in Children

Having studied the factors affecting drug treatment in children, let us look into other aspects of determining dose for pediatric cases. In order to help the doctors and pharmacists in deciding the dose for children various formulae (Page 228), charts and reference books are available. For example British National Formulary for children (BNF-C) gives the prescribing guidelines and drug monographs. Sometimes, the dose per day has to be divided into 3 or 4 equal doses and administered at correct intervals, which should be noted before giving drugs to children.

Calculating the dose according to the body surface area seems to be more scientific in arriving at children's dose. Charts are available to calculate the body surface area, however, getting the accurate height and weight of a sick child may be a problem to calculate the body surface area and drug manufacturers rarely provide dosages on surface area bases.

However body surface area method is used to calculate the percentage of adult dose to be administered to children of various ages. For example new born babies can be given 12.5%, 1 year baby 25%, 7 years child 50%, 12 years child 75% and 16 years 90% of adult dose, as per body surface area calculation. However, treating physicians and Clinical Pharmacists has to determine the dose required for each child according to its clinical status. Individualization of dose by Clinical Pharmacist plays an important role in this aspect.

Therapeutic Drug Monitoring (TDM)

It is the main tool used by the Clinical Pharmacist, to individualize the dose for each patient. This is, thus very essential for pediatric cases which require careful and continuous monitoring. Clinical Pharmacist usually measures the Blood Drug concentration of selected drugs and adjusts its dose according to the need of the patient. Thereby not only effective treatment is ensured, but also adverse drug reactions are avoided as far as possible.

The factors to be considered while monitoring the therapy, like time of administration of drug, time of withdrawal of the blood sample, and concurrent administration of other drugs are recorded carefully. It may not be possible or necessary to monitor all the drugs given to pediatric cases, however, drugs with narrow therapeutic window and other risky drugs must be monitored by TDM. For a detail review of this requirement refer the chapter on TDM elsewhere in this book.

Noncompliance

It is the phenomenon of not following the instructions of treating physician or pharmacist regarding the use of prescribed drugs and other advices by the patient. In the case of pediatric patients, it acquires different dimension that the drug is not directly used by the patient, but his/her parents or care taker has to administer the drug to this young patients. Usually parents forget the dose or delay the administration due to their busy house hold daily routines and the patient – the child – is not in a position to remind or ask for the drug. Thus the problem becomes acute.

Consequences of non-compliance are not difficult to guess, the foremost one being reduced efficacy of treatment and relapse or return of severity of disease. Antibiotics resistances by microorganisms, increased dose or requirement of more potent drugs are the other problems associated with non-compliance.

Problems peculiar to pediatric cases include, palatability of drugs, multiple Drug regimen, size of tablet or capsule, fraction of unit dose formulations etc. Usually parents commit mistakes while giving fraction of tablets or capsules to children. Breaking or opening tablets or capsules results in wastage, inaccurate measurement of dose and bad taste while swallowing. These problems can be solved by the pharmacist, by dispensing the needed dose by weighing or measuring and packing separately. The nauseating or bitter powders should be administered after mixing with honey, sugar syrup or Jam.

Moreover, pharmacists can help the patients by dispensing once a day sustain release formulations or combination drugs to reduce number of doses and number of drugs to be administered per day. Thus compliance or adherence to the treatment schedule can be improved.

Medication Errors and ADR

Most of the time, the former is responsible for the later. Hence medication errors should be prevented, especially in children as they are susceptible to ADR due to various unique factors. They are:

1. Dose calculation errors by doctors, pharmacists, nurses or parents which results in either excess (toxic) dose or less (ineffective) dose.
2. Lack of availability of pediatric formulations in suitable dosage forms and concentrations.
3. Heterogeneous nature of pediatric patients (Age 1 day to teen age)
4. Difficulties in measuring, weighing or administering pediatric doses.

5. Under development of internal organs of body and their functions resulting in ADR or ineffective results.

Apart from the above, some drugs are known to cause ADR in children. The well known example is discoloration of teeth by Tetracycline in children below 9 years of age. Other example is use of Aspirin, the very popular and common house hold drug which causes problem if used in children below 16 years of age during viral infections such as influenza or varicella. It causes Reye's syndrome, associated within drowsiness, hypoglycemia, seizures and liver failure. It may even results in coma or death. Hence Aspirin should not be used in pediatric cases.

A quarter of ADRs are preventable, if proper precautions are taken. Drugs which usually cause adverse drug reaction in children are antibiotics, anticonvulsants and analgesics. Corticosteroids and Phenobarbitone also produce adverse events in pediatric cases on prolonged use.

Gray baby or Toddler syndrome is reported due to Chloramphenicol toxicity which results in cardiovascular collapse in new born babies. Similarly absorption of Hexachlorophene or Boric acid through topical application also found to be toxic in infants.

Thus, to prevent medication error and consequent ADR, standard treatment procedures for pediatric cases should be prepared and followed sincerely. This protocol should start from the selection of appropriate drugs for the patient to its dose, administration and monitoring of therapy.

Even after all these precautions, if Adverse Drug Reaction occurs in a pediatric patient it should be sincerely reported to relevant authorities, including WHO cell on ADR. This is more important in the context of insufficient information available on ADR in pediatric patients. As pointed out in the beginning, no clinical trial is conducted on children, and hence any information about ADR in children is highly useful to worldwide health care team. Pharmacists have a special and important role in this aspect.

Questions

Short Answer Questions

1. List the formulae used to calculate doses for Children.

2. Write a note on Non compliance among pediatric cases.

Long Answer Questions

3. Write in detail about calculation of doses for children.

4. Explain the factors affecting use of drugs in children.

5. Explain how therapeutic drug monitoring play important role in pediatric pharmacy.

CHAPTER 27

GERIATRIC PHARMACY

Introduction

Due to scientific developments, rise in standard of living in the last of 50 years and other reasons, number of aged people among the population is steadily increasing in India. There are more then 7 crore peoples above 60 years of age living in our country. However this elderly population cannot be claimed to live in comfort. They are with many diseases because of age related failure of organs of their body and consequent physiological changes. No wonder they are the major consumer of medicines, on an average seven or more drugs per day like analgesics, anti-inflammatory, diuretics, hypnotics, anxiolytics and β-blockers. Thus even though the geriatric patients constitute less than 10% of population they generate more than 30% of all prescriptions. Hence we need to be vigilant in using drugs in these risky categories of people.

Pharmacokinetics in Geriatrics

Ageing brings in not only lot of visible bodily changes, but also corresponding or even more changes in the functions of internal organs. All these changes result in changes in pharmacokinetics and pharmacodynamics of the drugs consumed by the geriatric patients. Thus elderly patients are with less body surface area, muscle mass, liver size, digestive enzymes, gastro intestinal motility and renal functions, compared to normal young adults. They affect the absorption, distribution, metabolism and elimination of drugs.

Absorption

Rate of absorption of drugs is little less in geriatric patients; however, overall absorption is not significantly changed. GI disorders and concurrent administration of some drugs may alter absorption of drugs, same as in the case of any other patient. Presence or absence of food in GI tract has some role in the absorption of drugs. It should be checked for critical drugs as elderly patients usually forgo their food or take very minimum food on many occasions.

Distribution

As indicated above, aged patients have less body mass, less body water and less protein in their blood, hence, distribution of drugs is affected, resulting in large apparent volume of distribution. Free concentration of cimetidine, warfarin and other acidic drugs in blood may increase due to fewer albumins in the blood of aged patients. Similarly lipid soluble drugs are distributed more in fat of these patients and hence they have long half life or long duration of action.

Metabolism

Impaired first pass metabolism results in increased bioavailability of drugs like nifedipine, propranolol and verapamil. Consequently dosage of these drugs should be adjusted. Moreover in elderly patients decrease in blood flow to liver is observed and oxidative enzymes also found to be less in geriatric cases. This may lead to accumulation of drugs and its prolonged action. Hence while using drugs like phenytoin, theophylline, diazepam, warfarin, isoniozid, and rifampicin care should be taken.

Excretion

In general, glomerular filtration is reduced in elderly patients; hence the doses of drugs which are excreted through kidney should be reduced in geriatric patients. This is especially required for drugs with narrow therapeutic window like amino glycoside antibiotics, digoxin etc. As the renal function or impairment in individuals differs widely, they should be accessed before making decisions on the adjustment of doses. Antidiabetic drugs like metformin and glibenclamide should also be carefully given to these patients.

Pharmacodynamics in Geriatrics

Information on the changes in pharmacodynamics is not much available and hence decision has to be taken after studying individual cases. Clinical studies on the geriatric cases also very limited or almost nil and it is more difficult to answer what Pharmacodynamics changes could occur in an individual elderly patient.

However, there are few indications available on this, which a Clinical Pharmacist should take note off. There may be changes in response to drug, in receptors of those drugs and also modifications in homeostatic responses. The former affects CNS significantly. CNS depressants like morphine and barbiturates may produce hypotension in the geriatric cases. Cholinergic neurons start declining in number in elderly, resulting in loss of memory, confusions etc.and hence anticholnergic drugs should be carefully given to aged patients. The side effects of these drugs, constipation, dry mouth, urinary retention may be precipitated; hypnotics and β-blockers are the other group of drugs to be administrated carefully. Regulation of body temperature may also be affected due to pharmacodynamics changes in geriatric patients.

Ageing may affect the response of receptors of drugs. Since drugs produce their effects through specific receptors, any reduction in its number or affinity towards drugs, affect drugs effect after coupling with receptor. Even the target cells or organ's response may also change in aged patients. Benzodiazepines, warfarin and digoxin are drugs for which geriatric patients are more sensitive.

Antidiabetic drugs like glibenclamide, metformin, antibiotics like streptomycin, gentamicin, cotrimoxazole, analgesics, anti-inflammatory drugs, diuretics, antispasmodic and antihistamines are some of the other drugs that are required to be used carefully because of increased risk of toxic effects.

Geriatric Diseases

Anaemia, Arthritis including osteoarthritis, cerebero/cardiovascular diseases, hypertension, dementia, parkinsonism, osteoporosis, urinary incontinence, constipation, gastric ulcer, leg ulcers are some of the common geriatric diseases. Most of the diseases occur primarily due to ageing and require prolonged treatment with caution.

Anaemia

Due to pathological or nutritional reasons, anaemia may occur in elderly patients. Usually iron deficiency anaemia is noticed among this group of patients, though anaemia due to vitamin B_{12} and/or folic acid deficiency is also found in many patients. Iron deficiency usually results from poor absorption of it in elderly patients and also from blood loss. It should be treated with oral Iron preparations.

Similarly megaloblastic anaemia is treated with suitable formulations of vitamin B_{12} and folic acid.

Arthritis

It is the usual problem in elderly patient. Osteoarthritis the disease which affects the weight bearing joints is also common with geriatric obese patients. This affects the quality of life by arresting the movement of the patient and requires proper drug treatment and physiotherapy. Anti-inflammatory drugs including NSAIDs are used to treat these conditions along with exercise, massage and hot packs.

Cerebero/Cardiovascular Diseases

Myocardial infarction, cardiac failure and stroke are the major problems affecting geriatric patients. Thrombolytic agents, Anticoagulants, Diuretics, ACE Inhibitors and β-blockers, Digoxin are some of the drugs used to treat these conditions. Extra care should be taken while giving these drugs to geriatric patients.

Constipation

Due to age, gastrointestinal motility is declined in elderly patients. They tend to eat less and drink little water due to age related problems like immobility which results in constipation. Chronic constipation results in faecal impaction and then to faecal incontinence. Some medicines like opium derivatives, antacids and verapamil can also cause constipation.

Constipation is usually treated with laxatives for short periods, prolonged use leads to other complications like diarrhoea, electrolyte loss and even dependence.

Dementia

Loss of intellectual capacity is the character of dementia. It may be due various reasons, the major among them are Alzheimer's disease, and multi-infarct dementia. It starts with forgetfulness and progress slowly. It is occurring in patients above 60 years of age and also to the patients with the history of hypertension and stroke.

Confusion is one of the common problems in these conditions, which should be carefully treated. Confusion in elderly patients also lead to behavioural disturbances for which there may be many reasons like sight and hearing loss, pain, infection and medication. Medications which cause confusion in geriatric patients are barbiturates, cimetidine, diuretics, antidiabetics, steroids and opioids. Even deficiency of thyroid hormone, vitamin B_{12} or drinking habits can lead to confusion. Whatever may be the reason, it should be detected by careful monitoring of the patient and his medications and appropriate treatment should be given.

Gastric Ulcer

Due to many social causes and bodily changes, aged persons are not taking food in right quantity, quality or time. Social causes include worries and tension that is usually associated with uncertain future, helplessness and neglect by other family members. Hence there are many aged people with peptic ulcer. *H. pylori* infection is also common in this group of people. NSAIDs which are frequently and constantly used in excessive quantities by elderly patients, results in GI bleeding. Hence Clinical Pharmacists should give attention to these patients and the above factors. Along with proper treatment, counselling may be needed to remedy the problem.

Hypertension

Due to stress and worries, most of the elderly patients are with hypertension. It is also an important risk factor for cardiac diseases. Excessive intake of cholesterol containing food, sedentary life style with less physical activity and obesity, consumption of alcohol, smoking may also lead to hypertension and associated diseases. Such cases are advised to restrict consumption of above and also the salt intake 4 to 6 gm per day. Drugs for the treatment of hypertension in elderly must be selected carefully. Thiazide diuretics are found to be effective but used in low doses, as higher doses increases the adverse effects. β-Blockers can also be used for its diuretic value. Calcium antagonists like verapamil, diltiazem can be given along with ACE Inhibitors, the later with caution, as it may result in kidney failure in geriatric patients.

Osteoporosis

It is characterized by increased risk of bone fracture in aged patients, due to low bone mass and deterioration of bone tissue. Women, after menopause are usually affected by this condition. Hyperthyroidism, kidney failure, increased production of glucocorticoid or intake of steroids may lead to osteoporosis. The disease is more prevalent in women than man, as they loss up to 30% of bone mass by 75 years of age, compared to only 11% by men. Treatment is by giving vitamin D and calcium, biphosphonates like alendronate, etidronate etc. Hormone replacement using oestrogens is also beneficial.

Urinary Incontinence

It is a condition in which patients are passing urine involuntarily. There are many reasons for this condition. Important among them are Urinary tract infection, problems in urinary bladder, polyurea, constipation, neurological and psychiatric reasons. It may also be due to stress over flow.

In the first type small amount of urine is eliminated due to abdominal pressure while performing such activities. For example even coughing, sneezing may cause this. It occurs mainly in ladies due to weakening pelvic muscles. Overflow may be caused by incomplete emptying and often occur in diabetic patients. Before treating these patients with drugs, which are often either ineffective or risky, basic reason for the condition should be found. If it is due to use of other drugs, such drugs should be either reduced or replaced with less problematic one. Even placebo treatment was found to be useful in many cases.

Parkinsonism, leg ulcers, vision and hearing loss are the other problems often encountered by geriatric patients. They are treated appropriately with or without drugs following general precautions outlined below.

General Precautions in Geriatric Treatment

1. **Conduct Medication History Interview:** It is must for geriatric cases as these patients are with multiple complications and invariably under one or other treatment.

2. **Selection of Appropriate Drugs:** As mentioned above, due to physiological changes in the body of elderly patients, proper drug should be selected with less

chance for ADR. If possible non-drug treatment like exercises, food habits and life style changes should be tried.

3. **Treatment:** It should be started only after proper diagnosis. Symptomatic treatment must be for a minimal period. Polypharmacy or multiple drug regimens should be avoided. Right dosage forms, suitable for this category of patients should be prescribed.

4. **Monitoring:** Therapeutic Drug monitoring (TDM) must be carried out for elderly patient, as their pharmacokinetic and Pharmacodynamics profile changes vastly with age. Starting with low dose suitable dose must be determined and followed. Necessary advice must be given to the health care professionals regarding the special status and treatment of these cases. As most of the ADR in these cases are of type I and hence predictable, careful monitoring for ADR must be done.

5. **Patient Friendly Packages and Labels:** If the geriatric patient is treated as out patient, suitable packing, easy to recognise and open should be dispensed. Labels should be in large print so as to read easily with their poor falling eye sights. If necessary, supplementary labels should be pasted on the drug container.

6. **Noncompliance:** It is one of the significant problems with aged people. They often tend to forget their doses. Hence suitable calendar packing with day and time markings must be given. Some patients refuse or even voluntarily forgo their medicines due to depression and disappointment; such cases should be monitored by other family members or attendants of patients.

7. **Counselling:** Counselling by Clinical Pharmacists is proved to be an effective tool in successful treatment of geriatric patients. As these people feel isolation or negligence by relatives, they are always in depressed mood and hence a clinical Pharmacist's soothing words and deeds will go long way in ensuring speedy recovery of these cases. He must be made to understand the disease, its manifestations and the treatment. He should also be informed of any temporary inconvenient caused by drugs so that they will adjust with those medicines.

8. **Feed Back and Follow Up:** Once geriatric patients are discharged from hospitals they should be counselled for continuing treatment at home, return visit, prescription refilling etc. They should be encouraged to contact the treating physician and Clinical Pharmacist for their problems or doubt during the post discharge period. They can also be requested to send feed back to the treating team. Thus organised follow up measures ensure further success of treatment. It helps to avoid relapse of the disease and need for readmission.

Conclusion

With proper understanding of physiology, psychology, pharmacokinetics and pharmaco dynamics of geriatric patients, best possible treatment can be given to them. Clinical pharmacist has thus, a prominent role to play in these cases; and he should be ready to shoulder this responsibility by acquiring both theoretical and practical knowledge about geriatric patients.

Questions

Short Answer Questions

1. Name few diseases commonly found in geriatric patients.

2. Why we should be vigilant while using drugs in elderly patients?

Long Answer Questions

3. How the Pharmacokinetics and Pharmacodynamics of drugs are affected in geriatric patients?

4. Write an essay about Geriatric Diseases.

5. Explain the general precautions to be taken in geriatric treatment.

CHAPTER 28

USE OF DRUGS IN PREGNANCY AND LACTATION

Introduction

Use of drugs in pregnancy and lactation is complicated because of anatomical physioligical and biochemical changes that occur in the body of pregnant woman. Obviously the Pharmacokinetic and Pharmacodynamic properties of drugs are modified and that may result in damages to either mother or foetus or both. Hence a clinical Pharmacist must take precautions while dispensing, treating and monitoring such cases. This chapter deal with such requirements and make the pharmacist aware of his additional responsibilities.

Lack of Literature and Research

There are very few studies carried out on the effect of drugs during pregnancy and lactation. Many limitations are there even in the published papers. Animal studies are not always applicable to humans. They cannot be extrapolated directly to pregnant mothers, as Teratogenicity differs widely between species. For example, the infamous Thalidomide produces malformations in rabbits and humans but not on rodents. Hence studies using rodents may be misleading. Similarly sulphonamides and corticosteroids cause damage in animals but not in humans at therapeutic doses.

Even the data published after human studies are also not always accurate as the toxic effects of drugs are always undetected or under reported. Study subjects (patients) are not able to identify the drug related problem or not in a position to distinguish the drugs effect from those of disease manifestations. Moreover the patients are not able to accurately report the time of consumption or dose of OTC drugs they use concurrently with prescription drugs.

Thus we are not in a position to forecast fully or warn the toxic effect of drugs during pregnancy and lactation. Each case has to be individually monitored, if they use drugs during pregnancy and lactation.

Effects of Drugs during Pregnancy

The effects of drugs given to a pregnant lady may affect her as well as the foetus. Its effect may be direct or indirect. It may be toxic, teratogenic or fatal for the baby. Sometimes it affects directly the supply of oxygen and nutrition to the foetus by constricting the placenta. Indirectly, the biochemical changes that results from the administration of drugs, affect the foetus slowly.

But these damages depend not only on the dosage or potency of the drug but mainly on the foetal age. In the first fortnight after conception, it either kills the foetus or not affects it at all, because the foetus is resistant to teratogenic effect of drug during this stage. But after that period i.e. from 3rd week of pregnancy to the end of 2 months, it's highly susceptible. The effects produced during this period may be noticeable due to anatomic effect or manifest at a later stage by producing metabolic or functional defect. Even abortion is possible at this stage of pregnancy. But drugs given during later stages of pregnancy (6th month to 9th month) may not produce teratogenic effect, but affect growth and physiological or biochemical functions.

Teratogens

These are the agents which cause damage to the growth of foetus and results are anatomical changes in the body of the foetus which are observable after birth. These agents may be, drugs taken by mother during pregnancy or mother's illness like diabetes and hypothyroidism or her infection or irradiation. Any one of the above agents can cause congenital abnormalities that is, structural defects present at birth of the baby.

These teratogens acts on particular cell metabolism and they need not be affecting mothers, at the same time it may influence embryonic mortality. These damages depend on the extent they cross placenta. Thus drugs with less molecular weight (< 600), high lipid solubility, low protein binding and those that is non-ionized readily cross the placenta.

According to researches done on teratogenic potential, out of 1000 drugs only about 30 are found to be teratogens. They are antineoplastic drugs, androgenic hormones, bisulfan, coumarin derivatives, cortisones, anticonvulsants like phenytoin, thyroid drugs, oral antidiabetic drugs, narcotics, sedatives and other CNS depressants, antibiotics like tetracycline and aminoglycosides, anticoagulants, cardiovascular drugs, thalidomide, valproic acid etc.

This apart drugs used during labour and delivery may also damage the baby. Thus local anaesthetics like lidocaine may cause CNS depression or bradycardia. Similarly oxytocin given for uterine contraction may results in vasoconstriction, anoxia etc in babies. Analgesics like diazepam used during delivery can also have some effect on the baby though they are not teratogens. These drugs have to be eliminated by the foetus after the umbilical cord is cut, and when their metabolising enzymes and kidneys are not fully developed. Too much of cigarette smoking and alcohol consumption also have some effects on the development of foetus.

Conditions Commonly Treated during Pregnancy

The following are the conditions usually treated during pregnancy

1. Nausea and vomiting
2. Constipation
3. Common cold
4. Gastrointestinal disturbances
5. Pain
6. Edema
7. Asthma
8. Diabetes
9. Epilepsy and
10. Hypertension.

All these conditions require treatment during pregnancy. But as discussed above, drugs may produce some or other damage to the foetus during its developmental stages. Very little scientific studies were carried out on the effect of drugs on various stages of development and hence there is always risk in using drugs during pregnancy. It is better to avoid drugs and go for non-pharmacological methods of treatment if unavoidable.

For example, nausea and vomiting during early stages of pregnancy can be controlled by acupressure or lying down on the bed or even by smelling fresh lemon fruits according to traditional methods of treatment. If it is severe and not controlled by above measures, Meclizine at the dose of 25 to 30 mg oral can be given.

Similarly laxatives and purgatives are contraindicated during pregnancy; hence, constipation should not be treated with such drugs. Banana fruits are advised by traditional healers however, psyllium can be given in unavoidable cases. Diabetes should be controlled as far as possible as risk of congenital abnormalities is 3 times more in diabetic mothers. Pregnant patients with other disease like asthma, epilepsy, and hypertension should take their medications regularly and as advised by the physician. These diseases if present should not be allowed to go out of control at any stage of pregnancy requiring potent drugs and high doses. Thus pregnancy brings in lot of responsibilities and discipline to the couple, particularly to the expectant mother.

Drugs in Lactation

Drugs consumed by lactating mothers, reaches the milk depending on some conditions. They are pH of the milk, drugs solubility in milk, protein binding and drug's partition coefficient. Since the pH of milk is less than plasma pH, weak bases tend to have higher concentration in it. Weak acids will be equal or less than that of blood. However all these depends on many other factors, which should be taken into account while giving treatment to lactating mothers. These factors are listed below.

Factors to be Considered

1. While treating lactating mothers, the pharmacokinetic of the drug in question must be studied first. Mother's ability to absorb, metabolise and excrete the drug should be calculated. Especially amount of drug excreted in to the milk and also the amount of such milk given to the baby has to be arrived at. Full dosage regimen, dose, route of administration should be considered for safe use of drugs in lactating mothers.

2. Physical and chemical properties of drugs determine its crossing into the milk. Thus its solubility, protein binding and molecular weight play important role in its crossing into milk. Large molecules obviously do not pass into milk. Acidic drugs and those with high protein binding are also not passing into milk significantly.

3. *Time of Lactation*: Time of feeding milk to the infant is an important factor. If the mother gives milk, after she took the medicine and when its concentration is at peak, obviously, there is a possibility of more drugs being passed on to the baby. Hence mothers should be advised to feed on the baby just before taking medicines. Usually the peak concentration of drug in milk is reached after long time of its peak in plasma. Published research on this aspect is very much limited and hence individual patients should be monitored. On any account, breast feeding of the baby should not be interrupted because of mother's medication. It should be properly planned.

Drugs to be Avoided

The following drugs should be avoided by lactating mothers

1. Tetracycline
2. Ergot alkaloids
3. Antithyroid medications
4. Cascara and
5. Anticancer drugs

These apart, new drugs which are not tested properly should not be used. Minimum doses of drugs should be used as far as possible and at no point of time excessive doses should be taken. Mothers with suspected kidney or liver damages should be carefully monitored and for them doses of all drugs should be individualized. Other drugs contraindicated in lactating mothers are: Phencyclidine, Phenindione, Cyclosporin,

Amphetamine and Bromocriptine. Moreover, some drugs reduce the secretion of milk in lactating mothers and they should be avoided, Estradiol, Oral Contraceptives, Levodopa and Antidepressants Thiozide diuretics and even large doses of vitamin B_6 are the drugs that may suppress lactation.

Safe use of Drugs in Lactation

There are few safe ways of using drugs by lactating mothers, if drug therapy is unavoidable.

1. Safe drugs should be selected by studying its pharmacokinetic and pharmacodynamic profiles. For example if an analgesic has to be given, Acetaminophen can be given instead of Aspirin, as the later may produce salicylism in the infant. Drugs which are eliminated faster from the body, drugs which are not crossing into the milk, drugs which produce local action, rather than systemic absorption like pain balms can be used in minimum quantities.

2. *Lactating time*: Adjusting the time of lactating is another option. As pointed out earlier, feeding the baby before taking medicine or after a long gap between time of consuming the drug and feeding are some of the methods to avoid untoward effects of drugs on the baby. If need be, breast milk can be pumped using suckers, stored and given to infant later. This may be useful if the mother has to take a potent drug unavoidably.

3. Over the counter medications and other medications for existing illness should be taken in minimum effective doses and for a short term. Non-pharmacological methods of treatments should be followed as far as possible. External applications like plasters, pain relievers, hot water bags, should be tried first. No drug should be taken without consulting physician or pharmacist.

Conclusion

The pharmacokinetics of drugs are such that the absorption, distribution, metabolism and elimination processes of drugs leads to insignificant amount of drugs in the blood of infants. For example it was found in one study that isoniazid given to mother reached the infant only to the extent of about 1.5 mg per feeding of 250 ml approximately. The children's dose of isoniazid is 10 to 20 mg/kg. Hence drugs generally taken by lactating mothers are not considered toxic to the infant.

However, highly potent drugs which are toxic even at very low concentration or drugs which accumulate in the body should be carefully monitored. Drugs which are absolutely contraindicated like radio pharmaceuticals, lithium, thiouracil iodides and mercurials should be avoided. Even seemingly innocent drugs like caffeine (from coffee) in excessive quantities should be avoided. Alcohol consumption in large quantities is also harmful to infants. Vaccines, insecticides and other environment pollutants should also be prevented from lactating mothers.

Thus careful administration of drugs in minimum doses, if unavoidable, may save both the mother and the baby. The clinical pharmacist has an additional responsibility to ensure the safety of pregnant mother and also the baby.

Questions

Short Answer Questions

1. Write a note on effects of drugs during pregnancy.

2. What are Teratogens?

3. What are the conditions commonly treated during pregnancy?

Long Answer Questions

4. Write in detail about use of drugs during lactation.

5. How drugs can be used safely in lactating mothers?

CHAPTER 29

PHARMACOGENETICS

Introduction

We administer drugs to different group of people. We found, even at the same dose, many people are responding normally, some are responding less and some others are not responding at all, yet another small group, show excessive response leading to toxic effect of the drug. This inter-individual variation in drugs activity leads to many researches on the reason for these abnormal phenomena. Scientists could find many reasons like diseases, sex, diet, weight etc, but no single factor has a predominant effect. For example, some adverse effects of drugs cannot be explained by above factors. Further research lead deep into one's genetic makeup and thus originated the study of pharmacogenetics.

From the Human Genome Project, it was found that there is no difference between individuals, in the information gathered from 99.9% of their genes. There is a small difference in the balance 0.1% of genes, which is responsible for this variation in drugs action. These differences have no effect on human body, in its growth, development or function except drug's metabolism.

Thus, the study of relationship between genetics and therapy started and variously called as Pharmacogenetics or Pharmacogenomics. Earlier there was not much difference between the two terms and used interchangeably. However, recently the term pharmacogenetics is reserved for the study of genetic variation that leads to different response to drugs, whereas pharmacogenomics refers to "whole genome application of pharmacogenetics" (which deals with single gene interactions with drugs). Thus, pharmacogenomics is the broader application of genomic technologies for further characterization of old drugs and discovery of new drugs.

Definition

Pharmacogenetics is the word coined by combining two streams of science, pharmacology and genetics. It is defined by many authors in many ways: A few are given below:

The Australasian Genetics resource book defines.

"Pharmacogenetics is the study of genetic factors that influences how a drug works". It also describe, "Pharmacogenetics as the science that underpins understanding the role that an individual's genetic makeup plays, in how well a medicine works, as well as what side effects are likely to occur".

Yet another definition is,

"Pharmacogenetics refer to genetics differences in metabolic pathways which can affect individual responses to drugs, both in terms of therapeutic effect as well as adverse effects"

Most simple definition is

"Pharmacogenetics is a study which deals with genetic factors responsible for variations in drug response among individuals."

According to Bennell and Brown,

"Pharmacogenetics is the study concerned with drug responses that are governed by heredity"

All these definitions are given here, because they are well said and explain the subject in few lines, so that, students can have a better idea of the subject at the outset itself.

Inherited Factors that Affects Drug's Action

Many unexpected and peculiar adverse drug reactions occurring in a small percentage of individuals exposed to normal doses of drug is known as idiosyncrasy. This can be explained as genetically determined abnormal reactivity to a drug.

These genetic factors can affect the drugs action by two methods, either by altering drug metabolism or by modifying the individuals response to the drug, according to the Merck's manual. The quantitative abnormalities in the pharmacokinetic parameters (ADME) of the drug can be corrected by altering the dose or dosage interval or both, whereas, nothing can be done with changes in activity or pharmacodynamic of the drug, except to stop the drug altogether.

Though there are many factors that affect the pharmacokinetic of the drug (Chapter 34), we are concerned with inherited factors only in the study of pharmacogenetics. However, out of many pharmacokinetic and pharmacodynamic parameters like absorption, distribution, metabolism and excretion, research has been done mainly on the metabolism, which is considered single major parameter affected by inherited factors. Hence, a detailed study of metabolism of drugs is given below.

It was found most of the drugs that are involved in Adverse Drug reactions (ADR) are metabolized by enzymes with polymorphism. (Phillips, 2001). This and earlier research finding confirmed the role of enzymes in the metabolism of drugs. The quantity of those enzymes is controlled by particular gene and that leads to faster or slower metabolism of drugs. If that particular gene is affected and inherited by an individual, invariably the drugs action is diminished or increased.

Liver is the organ that metabolizes majority of the drugs and it is done by liver by various chemical reactions like oxidation, reduction, hydrolysis, conjugation, acetylation, condensation etc. These reactions are catalyzed and controlled by scores of liver enzymes and defects in them lead to following problems.

(a) *Problem in oxidation*: If an individual has defective gene and that lead to poor oxidation of drugs, he is highly susceptible to drug's toxicity. For example if CYP 2D6 is affected, even the standard doses of metaprolol, haloperidol and flecainide lead to toxicity. Similarly, Polymorphism of CYP 2C9 results in slow metabolism of warfarin and tolbutamide and increases the risk of toxicity.

(b) *Acetylation*: Many drugs are metabolized by liver by this route. N-Acetyl transferase is the enzyme responsible for acetylation of drug molecules to facilitate its elimination. However if the quantity of this enzyme is affected due to defective gene controlling the enzyme, the process of acetylation is affected and hence there are slow acetylators and fast acetylators of drugs. This results in different blood concentrations of drugs like isoniazid and procainamide. Slow acetylation of isoniazid may results in peripheral neuropathy and fast acetylation causes acute hepatocellular necrosis because of fast accumulation of hepatotoxic metabolites. Dapsone is another drug affected by this defect.

(c) *Deficiency of enzymes*: If a gene controlling particular enzyme is affected, the quantity of that enzyme may be deficient to complete the metabolism of drugs. For example glucose-6-phosphate dehydrogenase (G6PD) if secreted in less quantities results in haemolysis. Oxidative drugs such as Antimalarials, sulphonamides and certain analgesics are not properly metabolized because of G6PD deficiency, and results in an exaggerated sensitivity to the haemolytic effect of above oxidant drugs.

Similarly, deficiency of another enzyme Thiopurine Methyl Transferase (TPMT) increase the risk of severe bone marrow suppression and deficiency of the enzyme CYP2D6, which metabolizes codeine, may lead to respiratory side effects.

(d) *Other inherited factors*: Due to inherited factors a malignant hypothermia occurs in rare cases involving muscle relaxants and inhalation anaesthetics, starting with muscular rigidity, tachycardia, arrhythmias, fever, acidosis and shock may occur in those cases. As it leads to death, treatment should be initiated immediately. Anaesthetics should be stopped at once. Similarly about 5% of US population responds abnormally to corticosteroids leading to glaucoma. Genetic Warfarin resistance or sensitivity and porphyria which are precipitated by barbiturates, sulphonamides and phenylbutazone are other genetically inherited factors, to be monitored while treating such cases (Merck's manual).

If the gene responsible for receptors of drugs is affected the activity of drug is also altered. This inherited factor also plays important role in the treatment of patients.

Advantages of Pharmacogenetics

There are several advantages by the study of pharmacogenetics

1. Safer drugs can be used for treatment
2. Potent medicines targeting specific health problem can be developed
3. Individualization of dose is easier.
4. Better vaccines with reduced risk of infections can be produced and
5. Drugs can be produced to suit an individual (Personalized medicines).

1. *Safer drugs*: Now-a-days, drugs are prescribed and used by doctors by trial and error method. It unnecessarily increases not only the treatment period but also the risk of toxicity. If the genetic profile of the patients is known, safer drugs can be prescribed, thereby risk of adverse drug reactions are eliminated.

2. *Potent medicines*: More drugs that are potent can be developed for specific health problems. These drugs can be used to achieve maximum therapeutic benefits with less damage to other parts of the body. Target oriented drugs are recent innovation in the field of drug development where the study of Pharmacogenetics is very much useful.

3. *Individualization of dose*: Instead of determining the doses of drugs based on patient's body weight, age or surface area etc., doses can be calculated based on individual's genetic makeup. For example, slow acetylation or fast acetylation during metabolism of drugs can guide in determining the dose by reducing or increasing it accordingly. As such, it will be an additional tool in the hands of clinical pharmacist, who uses pharmacokinetic parameters of the patient for determining individual dose. Overdose and consequent toxic effects can be thus avoided.

4. *Improved vaccines*: Vaccines can be produced using genetic materials and used for activating our immune system. These vaccines will have the advantages of existing vaccines, at the same time its disadvantage of risk of infection will be considerably reduced.

5. *Personalized medicine*: As the study of pharmacogenetics reveal the role of individual's genetic makeup plays in drugs activity and toxicity, it is possible to produce drugs to suit that particular individual. Thus, medicines can be ordered to be tailor made, to the needs of an individual or group. By genetic engineering and manipulation, it is even possible to introduce a particular gene into a cow or goat to produce particular protein (drug or enzyme) containing milk to be used by patients. Thus, our own cow in the backyard of our home can be used as a drug factory!

Therapeutic Aspects of Pharmacogenetics

The goal of pharmacogenetics is, to use the knowledge for better therapy with drugs. By using this knowledge, not only drug's response and metabolism are studied extensively but also it is used to develop new drugs especially target oriented drugs. Therapeutic aspects, preciously, benefits of pharmacogenetics are detailed below.

1. *Metabolism of drugs:* How enzymes produced by liver control the metabolism of drugs and its deficiency leads to problems for the patient, are already seen above. If the gene responsible for this defective production of enzymes is identified for a particular patient, the treatment regimen can be modified. The doses of drugs metabolized by particular enzyme can be reduced or increased or stopped completely.

2. *Activity of drugs:* It is determined by the number of receptors and their ability to bind the drugs. If there is variation in the genes that has code for the receptors, the binding of drugs to it, is altered, consequently the activity of drug is reduced. For example, it was found, in those patients who were responding poorly for the antiasthmatic drug salbutamol. Similarly ACE Inhibitors work better in peoples of European origin than African origin, due to this genetic factor.

3. *Target oriented drugs:* In some patients, number of receptors varies due to defects in genes that control their production. In metastatic breast cancer, the gene called HER2 is over expressed, and hence, extra protein receptors are produced. This appears to stimulate the breast cells to grow and divide out of control and the cells become cancerous. A monoclonal antibody developed against this HER2 gene product, binds to these excessive receptor sites and thereby limit the cell division and growth of cancer. Thus, genetic screening of the patients can produce target-oriented drugs.

4. *Development of drugs:* Development of new drugs is very costly and time consuming. Pregenetic screening of the persons taking part in clinical trial can make the trial faster and hence less expensive. The national centre for biotechnology information of USA has revealed in its publication "The promise of pharmaco-genomics' the above benefits. In one clinical trial for developing drugs for Alzheimer's disease and other forms of dementia, the gene and its various forms were identified, that lead to development of drug, which is acting, on individual with Alzheimer's disease who have particular form of the gene.

Problems of Pharmacogenetics

It is clear from above discussions that different genes control drugs activities. Sometimes many genes may be involved in determining how an individual reacts to a drug. Hence targeting multiple drugs will become complex. More over very small differences exist in genes, between individuals; therefore identifying them will be very difficult and time consuming.

Drug's effects are also determined or influenced by large number of factors other than genes. Hence, excluding them and fixing particular gene responsible for particular drug's activity is problematic. Continuous and sincere research is needed to use pharmaco-genetics to the advantage of mankind. Moreover, discovering drugs to suit particular group or ethnicity of people many lead to criticism of bios and perception of stigma based on ethnicity. It actually happened during sickle disease screening in America during 1970's among American black population.

Above all, this route to discover new drugs is highly expensive.

Conclusion

Notwithstanding above problems, pharmacogenetics offers, yet another route to solve the problems of patients. It cannot be set aside as such, because, humanity has the history of struggling to achieve better life, throughout the evolution. One-day or other shortcomings and difficulties in research of pharmacogenetics will be solved; hence, we must continue to work hard for a prosperous, diseases free future.

Questions

Short Answer Questions

1. Define pharmacogenetics.
2. Define pharmacogenomics.
3. Differentiate between pharmacogenetics and pharmacogenomics.
4. What are the problems of pharmacogenetics?

Long Answer Questions

5. Explain the inherited factors that affect drug's action.
6. Enumerate the therapeutic aspects of pharmacogenetics. Add a note on advantages of pharmacogenetics.

CHAPTER 30

PATIENT COMPLIANCE

Introduction

If the patients fulfil or follow the instructions given by doctor and/or pharmacist while under treatment, it is known as patient compliance. It mainly depends on the understanding of the patient and to certain extent the severity of the disease. When the disease or troubling symptoms start receding after a few days of treatment, patient's compliance also start receding. Poor understanding of instructions also leads to non compliance. After all treatment is given for his welfare, then why would the patient not cooperate by following the instructions? It is discussed in this chapter.

Definition

"Non-compliance is the situation where the patient is not following the instructions by health care team regarding diet, exercise, rest, return appointment, refilling in addition to the use of drugs".

Self-regulated dose of drugs, as in asthma, diabetes etc, depending on the severity or condition of the patient cannot be termed as non-compliance. It is also true in the case of intermittent treatment with analgesics. Non-compliance by the patients may be due to inadequate instructions by the doctor and/or pharmacist or the failure of them to present the instructions in the manner he understands.

Evidence of Non-compliance

Though patients usually deny non-compliance, the following evidences point to the situation of non-compliance.

Omission of a dose, error in dose, error in the time of administration and taking the drug for wrong purpose, all coming under non-compliance. Also if the patient does not refill his prescription in time or discontinue the treatment prematurely they are described as evidences for non-compliance.

It is more among the out patients because of lack of supervision. It is also prevalent among paediatric and geriatric patients who cannot take their medicines on their own and depend on others for drug administration. These evidences can be used to device the methods of assessing non-compliance as well as the extent or level of non-compliance.

Methods of Assessing Non-compliance

The following are the various methods of assessing non-compliance:

1. Interrogation
2. Verification of left-out medicines on hand
3. Analysis of drugs in body fluids and
4. Use of markers

   1. *Interrogation:* Patients can be thoroughly enquired about their compliance to various instructions by asking clever questions. It is one of the easiest method, does not involve any cost but its accuracy is doubtful because patient may lie and hide the facts which cannot be verified. At the same time it is not feasible to interrogate all the patients every time we suspect non-compliance. Hence other methods have to be followed.

   2. *Verification of balance drugs with the patient:* It is possible to verify the residual medicines available with the patient, so that, his non-compliance can be detected, if excess or less of it is available with him. However it requires efforts as well as money as patient has to go home and bring the balance drugs and therefore the methods accuracy is doubtful.

   3. *Analysis of drugs in body fluids:* It is a feasible and accurate method however it is costlier compared to previous two methods. To analyze the sample, the services of analyst, chemicals, procedure and equipment are needed. By this method only the previous dose can be verified, not the doses of previous days.

   4. *Use of markers:* Some marker compounds are added to the drugs, so that they can be identified in the urine of the patient. Absence of such markers indicates non-compliance by the patient. Though it is a very accurate method, it has almost nil feasibility and cost involved is also prohibitive.

Though so many methods are available to assess the non-compliance they are not much used because it is considered complying with the instructions is the responsibility of the patient, if not, he will be the ultimate sufferer. If some drugs are to be administered compulsorily and non-compliance may lead to severe consequences to the patient as well as to the society, then the patients are admitted in the ward or quarantined, as in the case of infectious diseases, and then the drugs are administered by the nurses or doctors regularly.

In order to assess the seriousness of the problem the level of adherence to the instructions must be calculated. It is calculated using the following formula:

$$\text{Percentage compliance} = \frac{NDP - NME}{NDP} \times 100$$

Where NDP is number of doses prescribed,

NME is number of medication errors.

Less than 90% compliance is not acceptable and hence the reasons for non-compliance should be identified, before finding out the remedy for the problem.

Reasons for Non-compliance

There are many factors responsible for non-compliance. They can be classified into the following categories:

1. Diseases factors
2. Treatment factors
3. Medicine factors and
4. Health professional's factors

1. ***Diseases factors***: Non-compliance depends on the diseases, which require long time treatment like TB. After faithfully following the instructions for some time, patients start drifting willingly or unwillingly. However if the consequences of discontinuing the therapy is brought to their knowledge, they are motivated to adhere to the instructions. Some diseases subside after a few days of treatment and the symptoms disappear and hence patients assume that they are cured and stop taking drugs. The problem is further worsened by lack of symptoms even after discontinuation of drugs. Thus disease factor plays a major role in non-compliance.

2. ***Treatment factors***: Some doctors prescribe multiple drugs for the treatment which leads to non-compliance. Patients either forget one or other drug or willingly stop any of them found not suitable for them. Hence non-essential drugs should not be prescribed. Again if similar looking drugs are prescribed patients get confused and stop taking them or take double dose of the same drug by mistake. Careful prescription can prevent this problem.

Another important problem with treatment is frequency of the dose with single or multiple drugs. There are many chances of missing any of the doses in the course of a day. More the frequency of a dose more is non-compliance. Hence prescriber must go for once a day (sustained release) formulations and combination drugs. Moreover treatment must be finished as quickly as possible, long duration leads to less compliance. This doesn't mean doctor should prescribe highly potent drug for simple ailment.

3. *Medicine factors*: The medicines prescribed to the patient should be acceptable to him. He should be encouraged to bring to the notice of doctor or pharmacist any inconvenience or problem with any of the drug prescribed. Then the particular drug should be substituted with more suitable but equally potent drug. For example the nature of medicine prescribed may disappoint the patient leading to non-compliance. Thus unpleasant taste of liquid medicines, inappropriate package, poor labelling, staining ointments, very big size of the tablet, painful injections all lead to non-compliance.

Moreover, the cost of medicine is also an important contributory factor for non-compliance. Very expensive drugs should not be prescribed, if prescribed often, and not changed, then patient will try to change the doctor rather than adhering to his prescription.

Adverse drug effects of the prescribed medicine are another discouraging factor. If the patient feels sleepy throughout the day or if the drugs like anti psychotic lead to impotence, as and when they realize it, they stop taking the drug. Any amount of counselling will not help in those matters.

4. *Health professional's factors*: Sometimes the instructions given to the patient may not be understood by the patient or he may fail to comprehend the importance of therapy. In such cases they definitely slip to non-compliance. For example, there should not be any uncertainty in the instructions given to the patient. 'If' and 'buts', 'as directed' 'whenever necessary' are all such instructions, patients are unable to decide whether to take the drug or not.

If they are made to wait for a long time to see the doctor or pharmacist, they leave without waiting any further and take the drugs as they like or understood. They are not ready to come back even at a later date fearing this long waiting period. That is why many doctors are disposing the cases with quick diagnosis and prescription. Obviously they have no time to counsel the patients or to explain importance of each drug. Thus health professionals are also responsible for non-compliance by the patient.

Results of Non-compliance

There are many consequences of non-compliance and many are interrelated also. One leads to another problem. For instance, non-compliance first results in under utilization of drugs which not only deprive the patient of any therapeutic benefit, but also, may lead to recurrence of infection. Once relapsed, the infection may not respond to the earlier drug due to development of resistance by the microorganism. There are many examples of resistant microorganisms like Tubercle bacilli and malarial parasite, which are not responding to isoniazid and chloroquin respectively. These resistance organisms are dangerous to the patient as well as his neighbours and consequently society at large.

The situation warrants large doses of present medicament or more potent medicament than the present one, therefore the patients are exposed to greater risk. The problem does not stop here. Under utilization of one drug may result in an excessive response to other drug used simultaneously. For example if digoxin, furosemide, and potassium chloride tablets are prescribed and if the potassium Chloride tablet is not taken by the patient, it leads to more toxic effect of digoxin.

Similarly over utilization of drug is also dangerous due to the risk of side effects. Some patients forget one dose and double the next dose to makeup the loss! Some others think, if one tablet gives so much relief, why not 3 tablets at a time, to get quicker relief. That is their logic! They should be educated to realize how their logic is wrong.

The unused drugs lying in the patient's home leads to the following problems:

  (a)   They may be used inappropriately at a later date

  (b)   Their storage condition is a question mark

  (c)   They may be used accidentally later and

  (d)   They may be used to commit suicide or murder.

Thus non-compliance is not a simple problem as many think. It is a serious problem and hence doctors, nurses and pharmacists must pay required attention.

Remedy for Non-compliance

Having an idea how much serious the problem is, let us discuss the ways and means of tackling it. Non-compliance as such cannot be totally eradicated or stopped. At best compliance can be improved. If the reasons or factors for non-compliance are identified and removed, that leads to better compliance.

All the patients are viewed as potential non-compliers and we must identify the cause of non-compliance and find a solution. Simplification of regimen is one of the best solutions for the problem. If less number of drugs and less number of doses are prescribed, half of the problem will be over.

Patient education is another important tool to achieve better compliance, which can be given to the patient via counselling. During counselling:

  (a)   Patient should be made to realize, he is sick and that has been diagnosed.

  (b)   He should be educated on the consequences of that disease.

  (c)   How the treatment will reduce present or future severity of the disease should be told to him.

  (d)   How the cost of treatment and other disadvantages are nothing considering the benefits of the regimen should be explained.

If counselling on the above lines is carried out for the non-compliers or potential non-compliers, it results in better and successful treatment.

Moreover high standards of dispensing also help in better compliance by the patient, as many of their doubts are cleared by the process. For example if supplementary labels, warning cards, booklets, leaflets and calendar packing are used while dispensing, patients appreciate it and fall in line with the instructions of the pharmacist. But, at the same time excessive information given to patient may lead to self medication or even treatment of dependants at a later period. That must be kept in mind while counselling for compliance.

Conclusion

As pointed out in the forgoing pages, non-compliance is prevalent among outpatients only. By the very nature of their disease, the treatment may be for a short period or even if it is for longer period, their diseases may be of such nature they need not be admitted in the hospital. Only these later cases have to be monitored by the pharmacist for non-compliance. Examples for these cases are diabetics, hypertension, epilepsy, cardiac diseases, TB, asthma and leprosy etc. These people's condition worsens due to various reasons and seasons, one among them is non-compliance. Pharmacists are advised to look for such non-compliers and to take suitable action as detailed above.

Questions

Short Answer Questions

1. Define non-compliance.
2. List the methods of assessing non-compliance.
3. Write a note on effect of non-compliance.
4. How the problem of non-compliance is tackled?

Long Answer Questions

5. Write an essay about non-compliance, its effects and reasons.
6. What are all the factors affecting compliance? How it is solved?
7. Explain the methods of detecting non-compliance. How will you calculate the extent or level of non-compliance?

CHAPTER 31

DRUG THERAPY REVIEW AND THERAPEUTIC DRUG MONITORING

Definition

Drug therapy review is a process by which a clinical pharmacist reviews the patient's treatment regimen, to ensure an effective, safe and economical therapy.

Needless to say, it is the responsibility of the clinical pharmacist to ensure a best therapy possible for each patient. To do that effectively a Clinical Pharmacist must be knowledgeable in pharmacokinetics, pharmacodynamics, therapeutics, ADR, lab data analysis and clinical reasoning. All these require information from various sources and he must be able to interpret and utilize them properly. He should carry out this review daily for complicated cases and periodically for other cases. He must be ready with this review before participating in ward round along with treating physicians.

Purpose of Drug Therapy Review (DTR)

The prime purpose of DTR is effective, safe and economical therapy for all patients. However by undertaking DTR a clinical pharmacist is able to identify

(a) Patients who are in need of counselling

(b) Patients who require special attention and

(c) Patients with the risk of medication error.

To achieve these purposes, the DTR must be broad based and multicomponent in nature. They are discussed below:

Scope of DTR

Drug Therapy Review (DTR) is a broad function of which Therapeutic Drug Monitoring (TDM) is one of the components. In order to perform DTR the clinical pharmacist need to prepare pre hand. DTR is actually the review of the entire therapy of the patients with drugs. Hence, to arrive at a correct conclusion, clinical pharmacist should know the previous and present condition of the patient. He has to assess the treatment goals, and how far and how best it is achievable. He must be sure whether the present therapy is proceeding on the correct line to achieve the set goal.

It may not be easy for complicated cases and sometimes difficult even for cases with manageable problems as there are many chances of patients developing complications during the course of treatment. For example there could be drug related problems like non-responsiveness to standard drug regimen, sub therapeutic dose, over dosage, adverse drug reactions including drug-drug interaction, drug-food interaction or drug-disease interaction.

Hence therapeutic drug monitoring (TDM) by body fluid analysis or pharmacokinetic studies should be carried out wherever necessary. Using the data obtained from TDM, the dose of the drug should be individualized and a correct regimen arrived at.

Thereafter again the therapy must be monitored closely in order to find out treatment outcome. Thus the scope of DTR extends from patient medication history to TDM and beyond.

Duties Involved in DTR

As indicated above the first and foremost duty involved in DTR is collecting as much as information about the patient's previous and present condition. This includes collecting information about patients past medical history, including prevailing diseases before present illness and treatment undertaken or undergoing, allergy or sensitivity to drugs, habits, daily routines etc. Along with the above detail, present condition, treatment and clinical progress or otherwise will lay the foundation for drug therapy review.

This information can be gathered from various sources like patient's medication history interview, laboratory results, nursing notes, observational charts and case sheets. As described elsewhere in this book, value of medication history interview is well known that, it not only reveal almost everything about patient's present and past problems, it also helps in finding etiology or reasons for present problem and for arriving at a correct diagnosis and drug regimen. An interview conducted by a Clinical Pharmacist can also reveal the drugs already used by the patient, especially OTC drugs, drugs from alternative systems of medicine, house hold remedies etc.

The next important duty in DTR is setting and evaluating the treatment target or goal. Complete cure is what patients wanted but that may not be always possible. Hence a realistic target must be fixed like reduction of severity of disease, elimination of signs and symptoms of disease, slowing advancement of disease etc. The treatment goals are obviously patient-specific and vary patient to patient due to patient's age, weakness or susceptibility etc. This target or goal of therapy should be reviewed periodically and the progress evaluated. Suitable corrections can be made in that target and the reasons for failure analyzed. For this the entire team involved in the treatment of the particular patient is consulted and involved actively in the correction process.

Another crucial duty in DTR is identification of drug related problems occurred during the present therapy. If the treatment is in a hospital where, clinical pharmacist's services are available, problems like inappropriate drug selection, sub-therapeutic dose or over dosages are less. However even these problems may occur in few cases, hence a quick review must be carried out in these aspects also during DTR. More series problems like complications due to untreated indications or patients multiple diseases or organ failures, adverse drug reactions occurred during the course of treatment etc has to be reviewed carefully.

Once the drug related problems, if any, is identified and resolved, the next step is to correct the regimen to suit to the individual patient. This can be achieved by switching over to sustained release or once a day formulations, changing the route of administration, time of administrations etc. While changing the regimen to suit the individual, care must be taken to maintain cost effectiveness of the therapy and also ensure compliance of the regimen by the patient. Multiple drug prescriptions or poly pharmacy must be controlled as far as possible by including combination drugs wherever possible.

After carrying out all the duties during DTR, as detailed above, the results of the treatment must be monitored. For this the clinical review and tests carried out by and on the instructions of the treating physician are highly useful. The laboratory data such as the results of blood tests, x-ray, scan, liver function tests, kidney function tests, etc can be used for the purpose of monitoring. Some drugs may produce the desired results after a fairly long time. For example antidepressants require 30 to 40 days to produce response in patients. However if a drug does not produce the required result within a reasonable time, a careful review of drug prescribed must be made. Dose increase or replacement of a drug with some other drug or addition of one more drug to the regimen, may be needed.

Medication Chart Review

This is one of the important duties assigned to clinical pharmacists in developed countries, in order to prevent medication errors and to ensure best treatment possible to the patients. It has become an essential function in those countries, because patients sue the doctors and hospitals for a very huge sum as compensation in the courts, if anything goes wrong during the course of treatment. As, such a situation does not exist in our country, but slowly and steadily picking up, medication chart review is yet to be implemented here. However, the future pharmacists need to know the process of medication chart review as these duties will also be assigned to him in India, sooner or later.

Medication errors are preventable errors that may occur during prescription writing and/or drug administration. To prevent those errors, pharmacists must systematically review the medication charts. The following are the guidelines to carryout medication chart review:

1. Poorly written, illegible prescriptions should be returned to the prescriber and checked. It should not be guessed.

2. Identity of the patient must be clear, for which the name, age, sex, hospital number etc, of the patient should be clearly written on the medication chart. If not, check and write

3. If the patient is allergic to some drugs or tests it should be legibly written on the space provided in the medication chart with red ink. If no allergies are reported or identified it should also be mentioned in that place.

4. The name of the drug, dose and route of administration should be written by the treating physician and it should be checked. No abbreviations should be used to write the name of the drug. As far as possible, generic names should be written on the chart, if not written, pharmacist should write it, next to the brand name. Dose and dosage interval should be correct and as intended by the doctor depends on the patient's condition. Any extraordinary dose should be underlined by him, to indicate he mean it. Decimals should be avoided as far as possible, as it may lead to ten times more dose, if not seen. For example it should be 5 mg, not 5.0 mg and 0.5 gm, not .5 gm.

5. Time of administration should also be mentioned in the medication chart. If it is not suitable for the particular patient, for example, if there is possibility of Drug-Drug interaction or drug-food interaction, pharmacist can write annotation on the chart, recommending change in time of administration of the particular drug.

6. Prescriptions with instructions like SOS (as required or whenever necessary) should have minimum dose interval to be adhered, otherwise, there is a possibility of over dosage.

7. Additional instructions like after food, before food, with plenty of water etc., can be written by the clinical pharmacist wherever necessary.

8. The medications should be prescribed according to legal and local requirements of the government concerned. It should be signed and dated by the prescriber and any corrections in the medication chart should be endorsed by him.

9. The medication chart should also be signed by the nurse who administers the drug to the patient, in the space provided. Thus the medication chart will be a complete and authentic record of treatment given to the patient.

Model Mediation Chart
XYZ Hospital

Patient name: .... IP No: .... Unit: ....

Age: ....Sex: ....Height: ....Weight: ....

Allergy: ....

S. No.	Name of the drug	Dose	Route	Time of admn.	Day of administration (Nurse initials)							
					1st	2nd	3rd	4th	5th	6th	7th	8th
1.				8 am 2 pm 8 pm								
	Additional instructions											
	Signature of doctor with date											
2.												
	Additional instructions											
	Signature of doctor with date											
3.												
	Additional instructions											
	Signature of doctor with date											
4.												
	Additional instructions											
	Signature of doctor with date											
5.												
	Additional instructions											
	Signature of doctor with date											

Therapeutic Drug Monitoring

TDM is a process of monitoring drugs given to patients, by measuring the drug concentration in patient's body fluids and analyzing other vital parameters.

It is one of the important aspects of drug therapy review to monitor the drugs used in therapy. It is done by analyzing the body fluids of the patient periodically and regularly. Based on the pharmacokinetics of the drug used on the particular patient, critical clinical decisions are made. Drug concentration measured in the body fluids of an individual patient is used to give optimum drug regimen for the patient. Ideal therapy can be given to a patient only by individualization of dose and drug regimen and that is possible only by proper TDM.

Drugs Suitable for TDM

TDM cannot be undertaken for all the patients and for all drugs. That is impossible and unnecessary also. Cost of TDM is one of the prohibitory factors. Hence we have to select the drugs for which TDM must be carried out. The criteria for selecting such drugs are outlined below:

1. *Drugs with narrow therapeutic index*: Therapeutic index can be defined as the difference between safe therapeutic dose and toxic dose. Wider the difference, safer will be the drug. However, if there is narrow difference between the two doses, the drug has to be used with caution. In order to arrive at a correct dose that produces the desirable effect and to prevent it from reaching toxic concentration, therapeutic drug monitoring should be done. For example, drugs like, amino glycosides, antineoplastic drugs and cardiac glycosides must be monitored by TDM.

2. *Drugs with varying pharmacokinetic properties*: The amount of drug which reaches the systemic circulation – the bioavailability – differs not only between drugs but also between individuals and between different dosage forms of the same drug. Hence such drugs should be monitored. Absorption, distribution, metabolism and excretion of these drugs play major role in the variation of bioavailability of them in individual patients.

3. *Drugs that produce different amount of effect*: Some drugs produce huge effects on some patients or produce little effect on some other patients for the same dose. This variation is due to many factors, one among them is concentration of drug that reaches the site of action and consequent effect it produce. There may or may not be correlation between the amounts of drug at the site of action and in plasma. Drugs protein binding on tissue protein and diffusion rate through the membrane may also be the factors for the above difference. This inter individual variability in pharmacodynamic or effect of drugs, is one of the complication of TDM. However TDM helps in identifying such drugs and such patients, thereby necessary precautions can be followed, while treating such cases. E.g. Sodium valproate.

4. TDM is essential, if the patient is not responding to standard drug regimen for a considerable time.

5. This non responsiveness to standard drugs may be due to non-compliance or drug resistance. In order to find out the real reason, TDM must be performed.

6. Many times, drug toxicity symptoms are mistaken for disease manifestations. For example increase in creatinine level in patients may be due to disease or graft rejection. Cyclosporine which is used to suppress the patient's immunity may produce this toxic effect and hence TDM should be carried out for such drugs.

7. Some drugs produce huge effects even for a small increase in dose. Such drugs are said to have non-linear kinetics in its action. For example Phenytoin produces disproportionate effect for a small dose increase. These drugs should be monitored by TDM.

8. We know with certainty that some drugs if reaches toxic range in the body produce series side effects. Needless to mention, such drugs should be closely monitored.

9. If a drug's pharmacological effect cannot be measured by any means such drugs should be obviously watched.

10. Drugs that are given to infants and drug reaction cases under extra-ordinary circumstances have to be monitored.

11. Pharmacokinetics of drugs is certainly altered in some cases and conditions such as in anaemia, pregnancy, liver damage, kidney damage etc. Hence TDM is must for these cases and conditions.

12. Because of non-availability of alternatives, we may have to administer together the drugs which have potential to interact. For example anti T.B and anti epileptic drugs, if given together may interact and produce side effects. Even if measures like dosage interval are maintained between these drugs, TDM must be undertaken to ensure safety of the patient.

Thus, TDM has to be ordered by treating physicians for drugs like, digoxin, lithium, quinidine, propranolol, salicylates, phenobarbitone, theophylline, phenytoin, amino glycosides, procainamide and methotrexate.

Development of TDM Services

A. *Organization*: As the TDM involve many services like sample collection, sample analysis, interpretation of results and taking appropriate clinical and therapeutic decisions, specialists in all these fields must be employed. Thus the services of suitably trained physician, clinical pharmacologist, clinical biochemist, and clinical pharmacist are required to run an effective TDM service. Suitable analytical methods for sample analysis, expertise in analyzing those samples, producing results within a short period possible are also essential to perform TDM.

B. *Functioning*: First of all, a treating physician must request for TDM services for the patient, if the expected clinical results are not produced for standard or special drug regimen. Thereafter the sample is drawn (usually body fluids) from the patient and analyzed by clinical pharmacist or analyst. With his knowledge in pharmacokinetics of drugs, clinical pharmacist is most suitable for this job and also to interpret the results. Then the results are conveyed to the physician who requested the service, in writing, along with clinical suggestion on refinement of current drug therapy. Patient has to pay for the TDM service.

C. Information required for TDM service

1. *Information about patient*: All relevant information about the patient should be provided to the clinical pharmacist to interpret the results, to calculate the dose and to suggest refinement to the therapy. Hence not only the usual information like patient's age, sex, height and weight, but also other conditions, pharmacological status etc., should be provided in the request to TDM service. If not provided, this information should be collected at the time of drawing sample from the patient.

2. *Sample time*: Usually sample is drawn at an appropriate time depends on the body fluid to be collected, like blood, urine etc. If blood is collected from the patient, it should be between two doses, when the concentration is low. Care should also be taken that patient is in steady state while drawing the sample. However peak concentrations are to be measured in certain cases like IV administration of antibiotics, theophylline and antiarrhythmic drugs. This time of collection of sample should be mentioned in the analytical records.

3. *Interpretation of blood drug concentration*: Plasma concentration should be compared with therapeutic range for the given drug. If excess, reassessment should be carried out; if below range, appropriate corrections should be made in the dose to bring levels closer to the equated range. For doing this, knowledge of pharmacokinetics, pharmacodynamic and expertise are needed. Interpretation of results should be in the light of clinical situation of the patient, arrived at from the information provided.

Problems in TDM

1. *Analytical methods*: In order to save the cost many assays of TDM are carried out using low cost equipments or methods. For example most of the assays are done using Calorimeter or Spectrophotometer, rather than HPLC which is more accurate. Drugs which produce fluorescent metabolites should not be analyzed using spectoflurimetric methods, as in the case quinidine, as it gives twice the quantity as result, than HPLC method.

Similarly Radio Immuno Assay (RIA) is a problem in measuring digoxin concentration. Some, circulating natural substances in new born infants show positive result for quinidine concentration by RIA method, even though they are not given quinidine. Hence non-specific methods of analysis are great problem with TDM.

2. *Altered protein binding*: Protein binding of drugs and consequent free drug concentration in blood depends on many factors. It is altered due to disease conditions. Hence measuring plasma drug concentration become useless, if not correlated with other measurements.

3. *Quality control problems*:

   A. Interferences with drug assay by other substances: Combination of drugs is one of the major problem in analysis for example, gentamicin with gallium, phenytoin with phenobarbitone and digoxin with prednisolone interfere in analysis.

   B. Stereoisomer: Many drugs are administered as mixture if isomers. Though they are chemically same compounds, differ vastly in their pharmacological actions. Hence mere assay of mixture of isomers will not help in determining the pharmacokinetics and pharmacodynamics of the drug. E.g. Verapamil.

   C. Active metabolites: Some metabolites are also active; some times more than the parent drug, hence TDM should assay both these compounds while deciding corrections in regimen. E.g. Procainamide and its active metabolite. N-acetylprocainamide and 3-hydroxy quinidine and quinidine.

   D. Many TDM assay results are not accurate or reproducible hence difficult to rely upon.

4. Apart from this, factors that make measurement of plasma concentration useless also affects the TDM, they are:

   A. Drugs whose response is easily measurable: (e.g.) Diuretics, hypoglycemics

   B. Drugs that are activated in body (e.g.) Levodopa.

   C. 'Hit and Run' drugs, whose effects last much longer than the drug itself (e.g., Reserpine, MAO inhibitors) and

   D. Drugs with irreversible action (e.g.: Organophosphates and anticholine-starases)

Competence to carry out DTR and TDM

In order to carry out the above complicated services of DTR and TDM – the very important functions of a Clinical Pharmacist – he should have skill and competence. For that his clinical pharmacy services should be evaluated and its quality assured. How it is done is discussed below:

Quality Assurance of Clinical Pharmacy Services

Introduction

The words quality assurance themselves self explanatory that it is about guarantee of quality of any product or service. Clinical Pharmacy services can not be an exemption from the expectations of increasingly quality conscious world. The service requires demonstrating its competence as well as performance not only to the patients but also to the fellow health care providers. After the Bristol Royal Infirmary Enquiry in 2001 in Briton into pediatric cardiac surgery, there has been lot of importance given to the competence of health care providers. The questions raised, then were what the overall standard of care given to the patients and how well the consistency of these services were maintained? Hence these services are subjected to appraisal from then on.

Appraisal of Quality

In order to appraise something we need to have some standards against which the quality of service can be compared and evaluated. Hence for clinical pharmacy services we have to set some standards first. As this branch of pharmacy is new, just few decades old and yet to be introduced in many countries, fixing standards is not that easy. However few performance indicators were developed recently, among them rate of intervention in therapy by clinical pharmacist is considered significant.

Intervention just for the sake of intervention will not stand scrutiny of strict standards. Interventions which are really beneficial and corrected the course of treatment after acceptance by the clinicians are taken in to account. Similarly suggestions, comments and ideas given during the therapy by clinical pharmacists are recorded and taken up for appraisal.

Range of Services and their Appraisal

A clinical pharmacist is not only participating , intervening and evaluating drug therapy in the wards, he also conduct medication history interview, suggests medicines suitable for the patient, helps in individualization of dose, monitor treatment for ADR and offer counseling for the patient during and after the treatment. Hence all these services should be evaluated to appraise the quality of services from clinical pharmacists. For example a well taken, complete and accurate medication interview by clinical pharmacist not only helps the doctor to diagnose the problem quickly but also avoid unnecessary medications and tests on the patient. This results in less expenses, faster recovery and early discharge of the patient who appreciate the services of the hospital. Similarly prevention of repetition of ineffective drugs and ADR including drug interaction, consequently the sufferings of the patient speak volumes about the merit of clinical pharmacy services. Finally patient counseling take the clinical pharmacist to the patient's well wishers circle and the patient start developing rapport with clinical pharmacist and the health care team.

Patient start obliging with all instructions of health care team faithfully including sending feed back after his discharge.

Truly speaking, numbers of patients who are satisfied, partially satisfied or not satisfied are the real appraisers of the clinical pharmacy services of the particular hospital. However health care authorities have developed some tools for evaluation of clinical pharmacy services which are discussed below.

Ensuring Quality of Clinical Pharmacy Services – The Tools

1. Needless to mention, any service needs competent persons to provide those services without fault, as far as possible. Hence some regulations to maintain competence of the staff are framed by which some competencies like, patient care competency, problem solving competency and professional competency are tested by examinations. Clinical pharmacists must demonstrate competence in a range of clinical pharmacy functions by passing them.

2. Performance appraisal is done by various methods like mini clinical examination, Mini-peer assessment and case based discussions. They are given in "General Level Framework" [GLF] Hand book published by Competency Development and Evaluation Group [www.codeg.org] for pharmacy practitioners. Students in Clinical Pharmacy should go through such wonderful resources and qualify themselves.

3. Professional development is a continuous process; a clinical pharmacist should undertake such programs regularly during his career. These refresher courses definitely improve the quality of clinical pharmacy services in a hospital by satisfying expectations of the job.

4. Finally all the clinical pharmacy services must be revalidated at fixed time interval to improve them. These improvements should be brought to the notice of health care team. Subsequent revalidations, ultimately firm up these standards and thus quality clinical pharmacy services can be assured.

Questions

Short Answer Questions

1. Define drug therapy review.
2. What is the purpose of drug therapy review?
3. Write a note on scope of DTR.
4. Define therapeutic drug monitoring.
5. What is the information required for TDM service?
6. Write a note on the problems of TDM.
7. What are the tools to ensure quality of clinical pharmacy services?

Long Answer Questions

8. Explain the process of drug therapy review by Clinical Pharmacist.

9. How the medication chart review is carried out? Explain in detail.

10. How will you select a drug for therapeutic drug monitoring?

11. Enumerate the development of TDM services.

12. How will you assure the quality of clinical pharmacy services?

Chapter 32

Patient Data Analysis

Patient Data

These are the data collected from the clinical laboratory tests carried out on a patient. These data are very much useful in diagnosis, prevention and treatment of diseases. However in order to arrive at a decision, a reference standard is essential. This reference is usually available in the form of quantitative range which is obtained by testing normal disease free individuals. While interpreting this data, one has to be careful in that, they always not reflecting the true condition of the patient. If anyone of such parameter is in excess of the range, it does not mean the person has got a disease. Similarly if it is lower than the range, that also not indicative of any series problem with the patient. All these data has to be viewed along with other signs and symptoms. There are many individual variables also like age, sex, weight, body mass, disease etc., that affect the results of these laboratory tests. Hence, a series of tests is to be carried out before arriving at a conclusion and to eliminate errors.

Need for Analysis of Data

The main duty of a clinical pharmacist is to individualize the dose and drug regimen of the patient, for which he has to rely upon pharmacokinetic data, as well as routine haematological data. Hence he should possess at least a working knowledge of the significance of lab tests. Using that knowledge, he has to evaluate the outcome of the treatment so far given and recommend to the treating physician, the changes to be made in the drugs or doses or treatment itself.

Also, depends on these results he has to determine the appropriateness of the treatment, efficacy of the treatment and also the drug's toxic effect, if any, occurred. Thus patient data analysis plays a major role in safe and effective therapy.

Fluid and Electrolytes Balance

Fluid and electrolytes are the important component of any living organism and they have to be in constant concentration and in balance so as the body to function properly. The self regulatory, feed back controlled stabilization of body as a whole or any sub system like fluid and electrolytes balance is known as Homeostasis. [Homeo – of similarity, Stasis – stopping the flow]. Water or fluid, electrolytes and acid-base balance are interrelated and kidney plays an important role in their balance.

Let us discuss, what disturbs their balance, what happens, when they are in excess or less and steps to be taken to restore their balance, etc in this chapter.

Water: Human body has lot of water, that is, up to 50 to 60% of total body weight is water. It is required to maintain body temperature and in metabolic reactions. They are the vehicles to carry solutes from one part of our body to another part of our body. It is distributed as intercellular fluid [ICF] and extracellular fluid [ECF] at the ratio of 2:1. That is about 28 liter of water is present in ICF and 14 liter in ECF. The ECF is further classified into interstitial fluids [10.5 lit] and intra vascular fluid or plasma [3.5 lit]. Body regulates this balance by controlling water input and output.

Regulation of water intake: Depends on the climate and habit we drink 0.5 to 5 lit of water per day. This apart our solid food also contains some water. They are together called as exogenous water and mainly controlled by thirst center present in hypothalamus. It is stimulated whenever water level in our body goes down below the optimum level. Some amount of water is produced in our body itself by metabolic reactions which is known as endogenous water and about 100 ml is produced like this.

Regulation of water output: Water is excreted by kidney via urine, skin via sweat, lungs via exhaled air and G.I tract through feces. Out of these four, urine is the major source of elimination of water. About 1 to 2 liter of urine is excreted every day and it is controlled by vasopressin or antidiuretic hormone [ADH] secreted by pituitary gland. The secretion of this hormone in turn is regulated by osmotic pressure of plasma. Skin excretes about 400 ml to 450 ml of water through sweating which depends on climate [Temperature and Humidity]. Lung excretes water through exhaled air, almost the same amount as skin, i.e., 400 ml per day. Loss of water through GI tract via feces is estimated to be around 150 ml per day and needless to mention it is many times more in diarrhoea. Excess or less water intake or output leads to over hydration or dehydration respectively.

Over hydration: It is the retention of water in the body due to excessive intake of water, kidney failure or abnormal production of antidiuretic hormone [ADH]. This may lead to headache and even convulsions. It is treated with hypertonic saline solution and complete stoppage of water intake until patient recovers.

Dehydration: It is common in excess of loss of fluid during diarrhoea, dysentery and Cholera. There is loss of water from body after fire accident [burns] and in excess vomiting or sweating. Usually in these conditions not only body water is lost, also the electrolytes Na^+, K^+ etc. Dehydration is characterized by less urine output, shrunken cells of body due to excretion of water even from intercellular space and increased protein destruction. Protein and urea concentrations are thus increased in blood. Clinical symptoms of dehydration are low B.P, increased pulse, sunken eye balls etc. Usually dehydration is treated with oral rehydration salt [ORS], where plenty of water is given orally. If it is not possible for any reason, 5% glucose or Normal Saline or Glucose saline injections are given intravenously.

Electrolytes

Electrolytes are inorganic salts which undergo dissolution in solution and exist as positively and negatively charged ions in animal body. For example Sodium Chloride dissociate in to Na+ [cation] and Cl⁻ [anion]. They are measured in milliequivalents [mEq/l]. Number of gram of a substance required to combine or displace one gram of hydrogen is known as milliequivalents weight and also its one thousandth part known as milliequivalents. It is calculated by the following formula:

$$mEq/1 = \frac{mg \text{ per liter} \times valency}{Atomic \text{ weight}}$$

To maintain osmotic and water balance, electrolytes are well distributed in body fluids. As the electrolytes are in the form anion and cation, they have to be in equilibrium to maintain electrical neutrality.

To describe the electrolyte balance we need to understand some words like osmolarity and osmolality which are used to explain the concentration of these molecules. Osmolarity is about moles or millimoles of electrolytes per liter of solution. On the other hand osmolality measure the solute present in a fluid. It is defined as moles or millimoles per kg of solvent. If the solvent is pure water there is no difference between osmolarity and osmolality. But obviously body fluids are not pure water and have lot of constituents like proteins. Hence osmolality is invariably used to describe the concentration of molecules.

The electrolytes are important for proper functioning of cells. It has to be balanced not only in ECF but also in ICF, because the ratio between them is important. Though this ratio is critical their mechanism is very complex. We study mainly the concentration of electrolyte in plasma but to get a true picture of them we need to go for some ancillary studies also. For example, certain electrolytes like calcium and phosphate are present in hard tissues like bone and teeth.

Osmolality of Plasma, ECF AND ICF

Electrolytes are not equally distributed between ECF and ICF. For instance, Sodium is the major cation of ECF and Chlorides and bicarbonates are its anion. On the other hand Potassium is the predominant cation of ICF, phosphates and sulphates are its anions. Only water moves freely between cells but electrolytes require active transport mechanism for its movement between cells. Though electrolyte concentration differs between ECF and ICF, their osmolarity is equal.

The osmolality of plasma is measured by osmometer and it is from 285 to 295 milliosmoles per kg. Sodium and its anions are major contributors [up to 90%] for this osmolality of plasma.

Balancing Electrolytes

Electrolytes are balanced mainly by three hormones, Aldosterone, Antidiuretic hormone and Renin angiotensin and also by food intake. Aldosterone increase sodium reabsorption which increases osmolality of plasma. This in turn stimulates hypothalamus to release ADH which on its part increases water reabsorption. Thus all these hormones are interrelated and function in coordination to maintain normal fluid and electrolyte balance. Rennin angiotensin regulates the flow of aldosterone in this complex process.

Our body requirement of electrolytes is usually met by balanced diet. During summer months we may need to support our body with extra electrolytes. The normal range of these electrolytes and water are given in Table 32.1.

Table 32.1 Normal Values of Electrolytes

Electrolytes	In serum	In urine
Sodium	135 -155 mEq/L	150 – 197 mEq/ day
Potassium	3.9 -5.6 mEq/L	20 -64 mEq/ day
Calcium	8.8 -10.2 mEq/L	--
Chloride	95 – 106 mEq/L	180 – 270 mEq/day
Total anions	154 mEq/L	--
Total cations	154 mEq/L	--

Estimation of Electrolytes

Body fluids are analysed for the estimation of electrolytes using various instrumental methods. Flame photometry, x-ray fluorescence, Atomic absorption spectrometry and colorimetric techniques are used in the identification and estimation of anions and cations in the body fluids. Recent advanced methods determine both anions and cations simultaneously. Normally sodium and potassium in serum are estimated either by Flame photometry or specific Atomic absorption spectrometry. Chloride is determined potentiometrically using silver–silver chloride pH electrodes. Calcium in urine or serum is estimated by EDTA method of analysis or Atomic absorption spectroscopy or Flame photometry. Magnesium is measured by ion-specific electrode and trace elements like copper, zinc and iron are determined by flame photometric or colorimetric methods.

Uses of Study of Electrolyte Balance

The study of electrolytes balances are useful indicators of renal and cardiac failure, anuria, adrenal cortical insufficiency and excess of electrolyte excretion. Pancreatic cystic fibrosis is detected by excess of chloride ions in the perspiration of patients. Thus the study of electrolyte and water balance is useful as a valuable diagnostic tool. As the analysis of metabolic excretion rates are carried out in these studies, it is useful to evaluate the functions of various organs like, liver, kidney, thyroid and other glands, which are dealt with elsewhere in this chapter.

Disturbance of Electrolyte Balance

Severe excess or less of electrolytes in the body leads to various disorders/ diseases. They are indicated by many clinical symptoms and are treatable. The cause of disturbed balance of electrolytes are many and outside the preview of this chapter, however, as a Clinical pharmacist is concerned with effect of drugs which may be the reason for such conditions they are listed here in a tabular form.

Table 32.2 Effect of Drugs on Electrolytes Balance

Condition	Sodium	Potassium	Calcium	Phosphates
Excess	Hypernatraemia	Hyperkalaemia	Hypercalcaemia	Hyperphosphataemia
Symptoms	Muscle weakness, confusion, etc	Asymptomatic but fatal	Seen in Malignancy and Renal transplantation	Seen in renal failure, Hypo para thyroidis
Possible causative drugs for excess	Phenytoin, Methyl Dopa, oral Contraceptives, Clonidine, Corticosteroid, etc	Digoxin, Isoniazid, Tetracycline, NSAID, Cyclosporine, Penicillin, etc	Lithium, Tamoxifen, Diuretics, etc	All drugs causing kidney damage
Less [Deficient]	Hyponatraemia	Hypokalaemia	Hypocalcaemia	Hypophosphataemia
Symptoms	Nausia,Confusion, Drowsiness, etc	Muscle weakness, Hypotonia, Depression, Confusion, etc	Seen in Pancreatitis, Liver disease, Kidney disease, Vitamin D deficiency, etc	Muscle weakness
Possible drugs responsible for deficiency	Diuretics, Heparin, NSAID, Tolbutamide, Amphotericin, Miconazole, etc	Aspirin, Corticosteroids, Gentamicin, Insulin, Laxatives, Salicylates, etc	Phenytoin, Phenobarbitone, Aminoglycosides, Furasimide,etc	All drugs causing kidney damage

Haematology Data

Among the tests performed on a patient, blood test is the one which helps the physician more than any other test. The characters of blood cells and other components give first line of diagnostic features about the diseases, deficiencies or defects that affect the human body. Hence a Clinical Pharmacist must be thorough with these tests.

1. **RBC count:** The normal range of Red Blood Cells in males is 4.4 to 6.1 × 10^{12}/L and 4.0 to 5.5 × 10^{12}/L in females. If it is less, the condition is called anaemia and if excess it is known as hypoxia. Anaemia may be microcytic due to iron deficiency or macrocytic due to folic acid and vitamin B_{12} deficiency.

2. *Reticulocyte count*: It should be 0.5% to 1% of RBC. In haemorrhage and haemolysis it goes up to 40% of RBC. Reticulocyte count is useful to evaluate the response of bone marrow to iron, foliate, vitamin B_{12} therapy.

3. *Mean Cell Volume* **(MCV)**: It is average volume of single red cell. It is measured in Femto litres (10^{-15} L). If the MCV is low it is known as microcytic MCV and if it is high called as macrocytic MCV. The former MCV is due to deficiency of iron and the later is due to folic acid deficiency.

4. *Packed Cell Volume* **(PCV)**: It is the ratio of the volume occupied by red cells to the total volume of blood. Normal value is 45%. Now-a-days it is calculated by multiplying MCV and RBC. PCV is decreased in anaemia, haemolysis and haemorrhage, whereas it is increased in polycythaemia. Obviously it is altered in macrocytosis and microcytosis.

5. *Mean Cell Haemoglobin Concentration* **(MCHC)**: It is a measure of the average concentration of Haemoglobin in 100 ml of red cells. It is measured in grams/lit or as percentage. The normal value is 315 to 345 g/L. If it is low, iron deficiency anaemia is the reason and if it is on higher side, severe, prolonged dehydration is indicated.

6. *Haemoglobin*: It is one of the important measurements in blood tests. It differs depends on sex, man has more Haemoglobin than woman, due to presence of more RBC and menstrual loss respectively. The normal value of men is 13.5 to 17 g/dl and a woman is 11.5 to 16.5 g/dl. Less than these values indicate anaemia.

7. *Platelets* **(Thrombocytes)**: It is formed in bone marrow. If it is synthesized less in bone marrow or destructed after formation, less number is seen in blood analysis. As it has a short life of only 8 to 12 days, it is easy to evaluate drug induced thrombocytopenia (less number). It comes back to normal level once the drug is stopped. Less number of platelet may also be due to pregnancy, viral infection or bleeding. Increased number is seen in Malignancy and inflammatory diseases. The normal value of platelet is 150 to 450×10^9/l.

8. *White Blood Cells* **(Leucocytes)**: This is one of the very important blood components and its character and count in blood tests reveal lot of information about the condition of the patient. There are two types WBC, namely Granulocytes and Agranulocytes (Lymphocytes). Granulocytes are further sub-divided into monocytes and polymorphonuclear granulocytes which consist of Neutrophil, Basophil and Eosinophil. Usually WBC is measured and reported as Total Count (TC) and as differential Count (DC) which lists the number of various types of polymorphonuclear granulocytes.

   (a) *Neutrophils*: They form the majority of white cells. The normal range is from 50% to 70% of total white blood cells. If it is more there may be inflammation or tissue damage in patients, on the other hand, if it is less it indicates malignancy or hepatitis.

(b) *Basophiles*: It is less than 1% of white cells. Its function is not clear. However it is found less in malignancy conditions.

(c) *Eosinophils*: The normal value of Eosinophil is less than 6% of TC. It is increased in allergic conditions like asthma, Hay fever, drug sensitivity and malignant diseases.

(d) *Monocytes*: It forms 0% to 7% of total white cells. They are increased in infections like TB, typhoid etc.

(e) *Lymphocytes*: It is mainly found in spleen and other lymphatic tissue. However it is present in large numbers next to neutrophiles in the blood. The normal value is 20% to 40%, increased in viral infections like Infectious hepatitis, decreased in AIDS, Renal failure and cardiac failure.

9. *Erythrocyte Sedimentation Rate* (ESR): ESR is a measure of sedimentation rate of red cells in a sample of blood containing an anticoagulant over a period of one hour in a cylindrical tube. The normal value is less than 10 mm/hr. It is increased in rheumatoid arthritis, inflammatory bowel diseases, malignancies and infections.

10. *Bleeding time*: It is the time taken by the blood to stop from the bleeding wound. It shows the haemostatic efficiency of the blood. Normally blood should stop within 2 to 5 minutes. It is increased in thrombocytopenia, platelet disorders and prolonged use of aspirin and anticoagulants. Hence clinical pharmacist should take care in these conditions of the patient.

11. *Whole blood clotting time*: It is the time taken by the blood to clot when tested outside the body (*in vitro*). Normal range is 4 to 9 minutes at 37°C. Prolonged time indicates haemophilia or factor 8 deficiencies or presence of anticoagulants.

12. *Prothrombin Time* (PT): It is the time required to clot citrated plasma to which an optimum amount of thromboplastin and calcium has been added. Usual prothrombin time is 12 to 15 seconds. The PT is usually indicated as a ratio known as International Normalized Ratio (INR) which is the ratio of PT of the patient and the normal (disease free) man. The result of oral anticoagulant therapy can be monitored using PT. Also it is useful to evaluate liver function.

13. *Blood sugar*: Blood sugar level is an important parameter that is usually checked for patients. A fasting blood glucose level of 70 to 110 mg/dl is considered normal. It is usually increased in diabetes. However it cannot be confirmed by this elevation alone as other conditions like severe nephritis, pancreatic disease, hyperthyroidism and certain liver diseases also increase blood sugar level. Hence glucose tolerance test [GTT] should be done on the suspected cases. 50 gm of glucose is given to the patient. Blood sugar level reaches maximum within a short while and should return to normal within 1hour 30 minutes to 2 hours. If it is not, and more than 50% in excess of fasting sugar level, it is confirming diabetes. Similarly low sugar levels indicate hypopituitarism, cretinism or hypothyroidism.

14. ***Serum enzymes*: *Alkaline Phosphate* ALP (or) AP:** It is present in liver, bone, intestinal wall and placenta. Each of the above sites produce specific isoenzyme of AP. Normal range of AP is 30 to 90 IU/L. It is increased in jaundice, osteomalacia, rickets and in low absorption of vitamin D and calcium. It is decreased in low phosphate conditions of the body.

15. ***Creatine Phosphokinase*: (CPK) *or Creatin Kinase* (CK):** This enzyme is found in heart muscle, skeletal muscle and brain tissue. There are three isoenzymes of CPK known as CPK-MM found in skeletal muscle, CPK-BB in brain tissue and CPK-MB in heart muscle. Measurement of these enzymes indicates the source of damage. Usually CPK-MM isozyme is present in serum. CPK levels are increased in tissue damage conditions like fall, vigorous exercise, deep IM injection etc. Diagnosis of acute myocardial infarction is possible by measurement of CPK level.

16. ***Lactic acid Dehydrogenase*: (LDH or LD):** This enzyme interconvert lactate and pyruvate in the body and present in all metabolising cells. There are five isoenzymes of LDH, namely LDH 1 to LDH 5, out of which the first two are present in heart, third in lungs, fourth and fifth in liver and skeletal muscles respectively. Measurement of these enzymes point out where the damage is and this helps in the diagnosis of myocardial infarction, liver and lung diseases.

Other enzymes are discussed below under Liver Function Tests.

Liver Function Tests

Concentration of enzymes and other compounds in serum are measured in usual liver function tests. Specific function of the liver cannot be quantified by these tests. However they are useful in the diagnosis and watching the progress of liver diseases. Thus bilirubin is a measure to indicate the overall liver function whereas serum albumin level and Prothrombin time indicates synthesis of protein in liver. Similarly alkaline phosphate estimation gives an idea about obstruction in bile flow and the transminase levels indicate liver injury or cell death.

Albumin: It is a protein, synthesized in liver up to 10 to 15 g per day, of which 60% is found in ECF and the balance 40% in the serum.

If there are fewer albumins in the serum, edema may occur. As there is less protein (albumin) in the blood, less amount of drugs can bound to it and hence there is significant increase in free drug concentration in the blood. If it is not eliminated quickly as in kidney damage and other conditions, toxic effects of drugs may occur in the patient. Hypoalbuminaemia is due to damaged kidneys, skin damage as in burns, and increased catabolism due to many illness. Because of short life of Albumin (20 days) it cannot confirm the change in liver function however it has some prognostic value. Albumin level may increase rarely and after dehydration, shock or individual's peculiar reactions. [Idiosyncratic].

Bilirubin: It is tested to diagnose jaundice. If the serum bilirubin level is above 50 μ/mol/L, it indicates jaundice. In chronic liver diseases increased level of bilirubin is of prognostic value. Elevated level of bilirubin may be due to increased production, decreased excretion or impaired transport or combination of these factors.

Enzymes

The following components and enzymes are measured in liver function tests:

1. Albumin   -   38.50 g/L
2. Bilirubin (total)   -   < 19 μ mol/L
3. Bilirubin (conjugated)   -   < 4 μ mol/L
4. Alanine Transaminase (ALT) or   -   < 60 μ/lit
   Serum Glutamate Pyruvate
   Transaminase (SGPT)
5. Aspartate Transaminase (AST) or   -   < 35 μ /L
   Serum Glutamate Oxaloacetic
   Transaminase (SGOT)
6. Alkaline Phosphatase (AP or ALP)   -   < 35 – 130 μ /L
7. γ-Glutamyl Transpeptidase   -   < 70 μ /L

Usually enzyme concentration in healthy people is low, it is only when cells are damaged, the contents of them are released into the blood and the levels are increased. Before analysing the blood for enzyme, one must understands the principles involved in the assay. Actual enzyme concentration is not measured in assays, but only the catalytic activity. Many enzymes are present in more than one tissue and hence elevated levels of enzymes in blood may be due to damage to anyone of the tissue. Apart from this sample drawing time is also important, as these enzymes may not be present immediately after tissue injury or vanish from the blood if the sample is drawn after a long time.

Alkaline Phosphatase

It is one of the important parameter checked in Liver function test and discussed above.

Transaminases

There are two transaminases, aspartrate transaminase (AST or SGOT) and alanine transaminase (ALT or SGPT). They are mainly found in hepatocytes and muscle cells apart from some other tissues. AST levels are increased in liver diseases, myocardial infarction, surgery and injury, whereas ALT level is increased in viral and non-viral liver diseases. This is markedly increased in liver damages due to alcohol, paracetamol and viral infections.

γ Glutamyl Transpeptidase

It is present in more amounts in liver, kidney and pancreas. It indicates the hepatobiliary diseases. Hepatitis, cirrhosis, alcoholic liver disease, pancreatitis and congestive heart failure increase this enzyme level.

Some drugs like phenytoin, phenobarbitone and rifampicin also increase this enzyme level. Apart from the above in liver function tests, level of ammonia in blood and amylase in serum are also measured, if they are in excess, hepatic dysfunction and pancreatitis are indicated.

Renal Function Tests

Renal function tests are used to evaluate kidney and its functions. The disease of the kidney can also be followed by testing nephron functions like glomerular filtration, blood flow and tubular transport.

Glomerular filtration is clinically tested by the tests like creatinine clearance, serum creatinine and serum urea. Renal plasma flow is tested by Para amino hipparate (PAH). Similarly tubular transport is tested by serum phosphate urate, urinary amino acids, maximal urinary osmolarity and acid bicarbonate loading.

Creatinine Clearance

Glomerular filtration rate (GFR) is estimated using creatinine clearance. The normal value for men is 140 to 240 L/day i.e., 70 ± 14 ml/min/sq.m and for women is 120 to 180 L/day i.e., 60 ± 10 ml/min/sq.m. Creatinine clearance is not useful to detect earlier stages of kidney damage because glomeruli is not damaged but just increase in size, hence only after 50% to 70% damage to glomerular filtration surface, a decrease in creatinine clearance is clearly detectable. Because of this problem serum creatinine is also measured along with creatinine clearance because creatinine production and excretion are constant if there is no kidney damage.

Serum Creatinine

If the GFR increases, serum creatinine concentration decreases and vice versa. Hence serum creatinine concentration is a useful index of GFR. It is increased only when there is kidney damage, however depends on some other factors like muscle mass, age etc. The maximum serum creatinine concentration in man with normal GFR is 1.2 mg/dl and in women 1 mg/dl. The formula for calculating cleatinine clearance in men is as follows:

$$C_{L(creat)} = \frac{(140 - \text{Age in years}) \ (\text{Body weight in Kg})}{72 \times (\text{Serum creatinine in mg} / \text{dL})}$$

For women the value should be multiplied by 0.85.

Usually if the GFR decreases by 50%, serum creatinine increases by 100%. For example if the normal value of serum creatinine is 1.2 mg/dl with 50% reduction in renal function the value doubles to 2.4 mg/dl.

Serum Urea or Blood Urea Nitrogen (BUN)

Though the concentration of urea in blood depends on many factors like urine flow rate, production and metabolism of urea, a ratio between BUN and creatinine is useful to differentiate pre-renal, renal and post renal azotemia. Azotemia is a condition in which excess of nitrogenous waste products are retained in the blood.

If the ratio is more than 15, it indicates pre renal, post renal azotemia. The increase in ratio may be due to uncontrolled diabetes, infections, and glucocorticoid therapy. Shock, dehydration and GI haemorrhage induce pre renal azotemia. This ratio is less, in the cases of liver diseases, malnutrition, and in pregnancy.

Renal plasma flow: It is a difficult and costly test and not useful than GFR.

Renal concentration ability: It is a simple and helpful test. If there is less renal concentration ability it results in edema and fibrosis.

Pulmonary Function Tests

There are many tests to check the pulmonary function like spirometry diffusing capacity, flow-volume loops etc. However all are not essential to identify the deficiency in pulmonary function. There are two types of disorders of lungs one is restrictive disorder another one is obstructive disorder. The obstructive disorders are Chronic Obstructive Pulmonary Diseases (COPD), asthma, bronchitis and loss of lung's elastic recoil. In restrictive lung disorders due to increased diameter of airways during expiration, flow rates are increased.

Pulmonary Functions or Parameters

In order to understand the tests and their interpretation a clinical pharmacist must understand various pulmonary functions or parameters. They are

1. *Vital capacity* (**VC**): It is the maximum volume of air that can be expired slowly and completely after a full respiratory effort.

2. *Forced vital capacity* (**FVC**): It is same as above (VC) but utilize a maximum forceful expiration.

3. *Functional residual capacity* (**FRC**): It is the volume of air in the lungs at the end of normal expiration when all respiratory muscles are relaxed. FRC has two components. Residual volume (RV) – the volume of air remaining in the lungs at the end of a maximal expiration and Expirator Reserve Volume (ERV) i.e., FRC = RV + ERV. The RV is normally accounts for about 25% of the TLC (Total Lung Capacity).

4. *Forced Expirator Volume in 1 second* (**FEV₁**): It is the volume of air force fully expelled during the first second after a full breath and normally comprises less than 75% of the vital capacity (VC).

Pulmonary Function Tests Including Spirometry

Pulmonary disorders can be evaluated usually by simple spirometry tests. It is one of the important tests and provides sufficient information. Using spirometry VC, FEV₁ and Peak Expiratory Flow (PEF) can be tested. The test procedure is easy to learn by both operator and patient and yields permanent, reproducible and accurate data. Spirometry test is useful to differentiate between obstruction and restrictive disorders and to estimate the severity of the disease.

Spirometry with determination of FVC, FEV₁ and Maximal Voluntary Ventilation (MVV) is performed in all patients with respiratory problems. Patients with larynx or trachea infection are tested by flow volume loop (FVL) test. Similarly if weakness of respiratory muscle is suspected MVV, MIP, MEP and FVC (the lung mechanics) are carried out. If the clinical picture is not coinciding with results obtained by simple spirometry or when complete investigation of abnormal pulmonary process is required full testing may be done.

Interpretation of Pulmonary Function Tests

If the VC is less, even when there are normal flow rates, it indicates restrictive disease. Exponentially decreasing flows suggests Asthma. The severity of Asthma and the potential for response to bronchodilator can be adequately assessed by simple spirometry before and after inhalation of a bronchodilator aerosol. The response to treatment should be monitored by portable spirometry.

Retesting of pulmonary function after inhalation of a bronchodilator aerosol (e.g., Isoetharine) provides information about the reversibility of an obstructive process i.e., Asthma. Improvement in VC and/or FEV₁ of more than 15% is usually considered a bronchodilator response. Return of these parameters to normal following inhalation of bronchodilator aerosol indicates Asthma. Absence of a response to a single exposure to bronchodilator however does not preclude a beneficial response to maintenance therapy in patients with COPD.

Thyroid Function Tests

Introduction

Thyroid hormones are biosynthesized by iodinating the amino acid Tyrosine. For this biosynthesis iodine is collected and concentrated by thyroid gland from food and water we take. Tyrosine is iodinated either one or two sites and named monoiodothyrosine [MIT] or diiodothyrosine [DIT] respectively. One MIT and one DIT coupled to form

Triiodothyronine [T3] or two molecules of DIT coupled to form Tetraiodothyronine [T4] the later is otherwise known as Thyroxin. These T3 and T4 are embedded in a glycoprotein known as thyroglobulin as colloidal droplets in thyroid cells.

Later these thyroglobulin releases T3 and T4 in blood stream by the action of protease. Similar to drugs, these T3 and T4 also bind to proteins in the blood as Thyroxin binding globulin [TBG] [up to 80%] Thyroxin binding prealbumin [TBPA] and albumin [up to 20%]. Very less quantity of these [0.05 to 0.5%] is free in nature, not binding to any protein. The formation of T3 and T4 are influenced and controlled by a pituitary secreted hormone known as Thyroid Stimulating Hormone [TSH]. The physiological functions of thyroid hormone are to promote protein synthesis in all the body tissue and to increase oxygen consumption in liver, kidney, heart and skeletal muscles.

Tests for Thyroid Function

There are many tests available for testing how well thyroid gland is functioning. They are T3, T4, TSH and radio active iodine up take [RAIU] tests. Before the arrival of these modern tests, protein bound iodine [PBI] test was widely used which was less accurate and hence now a days not done. Thyroid scanning tests, Thyrotropin releasing hormone [TRH] test and T3 suppression tests are the other tests very rarely used for evaluating the function of thyroid gland. Hence the first four tests are described below.

1. *T3 Tests:* These tests are usually done to diagnose hyperthyroidism. Excess level of T3 [Triiodothyronine] will be present in patients who are hyperthyroid. However this test is not useful to study hypothyroidism, because it shows abnormal only after the disease reaches severe stage. Also during pregnancy and while using birth control pills, both T3 and 4 may show excess level due to the fact that estrogens present in these conditions, increase the proteins for binding. T3 also increases during the condition called Grave's disease which is an auto immune disorder. Hence usually TSH and free T4 tests are ordered together under these conditions.

   Serum Total T3 is measured by Radio Immuno Assay. Obviously T3 level depends on the circulating proteins TBG, albumin etc. In order to overcome the problem of variation in TBG, T3 resin uptake tests are performed. This test reveals the unsaturated thyroid binding on TPG. Normally around 30% of TBG binding sites are occupied by thyroid hormone. By *in-vitro* analysis, ^{125}I T3 is added to patient's serum when a part of it binds to unoccupied TBG sites. If a resin is added to it after equilibration, it binds the remaining ^{125}I T3. The value obtained is reported as ratio or percentage of bound or unbound. In hypothyroidism, there are less occupied and more unoccupied TBG sites whereas opposite is the case with hyperthyroidism.

2. *T4 Tests*: T4 is circulating in the blood either bound to protein or in unbound form as free molecules. Both these forms of T4 are measured in serum total T4

whereas only T4 is measured in Free T4 [FT4] or Free T4 Index [FT4I or FTI] tests. As already mentioned level of protein present in blood alter these values. For example in pregnancy and when using birth control tablets more protein binding sites are available for T4 to bind. Hence total T4 may be on the higher side but the patient need not be hyperthyroid as only the free T4 is physiologically active. Thus hyperthyroid patients will have excess of FT4 or FTI value and if it is less it indicates hypothyroidism. So measuring FT4 or FTI is important. However low levels of T4 always not indicate hypothyroidism, because severe illness and prolong steroid use also reduces protein binding sites in blood and shows decreased level of T4.

T4 is isolated by ion exchange column chromatography and determined by colorimetric method. FT4 is determined by a competitive protein binding method of analysis in which[125]I T4 and serum are incubated and dialyzed to find out percentage of dialyzable [125]I T4. However there may be some interference by the presence of inorganic iodides, mercuric compounds in T4 column chromatography method. Also highly protein bound drugs affect the results of competitive protein binding method.

3. **TSH Tests:** It is done to measure the amount of Thyroid Stimulating Hormone present in the blood. Normally TSH is more when there is less amount of thyroxin secreted as in hypothyroidism and it is less or nil when excess of thyroxin is produced as in hyperthyroidism. Rarely there may be less amount of TSH, if the pituitary gland which secrets it, is affected. TSH is actually secreted as and when thyroxin level goes down in the blood and reduce or stop secreting when levels are excess, just like a thermostat switching on or off in an iron box or geyser. TSH is measured by Radio Immuno Assay [RIA].

4. **Radio Active Iodine Uptake Test [RAIU]:** It is a non-blood test in which patient is given a small amount of radio active iodine and its uptake by thyroid gland is determined. If excess of that is absorbed by the gland it indicates hyperthyroidism and less up take indicate hypothyroidism.[Iodine is required for biosynthesis of T3 and T4 by thyroid gland]. This test has the disadvantage of cost, time, patient inconvenience and exposure to radiation. However, the above test is useful in T3 suppression tests and for calculating the dose when ^{131}I is used as a treatment modality as per Merck manual for medical practitioners.

The results of above Thyroid Function Tests are summarized in the following table:

Condition	T3	T4	TSH	RAIU
Hyperthyroidism	↑	↑	↓	↑
Hypothyroidism	↓	↓	↑	↓
Normal Value	85 - 185 ng/dl by RIA	5 - 11 µg/dl by RIA	0.4 - 4.8 µU/ml by RIA	At 5hr =5 -15% At 24 hr =10 -35%

KEY: ↓ = Below normal   ↑ = Above normal

Tests for Infectious Diseases

Infectious diseases are more dangerous and one of the important reason for death of patients. It is caused by all types of microorganisms like bacteria, fungi, viruses and parasites. Many specific antibiotics are used to kill or stop the growth of microorganisms depends on the causative organism and the severity of the infection.

Hence a clinical pharmacist can contribute much to the success of the treatment by suggesting appropriate antibiotic, its dose and route of administration to the treating physician. Above all, after the commencement of therapy, he can monitor the patient constantly and assess the success or otherwise of the drugs. For doing this the laboratory tests and the data obtained from it are critical. They confirm the suitability and effectiveness of antimicrobial therapy.

Staring from the confirmation of infection by non-specific tests to specific tests there are many areas where a clinical pharmacist should have at least fundamental and working knowledge. The non-specific tests are white cell count and its differential count (TC & DC) Erythrocyte Sedimentation Rate (ESR) and serum complement concentration. For example if the neutrophil is elevated it is indicative of infection, same as ESR. C3 component of serum complement concentration get reduced in serious infections.

This apart there are more direct tests like identification of pathogens by microscopic examination of body fluids and other samples and immunological tests. They not only confirm the infection but also identify the causative organism. Different infections require different tests like x-ray, sputum analysis, blood culture, stool examination etc to confirm the organism's identity and the extent of infection. Then the therapy is started using suitable antibiotics and the optimum dose.

Once the therapy is started, next important duty for the clinical pharmacist is to assess the suitability of antimicrobial therapy using various tests. The tests are,

1. Susceptibility or sensitivity of the organism to the drugs.
2. Determination of minimum inhibitory concentration required to prevent the growth of microorganisms and
3. Determination of minimum bactericidal concentration required to kill the microorganism.

For monitoring the antibiotic therapy the following tests may be performed.

1. ***Serum Bactericidal Concentration***: It is the maximum dilution of the patient's serum that kills a standard inoculum of infecting organism. This tests should be performed on the patients who undergo long time antimicrobial therapy and for whom the route of administration is switched over from parenteral to oral route

2. ***Antibiotic Assay***: It is essential for drugs with narrow therapeutic index like aminoglycoside antibiotics, chloramphenicol etc.; blood serum concentration is measured for these drugs.

3. Patients should be monitored for antimicrobial toxicity also. It should be remembered that many false positive results are observed during the course of toxicity monitoring.

Tests Associated with Cardiac Disorders

Patients may be affected by various cardiac disorders. The frequently encountered disorders are

(a) Angina pectoris

(b) Myocardial infarction

(c) Congestive cardiac failure

(d) Atherosclerosis.

There are many tests to diagnose and estimates extend of damage due to these disorders. They help the clinician to take decision regarding medical or surgical management of patients.

Types of tests: These tests are classified in to two categories, invasive and non-invasive tests. The non-invasive tests are

1. Auscultation

2. Blood tests

3. Chest x-ray

4. ECG

5. Echocardiography

6. MRI scans

7. Radio nuclide and

8. Stress tests.

The invasive test is cardiac catheterization [Angiography].

Diagnosis of Cardiac Disorders: Diagnosis starts from collection of medication history of the patient and his/her family. It is followed by assessing risk factors and physical examination. Finally patients are tested by few or all the tests mentioned above, as one or two tests cannot diagnose the cardiac disorders with 100% accuracy. The detail of each of above test follows:

I. Non-Invasive Tests

1. *Auscultation*: This is nothing but testing the patient's heart beat with stethoscope which helps to hear the normal and abnormal sounds of heart beat. Changes in heart beat associated with breathing and murmurs also heard with stethoscope. Variation in sound, rhythm and murmur points to the fact that something is wrong with the heart and that is identified and confirmed by various tests mentioned below.

2. **Blood Tests:** The first test ordered after physical examination of the patient with stethoscope is blood tests. Number of components of blood is measured and they give valuable hints about impending or ongoing cardiac disorder. These tests and their normal values and risk values are given in the following table.

Table 32.3 Blood Tests Value

Tests	Normal Value	Risk Value
Total cholesterol	< 200 mg/dl	> 240 mg/dl
LDL	< 100 mg/dl	> 160 mg/dl
HDL	> 60 mg/dl	< 40 mg/dl
Triglycerides	< 150 mg/dl	> 200 mg/dl
Fibrinogen	< 300 mg/dl	> 460 mg/dl
Lipoprotein [a]	< 14 mg/dl	> 19 mg/dl

Apart from the above electrolytes in blood are also measured which is described elsewhere in this book. Arterial blood gas determination also helps in diagnosis and treatment of patients with shock and myocardial infraction [MI]. Oxygen level and acid-base balances are also tested.

3. **Chest X-Ray:** A chest x-ray gives the pictures of internal organs like, heart, lungs and chest wall. It can reveal the signs of heart failure, enlarged heart and edema. Usually frontal and lateral chest views are filmed to detect heart diseases by evaluating heart size, heart shape and the lungs.

4. **Electrocardiogram:** It records the electrical activity and rhythm of the heart. It is recorded normally by a 12 lead electrodes from the skin surface in three planes, anterior, posterior and lateral. The electrical signal of each heart beat is recorded by the ECG machine. Slow heart rate [Bradycardia] and fast heart rate [Tachycardia] produces rhythm abnormalities which can be visualized by ECG. But we must remember an abnormal reading does not always indicate a problem with heart, similar to normal reading does not rule out heart problems. Hence ECG is combined with stress tests, that is, ECG is recorded while the patient is undergoing stress tests on a tread mill or exercise bike.

5. **Echocardiography [ECHO]:** It produces a moving picture of heart using sound waves that provides information about the structure [size and shape] and pumping function of the heart. It also reveals the movement of heart valves and heart muscle thickness. After applying a lubricating gel over the chest, a hand held device called transducer is passed over it, so that there is continuous contact between the transducer and skin. The images produced can show the damages to heart muscle due to poor blood supply and non-functional area of heart. Thus echocardiography is the method of choice for diagnosing abnormalities of heart at birth, valve dysfunction etc.

Echo tests are carried out by more than one method. M.mode echo cardiography, Two-dimensional echo, Doppler echo and Contrast echo are often used methods to diagnose cardiac disorders. M.mode echo use pulsed-reflected ultra sound to look at the internal cardiac structures. Two-dimensional [2D] echo produce spatially correct images of the heart and can be recorded as video images. Doppler echo is the method of recording the flow of blood in around the heart using ultrasound. Contrast echo is nothing but M.mode and 2 D tests only, the difference being they are conducted after injecting contrast medium into cardio vascular circulation.

6. **MRI scan**: Magnetic Resonance Imaging [MRI] produces detailed pictures of heart. Patients are scanned using magnetic and radio waves when lying inside a tunnel like scanner. The computer attached to the scanner creates the picture – both still and moving – of the heart and major blood vessels. The disadvantages of MRI scan are it is expensive and images are formed slowly. It cannot be used on patients with metallic prostheses or implants. However it is safer than CT scan, because it does not use ionizing radiation for image formation. It is a valuable tool in diagnosing cardiomyopathies, myocardtitis, myocardial ischemia, iron overload, congenital heart diseases and vascular diseases.

MRI uses a strong and uniform magnetic field. Its field strength is measured by a unit called 'Tesla' [T]. Usual MRI machines are of 1.5 T, but other machines with 0.2 to 7 T are also available. A special type of MRI for using in specifically in cardiac disorders is used now-a-day. It is known as cardio vascular Magnetic Resonance Imaging [CMR] or cardiac MRI. Here basis MRI is optimized, so that they use ECG gating and rapid imaging techniques or sequences. In this CMR a sequence called spin echo is used in which the blood appears block in colour so that a contrasting agent need not be used.

7. **Radio nuclide test**: Here a small amount of radio active substance [an isotope] is injected into the blood of the patient. A camera is held near the chest which picks up the radiation released by the isotope as it passes through the heart, indicating the areas where there is poor blood supply. Thus they provide more detailed information than the Stress ECG test described below. From the collected information Clinician can assess how strongly the heart pumps and the blood flow to muscular walls of heart.

8. **Stress tests**: These tests are carried out using a tread mill and/or exercise bike. During this test the heart of the patient work hard and beat faster. An ECG may be connected to the patient so as to record the cardiac activity. If the patient cannot exercise he or she may be given drugs to increase the heart rate. If the patient' coronary arteries are deposited with plague and thus narrowed it cannot supply enough blood with oxygen to meet the increased need during these stress tests. Hence the following signs and symptoms can be detected:

   (a) Breathing Difficulty

   (b) Chest Pain

(c) Abnormal heart rate or blood pressure and

(d) Abnormal changes in heart rhythm and electrical activity which are measured using ECG and other equipments.

During stress tests pictures of heart are taken and that is compared with pictures of heart taken while the patient is at rest. They give an indication of heart's functions.

II. Invasive Tests

1. ***Cardiac Catheterization or Coronary Angiography:*** It is a technique in which a thin, flexible catheter is passed along vein or artery into the heart and connected vessels either for diagnosis or treatment of cardiac disorders. The catheter is put into the blood vessel in arm or upper thigh or neck. It is then threaded into the coronary artery with the help of x-ray images. A dye is injected through the catheter to visualize the arteries supplying blood to the heart. All these procedures are done under local anesthesia.

Then numbers of x-ray pictures are taken which indicate any block in the arteries. However this test cannot detect blockages in micro vascular diseases because they usually do not cause any blockage in large coronary arteries. Nevertheless cardiac catheterization or coronary angiography is relatively safe procedure and serious complications are rare. Possible problems, 1or 2 in 1000, are cardiac arrhythmias and ventricular fibrillation. If angina develops during the test, it is treated with sublingual nitroglycerin tablets.

During catheterization, intra cardiac pressure, blood gas saturation and pressure pulse tracings can also be measured. B.P can be measured at various points of heart by which pressure gradient across the valves can be calculated. Cardiac output and vascular resistance are also calculated which are useful quantitative information for further procedures. These tests are avoided in patients with severe infections or brain damage. Nausea, vomiting, cough, sense of warmth are the side effects of these tests.

Microbiological Culture Sensitivity Tests

Introduction

A microbiological culture sensitivity test is a laboratory procedure to identify the microorganism present in the patient's body fluids or other samples and to determine which antibiotic kill or prevent the growth of them. It is to select the antibiotic effective against the microorganism causing the patient's problem. The species and strain of the bacteria or the pathogen present in patient's body is first identified and then the drug most effective in killing or inhibitory in its growth is determined. The tests used for the purpose is known as culture and sensitivity [C&S] tests.

Basics of C&S Tests

These tests are performed in two stages. In the first stage the microorganism present in the sample are grown suitably and identified. In the second stage they are tested against the range and dose of antibiotics to determine their susceptibility to the particular antibiotic.

After the culture of microorganism, when they are sufficiently grown on the surface of the medium they are identified by using various techniques. They are studying surface characters like, colour, texture, and growth pattern, gram staining, microscopic examination, metabolic requirement 'foot prints' etc. Now-a-day they are identified by genome characters in well equipped labs.

Once identification of microorganism is over, they are tested for their sensitivity to a range of antibiotics and their doses. This is usually done by antibiotic disk diffusion test where the zone of inhibition of growth of microorganism is measured and compared with known standard strains and antibiotics.

Need For Culture and Sensitivity Tests

If the identity of microorganism is established by microbiological culture tests, its sensitivity to antibiotic can be predicted. Hence, treatment can be started without delay. For example, Streptomyces pneumonia, Streptomyces pyogenes are sensitive to penicillin, S.aureus to Cloxacillin, Candida albicans to Nystatin and so on. However these are preliminary interim measures till the report of more reliable and accurate results from sensitivity tests are supplied in two or three days. Sometimes these results could be delayed either due to slowly growing organisms or due to repeat tests. Any how as the strains of many pathogens differ from one another in their sensitivity to antibiotics, sensitivity tests are a must and performed carefully.

Other Purposes and uses of C&S Tests

Apart from identifying the microorganism and its sensitivity to antibiotics there are other uses for C&S tests.

1. It help the clinician to test the dose of antibiotic, as he is concerned with a dose which is high enough to kill the microorganism at the same time it should not produce any toxic effect on the patient.
2. If the sensitivity profile of microorganism reveals any change in its resistance, doctor has to change or control his antibiotic prescribing pattern.
3. Above all the C&S tests are useful to study the value of new antibiotic before the clinical trials.

Thus culture and sensitivity tests play an important role in usual treatment, change in treatment and discovering new treatment with antibiotics.

Limitations of C&S Tests

However there are few limitations in the use of C &S tests. These tests are performed '*in-vitro*' and they need not produce the same results '*in-vivo*' because of many variables working in patient's body. For example a pathogen which is sensitive in-vitro, may fail in 'in-vivo' because of inadequate absorption of drug indicating the role of pharmacokinetics of drug. Similarly an antibiotic found to be not useful in C&S test may work in patient's body due to high dose and/or patient's immune response. Nevertheless C&S tests are performed to get an idea about the line of treatment to be adopted by avoiding drugs which may out work against particular microorganism. For instance, Polymixins may not work with gram positive organism and Vancomycin is ineffective with gram negative pathogens. Similarly first generation Cephalosporins are not useful with H.influenzae. Thus C&S tests though have some limitations, guide the clinician to select a better drug for the patient.

Tests Procedure

Culture and sensitivity tests have two stages, microbiological culture and testing its sensitivity to antibiotics. First culture test is discussed below:

*Microbiological Culture***:** It is a method of growing and multiplying microorganisms by reproducing them in predetermined culture medium under controlled lab conditions. It is one of the primary diagnostic methods to find out the cause of infection. There are two ways by which microbial culture can be carried out.

1. In petriplates with solid medium and
2. In culture tubes and flasks with liquid medium [broth]

Whatever may be the way of performing these tests, aseptic technique must be followed. Aseptic technique is the procedure carried out in an aseptic area to prevent contamination by microorganism and thereby maintain the sterility of test materials.

If the purpose of culture test is to identify the organism responsible for the infection of the patient, culture in liquid medium will not be useful, as they grow microorganisms in different depth of the medium in the tube which makes the separation, isolation and identification of them difficult. The body fluid or other sample from the patient may contain multiple organisms; hence growing them in a solid medium in a Petri plate is the ideal method. Thus bacterial culture in petri plates using agar as solid of the medium is explained below. For other methods students are advised to refer books on Microbiology.

Requirements and Stages of Microbial Culture

To carry out a successful microbial culture, the first requirement is a suitable medium, followed by a proper procedure. It starts with preparation of medium [if not a ready made medium is used] and preparation of plates. Then the various stages of microbial culture are four 'I's – Inoculation, Incubation, Isolation and Identification of microorganisms. The detail of all these things follows.

Medium: For bacterial culture though many media are available, Soya bean – casein Digest medium to be incubated at $20°$ to $25 \ °C$ and Fluid Thioglycollate medium incubated at $30°$ to $35 \ °C$ are much used. Agar is used in medium as it offers many advantages. If individual colonies of bacteria or fungi are needed agar gives a best solid surface. It also permits separation of various species of microorganism, if there are more than one species in the sample, as they allow growth of partially identifiable colonies on its surface. Also it can be inoculated by any of the following methods:

(a) Streak plate dilution technique

(b) Lawn technique and

(c) Pour Plate technique.

A successful bacterial culture can be produced by following three important criteria:

1. Appropriate sample

2. Correct method of sampling and

3. Proper handling procedure.

To get a sample suitable for culture it should be approximately estimated weather the body fluid or other sample from the patient has sufficient microorganism to grow. If not it should be grown first in a liquid broth medium in culture tubes and then samples from it should be used for culture in agar plates. As sample of suitable dilution is required, series of dilutions are made and then inoculated on agar. Thus appropriate and correct sampling is important. To perform culture tests, handling procedure is also equally important. These procedure starts with preparation and aseptic transfer of sterile nutrient agar to plates.

Preparation of Agar Plates

The culture medium should be prepared as per the composition and method given in standard books like Pharmacopoeia. Now-a-days ready made commercially available media are used to save time and delay due to error or contamination. In culture and sensitivity tests quick reporting of results are expected, as they are vital for treatment of patients.

The media used must be sterile and molten for pouring it from flask to petri dish. It should be done when the media is having a temperature of around $45°c$. Both excess and less temperature leads to problems like moisture condensation and solidification respectively hence it is transferred ideally at $45°c$. For transferring the media, after the closure the neck of the flask is heated on a Bunsen burner. Then the empty sterile petri plate is placed on the laminar flow table and its lid is half lifted. Molten agar media is transferred to the petri dish and immediately closed with lid. The petri dish is rotated clockwise and anticlockwise and up and down three times each, at slow speed, so as to disperse the medium through out the dish uniformly. The neck of the flask is heated again and closed immediately. The petri plate is allowed to cool to solidify the medium. Then it is inoculated with the sample collected from the patient as follows.

Inoculation

The sample collected from the patient may be any of the body fluid or solid or semisolid like sputum. They are suitably prepared for inoculation by serial dilution or by growing in liquid broth medium as mentioned earlier to have the microbes of sufficient number. It is then inoculated by any one of the various techniques described below:

1. *Streak plate dilution technique:* In this method series of streaks are made on the surface of the medium using sterile loop dipped in the inoculums. The loop is sterilized by passing through the flame after each streak, so that the amount of material in each set of streak is reduced. It helps in the formation of well isolated colonies of microorganism in the final set of streaks, thereby bacteria are separated. Then they grow to form colonies and thus various species of bacteria are isolated from the sample if available.

2. *Lawn technique*: Here, aliquot of liquid sample is applied on the surface of medium to produce continuous growth of bacteria as grass grows in a 'lawn'. Actually the lawn is nothing but growth of numerous colonies very close to each other. Among the all methods this is the most suitable method of inoculation to study the effect of antibiotics on the microbes, i.e. to test their sensitivity to antibiotics.

3. *Pour plate technique*: This is the technique in which liquid sample prepared from the patient's body fluid is mixed with molten agar and then poured into the petri dish. Obviously the microorganism present in the sample is uniformly dispersed throughout the diameter and depth of medium unlike the above two techniques, where the inoculums is applied only on the surface of the medium. Similar to this there are two more techniques in which inoculums is added to the tube containing medium or petri plate with medium is kept upside down respectively.

4. *Incubation*: After inoculation, the petriplates are incubated in an incubator at around 35°c for 2 to 7 days or more depends on the requirement. Some media require less temperature which should be verified from manufacturer's literature.

5. *Isolation*: After incubation as above, the plate may show mixture of microbes. Before attempting to identify them as such, they are separated so that their identity can be easily established without doubt. Subsequent sensitivity tests can also be performed confidently. Isolation of pure culture is done by pour plate or dilution method. This method has the advantage of colonies forming throughout the plate unlike the streak method where they are formed only on the surface. Thus the pour plate method offers easy isolation of microbes due to its good distribution.

Pour plate or dilution method of isolation is carried out as follows:

1. 10 ml of molten agar is taken in 4 tubes, serially numbered and maintained at 45-50 °C

2. One loopful of sample from mixed culture is added to tube number 1.

3. It is thoroughly mixed by rotating between hands for proper mixing.

4. One loop of culture from tube number 1 is transferred to tube number 2 and mixed by rotation as above.

5. Again one loopful from tube number 2 is added to tube number 3 and mixed.

6. Once more a loopful of culture from tube number 3 is transferred to tube number 4 and mixed.

7. The contents of all the above tubes [1 to 4] are then poured into separate petri dishes and numbered 5 to 8.

8. They are all incubated at 30 °C for 2 days [48 hours].

9. All the above steps are carried out aseptically without any cross contamination.

10. Inoculation of culture from one tube to another must be done at the centre of medium in the tube, not on the surface.

At the end of incubation of above tubes different colonies of microbes are obtained which are used for subsequent identification and sensitivity tests.

Identification of Microorganism

Microorganisms are identified by two methods, by microscopical identification after staining and culturing as above.

When bacteria grow by binary fission they form colonies of genetically identical bacteria and hence genetically pure in nature. Their shape, consistency, colour, margin etc are verified from which some identification is possible. This can be confirmed by using chemicals [stains], pH, nutrients, temperature, salinity and other conditions of incubation. Once the organism is identified treatment can be started immediately. However different strains of some species of microorganism have different resistance. Hence we need to undertake sensitivity tests on the isolated and partially identified microorganisms.

Sensitivity Tests

This is usually carried out by disc diffusion method. In the direct [primary] tests, antibiotics of varying concentration are placed directly on the agar plates that have been inoculated with clinical samples like pus or urine. The results of sensitivity of microorganism to the particular antibiotic can be obtained after over night culture of those petri plates. The antibiotics required for the test is usually selected after gram staining of the sample.

The indirect [secondary] test results of 'pure culture' are usually available after 48 hours of receipt of sample collected from the patient. While performing sensitivity tests, the inoculums, the medium and the antibiotic discs are carefully selected so as to give a uniform growth and inhibition.

Disc Diffusion Tests: There are many methods of disc diffusion tests depends on its standardization, reading and control. US FDA recognizes the 'Kirby Bauer method' in which single, high concentration antibiotics are used on the inoculums of standard density on Mueller-Hinton agar. In India a comparative method is used, where the diameter of zone of inhibition of organism isolated from patient's sample is compared with that of various concentration discs of single antibiotic or different antibiotics. In this method antibiotic discs of high or low concentrations are used depends on the sample. For example, urine samples usually have high concentrations of microorganisms, hence antibiotic discs of high content are used to test their sensitivity. The advantage of this method is different antibiotic discs are used in the same plate hence not only many variables which may affect the accuracy of the test is taken care of, but also suitable antibiotic can be selected among the many.

Same plate comparative disc diffusion tests are thus widely used where suitable medium, proper inoculums and its application are critical to get the best result. Normally commercially available medium are used and it is prepared for the test according to the instructions of the manufacturer. It is customary to have a 4 mm depth of the medium in petri dishes 8.5 cm diameter. Proper inoculums preparation and its spreading are next critical requirements for the sensitivity tests. While too heavy inoculums reduces the size of zone of inhibition, too light inoculums produces a zone which is difficult to measure or no zone at all due to drug resistance developed by microorganism. Hence how many number of colony forming units needed to inoculate should be ascertained. It is done by suitable dilution of sample, its method of spreading and the species being tested. Various methods of applying inoculums are explained earlier. Normally, by placing a standard loopful of suspension of inoculum on the plate and then spreading with dry sterile cotton swab is followed in most of the laboratories.

After proper inoculation the antibiotic discs are placed on the surface of the medium, so that they are in firm contact with them. This is done within a short and standard time. In some laboratories the petriplates are kept at room temperature for some time so as to allow the antibiotics to diffuse into the medium from the disc before incubating. This is not required except for few tests. Up to six discs can be placed in the petriplates depends on its size, taking care to leave enough space between the discs as well as the edge of the plate to develop the zone of inhibition.

Standard control strains of microorganisms and antibiotics are essential for better results of sensitivity tests. These standards are explained in the publications by WHO, by name "Expert Committee on Biological Standardization." Series of these books are published by WHO now and then, and they should be consulted before doing sensitivity tests.

Selection of Antibiotics for Sensitivity Tests

Usually antibiotics often prescribed locally by the doctors are selected for sensitivity tests. However in some exceptional cases other antibiotics may have to be used. Gram stain gives an idea what antibiotic should be used and what not to be used. If the microorganism's identity is established by microscopic observation and other growth characters on the surface of the medium, it is easy to select suitable antibiotic. Only in doubtful cases many antibiotics has to be used to select the best among them. We have to keep it in mind that different strains of the same organism respond differently for same antibiotic. One representative antibiotic of a class of closely related antibiotics is sufficient to test the sensitivity. Thus any one of the Tetracyclines or Cephalosporins [First generation] can be used to represent the group.

Reporting Results

After incubation, the petriplates are taken out and the zone of inhibition on the surface of the medium is measured. Some people measure the distance in mm from the edge of the disc to edge of the zone, some others measure the diameter of the circular zone of inhibition including the antibiotic disc. Whatever the method adopted the zone of inhibition is compared with different zones produced around different concentration of single antibiotic or different antibiotics. The minimum inhibitory concentration [MIC] is taken into account which indicates the minimum amount of antibiotic required to prohibit the growth of microorganism.

The MIC is measured by three methods:
1. Tests with series of discontinuous concentration of antibiotics
2. Tests with break point concentration and
3. Tests with concentration gradients of antibiotic.
1. *Tests with series of discontinuous concentration of antibiotics:* This is performed by placing commercially available antibiotic discs of different concentrations. After measuring the MIC the test can be extended to measure the minimum bactericidal concentration [MBC] of the antibiotic. It is done by preparing sub cultures from each test culture and recording the lowest concentration of antibiotic required to inhibit the growth in the sub culture.
2. *Tests with break point concentration:* Here the test organism is compared with control organism of known MIC. They are exposed to only 2 or 3 important 'break-point' concentrations of the antibiotics. These concentrations are selected, keeping in mind the achievable level of antibiotic in patient's body fluids.

3. ***Tests with concentration gradients of antibiotic:*** In this method the antibiotic discs of series of concentrations are selected which are geometrically progressing in their concentration. The microorganism is prevented from growing around the disc and the lowest concentration of disc which has prevented the growth is recorded as MIC. It is compared with the control test.

After measuring MIC, the result of sensitivity test is reported sensitive or intermediate or resistant. If the organism is reported as sensitive, the MIC is less than 50% or even 25% of the concentration of antibiotic likely to be present in the infected site of the patient when given the usual dosage regimen, i.e., the infection can be treated with the reported antibiotic.

On the other hand if the organism is reported to be 'resistant', it means that it cannot be treated with the particular antibiotic within the maximum safe concentration of the drug achievable in the tissue of the patient. As the name indicate 'intermediate' sensitivity is nether acceptable nor to be rejected out right, as there is still some chance left, if it is retested under different conditions. Some laboratories used to report intermediate sensitivity as 'moderately sensitive' which means the organism might respond, if the dose is increased to more than usual dose.

As these terms are little vague in description, an idea can be of useful to students to understand how and when these terms are used. If the zone of inhibition size is similar to that of control sensitive strain, the test is reported as 'sensitive.' If the test organism grows within 3 mm of the disc and the control strain shows bigger zone of inhibition, the test organism is reported as 'resistant'. If it is not falling under the above two definitions it can be indicated as 'intermediate.'

Conclusion

Students must understand that, none of the above sensitivity tests are 100% satisfactory. They are affected by many factors like nature of medium, size of the inoculum, conditions of incubation, amount of antibiotic diffused and the organism's ability to resist the antibiotic. Thus the accuracy and reproducibility – the very important aspects of any scientific experiment – are affected. Nevertheless, at least they give some approximate idea to proceed while treating the patient; otherwise one has to struggle to start.

Because of these short coming of culture and sensitivity tests newer, more sophisticated methods are being developed, including DNA profile, Micro-colorimetry, Radiometric methods, bioluminescence etc. They are yet to be used in large scale.

Questions

Short Answer Questions

1. Write a note on 'Patients Clinical Data'.

2. What are the needs for patient's data analysis?

3. Write a note on Biochemical data.

4. What happen when electrolytes balance is disturbed?

5. Write the role of drugs in disturbing electrolytes balance with examples.

6. Write a note on biosynthesis of Thyroid hormone.

7. What are T3, T4, and TSH? Write few lines about each.

8. Write a note on an invasive test for cardiac disorder

9. How microorganisms are cultivated?

10. List various techniques of inoculation. Explain any two of them.

11. How the results of sensitivity tests are reported?

Long Answer Questions

12. What are haematological data? Explain important tests and the range.

13. What is the significance of Liver function tests? Explain how they are carried out.

14. Write short notes on: A] Renal function tests B] Pulmonary function tests

15. Discuss the importance and methods of tests for infectious diseases.

16. Explain various Thyroid function tests.

17. Enumerate the tests associated with cardiac disorder.

18. Explain the importance of microbiological culture and sensitivity tests. Write the procedure for sensitivity tests.

CHAPTER 33

DRUG UTILISATION EVALUATION AND REVIEW

Introduction

Diseases and their manifestations consequently drugs used and their effects on a patient are complex and cannot be predicted with 100% accuracy. Hence a constant vigil by the way of drug utilization evaluation [DUE] and review [DUR] is essential to achieve best results of the treatment given. So DUE is a **quality improvement program** of a hospital. It assesses the utilization of drugs continuously in order to improve the outcome. The program is variously called by different names like DUE or DUR, though, essentially they mean the same.

In this connection we should be clear that it differs from Drug Therapy Review [DTR] and Therapeutic drug monitoring [TDM] which are patient specific and about the entire Drug Therapy or on the use of particular, suspected to be problematic one or two drugs, used by a patient respectively. But DUE is about the use of all drugs given to many patients admitted in different wards of the hospital at different point of time. Thus DUE is useful to arrive at a conclusion about drug's use, safety etc, which obviously cannot be determined by conducting DTR or TDM on a single patient. DUE is carried out before, during and after the treatment is given to the patients whereas DTR and TDM can be done only after the drug is administered i.e., during the treatment.

Drug utilization evaluation review drug use and prescription trends and the result obtained by the study are communicated to clinicians, so that new guidelines are developed, if necessary, for the better use of drugs. Hospitals device appropriate education and intervention programs to correct deficiency, if any, found during DUE. DUE can be based on particular disease also instead of particular drug where use of drugs for a specific disease is evaluated. Contrary to TDM which is carried out by a individual Clinical Pharmacist, DUE is performed by a group of people formed into a committee, usually constituted by Pharmacy and Therapeutic committee [PTC] of the hospital. Normally Clinical Pharmacist is given a major role in this committee.

Aim or Objectives of Drug Utilization Evaluation

Before studying in detail about DUE, let us first define it. WHO define DUE as a system of ongoing, systematic, criteria based evaluation of drug use that will help ensure that medicines are used appropriately [at the individual patient level].

The overall purpose of DUE is to evaluate the hospital's performance. However in order to analyze that performance some parameters need to be met. Such parameters are set as goal or aim of DUE. The health care team has the responsibility to fulfill these objectives, as it enhances the reputation of the hospital they work. The objectives are listed below:

1. To evaluate the effectiveness of the treatment.
2. To prevent medication related problems
3. To fix responsibility and accountability among the members of health care team in medication use process.
4. To develop guidelines for proper drug use
5. To reduce cost of treatment
6. To identify areas for improvement and
7. To create and conduct further education and information program to the health care providers.

Benefits of D.U.E

DUE helps the health care professionals to understand the pattern of prescription, administration of drugs and use of drugs better. If it is found deficient, it makes the hospital to intervene to device educational program for its staff. It also supplies physicians with feed back data from DUE and thereby helps them to identify their weakness and strength. Doctors can gather lot of information about drug utilization by other senior doctors and that provides them an opportunity for course correction. Obviously with out DUE these benefits are not available for doctors and other health care professionals.

DUE System

DUE can be carried out before, during and after the treatment is given to the patients. Thus an ideal DUE system should permit, evaluation of drug use by prospective, current or retrospective review. Prospective review is carried out just after the writing of prescription but before administering the drugs written in it. This review helps to avoid problem before a particular drug is administered to the patient which is either contra indicated or unwanted. Current review is undertaken during the course of treatment. Treatment outcomes are monitored daily using lab tests and other vital parameters like, body temperature and B.P recorded by nursing and medical staff. If any ADR or drug interaction or non responsiveness to standard drug regimen is noticed during this review, a full pledged TDM is undertaken by Clinical Pharmacist. Then any problem identified by TDM data is brought to the notice of treating clinician and needed remedial measures are taken. Thus current DUE is fully useful to the patient.

During retrospective review of drug utilization, treatment outcome is evaluated after the completion of treatment. Though it is of no use to the particular patient, it helps the health care team to decide whether to follow the same line treatment to other patients or to carryout corrections in it. As this is done away from the patient, his doctor and others in the ward, there cannot be any bias or influence on the result of the review. This review is done at the convenience of the DUE committee and the biggest drawback is if any information is missing it can not be traced easily after the discharge of the patient. As pointed out above retrospective review is beneficial only to the health care providers rather than the patient concerned.

Prospective and current review is undertaken routinely but retrospective review is done as and when necessary or if specifically requested by hospital authorities like PTC.

Documents useful for DUE

To carry out DUE effectively the DUE committee requires some records and reports. Usually medication history of the patient, his medication profile and laboratory procedures profile are compared to complete the DUE. Medication history of every patient admitted in the ward is collected by clinical pharmacist. If necessary, some out patients are also interviewed for medication history by him. Patient is either interviewed personally or asked to fill computerized questionnaire designed for the purpose. It gives detail about the patient's concurrent medication including OTC drugs and drugs of alternative system of medicine, his allergic status towards drugs or food, and lab test undergone just before the present visit to the hospital.

Similarly patient medication profile is also prepared by the pharmacist to serve the purposes like, preventing drug-drug interactions, avoiding duplication of drugs, to detect lab test abnormalities due to drugs and above all to avoid ADR. It also helps to identify drug induced diseases and to adapt safe and rational use of drugs by better prescribing. Model patient medication profile form is given in the chapter on Records and Reports.

Apart from the above two documents, laboratory procedure profile of the patient is also useful to review the drug utilization. There are two broad categories of lab tests. One is diagnostic tests and the other is monitoring tests, while the former helps to identify the disease and consequently the drug required the later is useful to continue, stop or change the drug given to the patient depending on the outcome of its use confirmed by lab tests. Thus DUE requires all the above three documents for best results.

When to Conduct DUE?

The DUE team should first determine when to conduct its evaluation. Though it can be carried out any time to evaluate health care team's performance, it is usually undertaken under the following circumstances:

A. Whenever an ADR or serious medication error is noticed.

B. On occasions when clinical pharmacist has to intervene

C. During the use of new drugs or drugs not listed in the Hospital formulary

D. As and when signs of treatment failure appear and

E. On patient's complaint or deteriorations of his condition.

Procedure or Method of DUE Process

There are many steps involved in DUE process. They are

1. Appointing or nominating the head and members of DUE team,

2. Aim or objective,

3. Selection of drug[s],

4. Criteria and Standards,

5. Data collection,

6. Data analysis,

7. Feed back,

8. Follow up and

9. Evaluation of above steps.

Only when systematically carried out DUE ends in success, otherwise it is useless and results in waste of time, energy, resources and sometimes even in bitter feeling among the colleagues of the hospital. Hence a careful planning is the prerequisite for the DUE process. It starts with **appointing or nominating the head and members of DUE team**. This team is given authority and responsibility to undertake DUE in the particular hospital. Then they conduct, supervise and follow up the DUE. This team or committee is appointed usually by PTC of the hospital. Under special circumstances, higher authorities of health ministry of state or central governments form such committees.

As with any project or procedure, the second important step is to define the **aim or objective** of DUE study. This can be narrower or broader as required. **Selection of drug[s]** for the study is the next important task, as hundreds of drugs are used in a hospital. Criteria for selecting drugs are almost similar to the one for selecting drugs for TDM which is elaborately given in chapter on TDM. Let us have a glance of those criteria with out going into the detail.

1. Drugs with narrow therapeutic index. E.g. Amino glycosides, Cardiac glycosides

2. Drugs with varying pharmacokinetic properties.

3. Drugs that produce different quantum of effect. E.g. Sodium valproate

4. Non responsiveness for standard drugs regimen due to suspected drug resistance. E.g. Antibiotics, Anti malarial.

5. Drugs that is suspected to have produced toxic effects. E.g. Cyclosporins

6. Drugs whose pharmacological effects cannot be measured.

7. Drugs with non linear kinetics in its action. E.g. Phenytoin

8. Drugs administered to infants.

9. Drugs given to pregnant women and patients with liver and/ or kidney damage &

10. Drugs with potential for interaction E.g. Anti TB and Epileptic drugs.

Apart from the above, over use of expensive drugs, use of higher antibiotics when lower antibiotics are sufficient to treat and poor dispensing practices can also be evaluated during DUR.

Next, during the DUE the following **Criteria and Standards** should be verified in order to justify the entire treatment, starting from the diagnostic procedure to selection of drugs to its effects.

A. Verify choice of drugs

B. Verify choice of dosage form

C. Verify choice of route of administration.

D. Verify drug allergy, if any.

E. Verify drug idiosyncrasy or pharmacogenetics.

F. Study effect of treatment procedure on hospital services and

G. Evaluate follow up done after discharge of the patient

The above works are variously described as **Criteria and Standards or Method of DUE**. They are actually pre determined documents detailing optimum drug use against which present treatment's quality can be compared. Slight variation or deviation is permitted within a range, from standards set earlier. These criteria or standards can also be developed by DUE team on its own based on published standard literatures or it can simply follow the already available one.

To arrive at a decision at the end of DUE, data are required which are collected during DUE. **Data collection** must be from at least 30 to 100 patients and entered in computer. The important sources of data are patient medication profile, case sheet entries, laboratory reports, patient medication interview, patient complaints etc. Relevant data regarding drug utilization should be collected, if any data is not available or not clear, they should be obtained from people concerned. Without proper, sufficient and reliable data any decision made at the end may not be reliable, biased or inaccurate. Hence due importance should be given for data collection part of DUE.

The sixth step in the process of DUE is **data analysis**. It can be carried out using computer, as data are already entered and available in it. First they should be summarized and then deviation from standards calculated. The reason for deviation should be identified and discussed. If it is found logic and true even the criteria or standard itself can be amended.

Feed back of the results of data analysis is the next step in DUE. The results should be conveyed first to treating doctor and each member of his team including pharmacists and nurses. Later the same can be communicated to other health care staff of the hospital through News Letter, meetings or seminars.

As a **follow up** measure to DUE, future plans should be prepared and implemented. Few months later, everything should be revalidated to find out whether DUE has helped in improving treatment procedure. This is done exactly in the same way as the first evaluation. Data collection and its analysis etc are followed as above. If any problem is found in revalidation, it can be given special attention.

Finally, after all these procedures are completed, the procedure adopted for DUE itself should be evaluated. Any deficiency found in it can be rectified in the light of DUE already done. Thus new criteria for DUE can be included or conflicting criteria removed.

Factors Affecting DUE Program

DUE program should be well organized as described above. Nevertheless failures do occur due to the following factors:

(i)   Starting DUE program without higher authorities' permission and support.

(ii) Conducting it with out proper organization and defined roles for its members.

(iii) Communication gap between members of DUE team

(iv) Lack of interest and involvement by team members.

(v)   Poor documentation of data and consequent problem in its retrieval and management.

(vi) Deficiency in follow up action and

(vii) Poor methodology which results in interference with patient care.

If all these factors are addressed before, during and after DUE program, a successful evaluation can be done.

Questions

Short Answer Questions

1. What are the documents needed for DUE? Why?

2. Define DUE and list its aim and need

Long Answer Questions

3. Explain the method of DUE process and the factors affecting it.

CHAPTER 34

INDIVIDUALIZATION OF DOSE AND PHARMACIST INTERVENTION

Need for Individualization of Dose

It is common sense that there is lot of variables between individual patients like age, weight, sex, disease and its severity, body mass, genetic makeup, kidney damage, liver damage, concurrently administered drugs and environment. All these variables affect the effect of drug on particular individual. Hence a common dose or a dose guessed to be suitable cannot be expected to produce the desired effect. This is the important problem of any therapy; however it is ignored in short time therapy like the one given to out-patients of the hospitals, who are treated for short term illness. But for the patients who require prolonged therapy this problem cannot be set aside, just like that.

Among the variables listed above co-administration of many drugs to a patient causes problems. We can predict the action of one drug if given alone to a patient but if two or more drugs are administered to a patient, at the same time, there bound to be unexpected effects. For example ketaconazole, an antifungal, potentiate the effect of cyclosporine-- an immunosuppressant. Thus pharmacokinetic and pharmacodynamic properties of one drug is affected by completely unrelated another drug if given together.

Thus normal dose of a drug may produce normal effect in some patients, toxic effect in some other patients and altogether ineffective in yet another patients. Hence, the need for adjusting or optimising the dose for an individual is evident.

There are some drugs which have narrow therapeutic index; hence there is a danger of toxic effect to the patient if the dose is not proper. Similarly some drugs produce huge effects even for small change in dose and some other drugs, though dangerous to use in a given situation, critically needed for therapy and hence used with probable risks involved. For all these drugs, a dose suitable for the individual patient should be calculated and used. Examples for these drugs are digoxin, phenytoin, theophylline and cyclosporine.

Parameters useful in Individualization of Dose

The following are the important parameters, otherwise known as pharmacokinetic data useful in the individualisation of dosage regimen:

1. Bioavailability
2. Protein binding
3. Volume of distribution
4. Clearance and
5. Half-life

Clinical pharmacist must be thorough with all these parameters and able to calculate them accurately by performing necessary tests on the individual patient. He should able to correlate and interpret these data and arrive at the correct dose by necessary calculations.

Hence above parameters are explained below in detail.

1. **Bioavailability:** After an oral dose, a fraction or certain percentage of that drug reaches the systematic circulation and produces therapeutic effect. This fraction or percentage of the drug is known as bioavailability of that particular drug.

   Not all the 100% of drug administered is absorbed into the circulation, a part is inactivated in the GI mucosa or metabolised by liver (First pass metabolism), only the remaining percentage is available for pharmacological action. This is due to many factors given below:

   (i) Factors that affect absorption: It is obvious that if the absorption of drug is affected, it naturally affects the bioavailability. Hence the factors like, solubility of a particular drug, its physical chemical properties, concentration of the drug, surface area of absorption, circulation to the site of absorption, presence of food or water in the stomach etc affect bioavailability.

   (ii) Anatomical site from which the drug is absorbed also has important role to play in bioavailability. For example, if taken by oral route, it is first metabolized in the liver and excreted in the bile, hence bioavailability is altered.

   (iii) Diseases that alter the structure and function of GI tract, also affect the bioavailability.

2. **Protein Binding:** All drugs are bound to some extent to plasma and/or tissue proteins. Protein binding is the percentage of drug that is bound to plasma protein to concentration of drug in the blood. If something disturbs the protein binding of a drug, then more drugs may be freely circulating in the plasma. As we know only the free drug concentration is responsible for pharmacological action, this phenomenon should be monitored. Change in protein binding also

alters distribution and excretion of the drug. Hence, before attempting to individualize the therapy of a patient this factor should be considered seriously.

3. **Volume of Distribution (V_d):** It is the total fluid volume, required for the dose of the drug given to patient to be distributed throughout the body at the same concentration as in plasma. But it is not so simple like this statement. It requires detailed explanation, starting from the administration of an oral dose. The dose of the drug given to the patient is distributed in the body through the vascular system. Majority of the drugs have sufficient lipophilicity and hence they are able to distribute both in the intra and extra cellular compartments of the body. Thus the drug reaches to tissues and the process is called distribution.

The volume of distribution as mentioned above is not an identifiable physiological volume, but an imaginary volume that is required to distribute the given drug at the same concentration as in the blood or plasma.

If we take body as a single compartment, the body fluids are:

Blood volume	:	5.5 L
Plasma volume	:	3.0 L
Extra cellular fluid	:	12.0 L
Total body water	:	42.0 L

Distribution of the drug may be in blood and/or extra cellular fluid and/or into the tissue. Drugs that are distributed only in the blood will have the volume of distribution close to blood volume 5.5 L. For example volume of distribution (V_d) of Furosemide is 7.7L. Similarly drugs that reach extra cellular space but not the tissue will have a V_d of around 20 L. e.g.: Atenolol, Theophylline etc (V_d = 20 to 40 L) and drugs that enter tissues will have still larger volume of distribution.

e.g.: V_d of chloroquin = 13,000 L; Digoxin = 700 L

This unrealistic value is obtained because of this drug's low concentration in blood (and majority of drug distributed up to tissue). The volume of distribution of a drug is calculated by the following formulae:

$$V_d = \frac{f_D}{C_p} \text{ [For oral dose]}$$

where f is the fraction of drug available (Bioavailability)

D is the amount drug given (Dose)

C_p is the concentration in plasma

$$V_d \text{ (For Inj)} = \frac{\text{Total injected drug}}{\text{Plasma conc.}}$$

4. **Clearance:** It is the volume of plasma freed of the drug per minute. The organs of clearance are kidney and liver. However it takes place at other places also like in sweat, saliva, bile, into stomach, faecal loss, loss in lungs and at other sites of metabolism. Total systemic clearance is obtained by adding all these separate clearances.

$$C_L \text{ Renal} + C_L \text{ Hepatic} + C_L \text{ Others} = C_L \text{ Systemic}$$

Clearances by main organs like kidney or liver is calculated by the following formula:

$$C_{LR} \text{ (Renal clearance)} = \frac{UV}{P}$$

where

U is concentration of drug in urine

V is the average volume of urine/minute

P is concentration of drug in plasma

$$C_{LH} \text{ (Hepatic clearance)} = \frac{Q \times (C_{in} - C_{out})}{C_{in}}$$

where

Q : Blood Flow

C_{in} : Concentration of drug going into the liver

C_{out} : Concentration of drug coming out of the liver

Clearance can also be calculated by another formula

$$CL = \frac{V_d}{t_{1/2}}$$

where V_d is volume of distribution, $t_{1/2}$ is half life

If clearance is more, naturally the half life will be less. Only when the fractional availability of the drug is known, clearance can be calculated. Hence, to accurately calculate the clearance, oral dose is not reliable, and therefore it is determined following I.V dosage where the availability is 100% of the dose given.

Use or value of studying clearance

There is up and down in the plasma concentration of drug due to various factors. But the physician wants to achieve more or less a steady state concentration of drugs in patient's plasma, so as to achieve the goals of the treatment. This can be achieved only when the rate of elimination is equal to rate of administration of the drug. Simply, the input should be equal to output. i.e.,

The dosing rate $= C_L \cdot C_{ss}$

where C_L is clearance and C_{ss} is the steady state concentration of the drug.

Thus if we know the desired steady state concentration of the drug, the clearance dictates the rate at which the drug should be administered. Then the maintenance dose and dosing interval can be determined. Study of clearance is also much useful in clinical pharmacokinetics as it is constant over a range of dose and consequent plasma concentrations.

5. **Half-life:** Half life can be defined as the time taken by the body to eliminate half of the amount of the drug in the body. The following table is self explanatory.

At the end of	Plasma Conc. in mg	Total Drug Eliminated
0 Time	100	NIL
1st Half life	50	50%
2nd Half life	25	75%
3rd Half life	12.5	87.5%
4th Half life	6.25	93.75%
5th Half life	3.125	96.875%

Thus after the 5th Half life almost all the drug is removed from the body. To compare pharmacokinetic of drug in normal person and diseased patient, this parameter, half life, is very much useful.

Alteration of the Pharmacokinetic Parameters in the Individual Patient which require Attention and Intervention by Pharmacist

Pharmacokinetic parameters discussed above are altered or determined by many physiological or biochemical events that occur in normal persons and pathological conditions that may exist only in particular disease. Hence a clinical pharmacist must be thorough with those conditions and intervene as and when necessary.

I. Bioavailability

The following factors affect bioavailability of a drug that requires monitoring by the pharmacist.

1. Patient's non-compliance to drug regimen
2. Poor formulations like tablets with less solubility
3. Drug-Drug interactions
4. Drug-Food interactions

5. Metabolism of drug in GI Tract

6. First pass metabolism by liver

7. Biliary excretion

8. Poor Metabolism of certain drugs by liver (e.g., lidocaine)

9. Surface area of absorption

10. Pathological conditions of stomach

11. Physical and chemical properties of drug

12. Amount or concentration of drug in the GI tract

As so many factors affect the bioavailability, frequent checking of this parameter helps in continuation or modification of the drug regimen.

II. Protein Binding

Protein binding is mainly affected by the liver damage which in turn affects the production of albumin and other proteins. If the nitrogenous waste materials are not properly removed from the body then also the protein binding is affected (The condition is called Uraemia). Once protein binding is affected, it leads to huge changes in volume of distribution due to increase in free-drug concentration or binding of drugs in tissue proteins.

III. Volume of Distribution

The following factors affect the volume of distribution:

1. pk$_a$ of the drug (Log of dissociation constant of weak acid)

2. Degree of binding to plasma proteins

3. Partition co-efficient of the drug in fat

4. Degree of binding to tissue proteins

5. Patient's age, sex and body composition and

6. Disease of the patient

If the plasma concentration is very low and when the fraction of the drug available in the body is divided by it, a huge volume of distribution is obtained. Sometimes it may be thousands of litters as in the case of chloroquin and hence highly unrealistic. However volume of distribution thus obtained is also useful as it indicates the extent of binding of drug to the tissue protein. This knowledge is again very much helpful in the treatment of drug over dose cases, when any amount of haemodialysis or haemoperfusion will not be useful as that will reduce plasma concentration only temporarily and the drug will redistribute from tissue to plasma after the dialysis. Thus alternative methods of treatment should be given to the patient as quick as possible.

IV. Clearance

The following factors alter the clearance of a drug by an organ

1. Blood flow to the organ
2. The fraction of the drug unbound in the blood (free drug concentration)
3. The ability of the organ to remove the free drug

If any one of the factors is affected due to disease, the clearance is altered. Thus liver damage and kidney damage play important role in clearance.

V. Half-Life

Though half life is not depending on the body mass of the patient, indirectly it is affected because it is depending on volume of distribution which is proportional to body size. If the clearance decreases due to disease, half life increases, similarly if the volume of distribution is reduced due to age (less body mass) clearance is increased and consequently half life is affected. Thus these problems start from the quantity of proteins available for binding by a drug, and continue to affect, the volume of distribution, clearance and finally the half life. These parameters are thus interdependent and well connected with each other and hence should not be viewed in isolation.

Pharmacodynamic Parameters

The parameters described above are all pharmacokinetic parameters depend on the absorption, distribution, metabolism and excretion (ADME) of the drug. However, there are other parameters that affect the pharmacodynamics of the drug. Pharmacodynamic is the study of effects of drug on the body. While pharmacokinetics describes "What the body does to the drug, pharmacodynamic deals with "what the drug does to the body".

For many drugs, the effect cannot be quantified. Similarly the amount of drug required to produce certain effect in the site of action is also difficult to estimate. It is because there is little or nil information about the receptor number or drugs affinity or subsequent coupling of drug with receptor or effect of disease on these factors, etc. Hence the relationship between effect and plasma concentration is unknown. This relationship is so complicated and disturbed by many factors, for example, the effective concentration of an antibiotic depends not only on the dose but also on the type of microorganisms. Apart from it, the drug effect is ultimately affected by the pharmacokinetic factors. Hence if we want to correlate both these pharmacokinetic and pharmacodynamic factors, time of distribution of drug to the site of action must also be taken into account. All these make the study complicated.

Pharmacist's Intervention

Hence clinical pharmacist has to adjust all mean parameters for individual patients carefully. To calculate the desired steady state concentration of a drug, free drug circulation in the blood (bioavailability) should be known. To arrive at the maintenance dose, fraction of the drug absorbed and clearance must be estimated. To compute the loading dose and to estimate half life and dosing interval, volume of distribution is needed. Thus bioavailability, clearance and volume of distribution are the important parameters in adjusting or individualizing the dose for a patient which a clinical pharmacist must keep it in mind while intervening in therapy.

Questions

Short Answer Questions

1. Explain the need for individualization of dose briefly.
2. Write short note on factors affecting bioavailability.
3. List the parameters useful in dose adjustment.

Long Answer Questions

4. How will you individualize the dose for a patient?
5. Explain how pharmacokinetic parameters are interconnected?
6. Describe how volume of distribution and clearance are calculated.
7. How and what affect the pharmacokinetic parameters? Why a pharmacist should intervene in those situations?

CHAPTER 35

ADVERSE DRUG REACTIONS

Introduction

Due to many reasons listed below, drugs may produce unwanted reactions in patients. These effects occur at normal accepted dose and not at excessive dose hence require careful monitoring of the patients who are under long time therapy. Some drug's Adverse Drug Reactions (ADR) are documented and hence known to the treating physicians, nevertheless they are also counted as ADR. Some other reactions which occur due to accidental over dose, prescribing or dispensing error and intentional overdose are not included in Adverse Drug Reactions. Thus ADR can be defined as the reaction that is harmful, unintended and occur at doses normally used in humans for prevention or diagnosis or treatment of diseases.

Reasons or Predisposing Factors for ADR

1. Midway stopping of drugs: Patients often stop taking medicines due to various reasons like cost, ignorance, non-availability of drugs etc. There is a possibility of ADR if the drugs like steroids and hormones are suddenly withdrawn.

2. Patient factors like age, Idiosyncrasy and disease conditions also cause unwanted reactions in some patients.

3. Bioavailability Problems: Due to poor formulation of drugs, their blood concentration is affected and hence they may reach toxic level in some patients and subsequently ADR may occur.

4. Intake of drugs should be stopped at an appropriate time; it should not be continued indefinitely unless otherwise indicated. Failure to set therapeutic end point is one of the reasons for causing ADR. Drugs like digitalis, diuretics, steroids and antibiotics are to be stopped as and when their continuation is not necessary.

5. Self Medication by patients and over prescription by Doctors may produce ADR. If any problem or disease occurs due to doctor's treatment it is known as Iatrogenic or Drug Induced Diseases (Chapter 36).

318

6. Sex: It is a general perception that women are more susceptible to ADR than men. Though the reason is not established it is suspected that may be due to hormonal factors or pharmacokinetic or immunological factor. One known example is adverse effect of Chloramphenicol [Blood Dyscrasias] is more in female population than men.

7. Age: Chances of drugs producing ADR on the infants and young children, as well as on elderly people is more due underdevelopment of internal organs in the farmer and improper functioning of them in the later. Chloramphenicol produce 'gray baby syndrome' on the neonates whereas nitrates and ACE inhibitors causes hypotension in geriatric cases.

8. Apart from above, drug interactions is one of the major reasons for ADR (Chapter 36)

Reducing or Preventing ADR

Though Adverse Drug Reactions cannot be eliminated, it can be reduced if the drugs are used with caution and by following the safety aspects listed below, by the patient and health care team.

1. Patient medication history should be obtained before prescribing and drugs should be prescribed accordingly.

2. Drugs should be administered only when required. If there is no indication such drugs should not be used.

3. As far as possible minimum number of drugs should be prescribed. Poly pharmacy or multiple drug regimens should be avoided.

4. Children and old people are susceptible to ADR. Hence they should be monitored while under therapy.

5. Continuous review of need for the drug should be undertaken and the dose should be reduced or drug altogether stopped at an appropriate time.

Classification

There are 2 types of Adverse Drug reactions. They are:

Type I : Predictable and dose dependent

Type II : Unpredictable and independent of dose

Type I: This type of ADR is more common and they are due to pharmacological activities of the drug based on which it can be further classified into three:

A. Excess pharmacological effect or toxic effect

B. Secondary pharmacological effect or side effect and

C. Return effect on stopping the drug

Type II: This type of ADR is not common; occur only in some patients due to their peculiarity. It has nothing to do with drugs pharmacological action, at the same time it is more dangerous and hence require stopping of the drug concerned. This type can be further classified into.

    A. Idiosyncrasy

    B. Allergy including anaphylaxis and

    C. Genetic related

I.A   ***Toxic Effects:*** It is due to excess activity of a drug, which may be due to long time use of the drug or over dosage. Over dosage may be absolute or relative. Drugs are usually given in a range of dose. Sometimes the upper range of permitted dose is prescribed for the patient, which may produce toxic effect in some patients. Similarly due to patient's kidney failure or liver diseases or anemia some drugs cause excessive pharmacological effect even in normal doses. Examples are gentamicin in the case of kidney failure and paracetamol in liver diseases. Toxic effects of almost all the drugs are documented for ready reference and monitoring. Some are given below:

    1. Heparin induces bleeding

    2. Streptomycin causes deafness

    3. Emetine causes myocardial damage

    4. Coma by barbiturates

    5. Digoxin causes atrioventricular block and

    6. Corticosteroids and anti-inflammatory drugs suppress response to injury and infections.

I.B   ***Side Effects:*** Drugs may have two or more activities even though they are prescribed for its primary activity only. The secondary effects are nullified by various means like prescribing corrective drugs or formulation techniques. However, some side effects cannot be corrected from outside. For example, steroids weaken defense mechanism of the patient, hence latent diseases like tuberculosis gets activated. Sedation by antihistamines is another common example for secondary pharmacological or side effect.

I.C   ***Rebound Effects:*** Adverse effects are noticed not only for the drugs which causes dependence, but also for other drugs, when they are stopped suddenly. Usually the diseases, for which they were used gets further activated or return. For example, if an antiepileptic drug is stopped suddenly, seizures may increase in those patients. Similarly if the β.blockers are stopped angina pectoris worsen, and hypertension results if clonidone– a hypotensive agent is discontinued.

Another example is stopping of addiction forming, CNS depressants which results in tachycardia, confusion, delirium, agitation and convulsions. They are all called, rebound response on discontinuation of therapy. These drugs should be stopped gradually, not abruptly, and/or with proper substitutes or alternative drugs to prevent ADR.

II.A *Idiosyncrasy*: It is defined as a reaction due to certain, unexpected effects of drugs because of peculiarities of an individual. It is an unusual, individual response to certain drugs by the patient. As mentioned earlier it is unexpected, unpredictable and not depending on the dose. For example, cinchona alkaloids like quinine and quinidine produce cramps, diarrhoea or vascular collapse in some patients. Barbiturates instead of causing depression produce excitement and mental confusion in some individuals.

II.B *Allergy*: This is also called drug hypersensitivity. All patients are not experiencing allergic reactions for the drug and only a small percentage of them suffer, that too, it is not a sudden development as believed by many. Prior sensitization is needed and at least 7 to 10 days require to produce the effect, after first exposure. They may tolerate the drug later and who tolerated it earlier may develop allergic reactions subsequently. Different types of allergic reactions are produced in different individuals for the same drug and sometimes completely different drug may produce same type of reactions. Thus as already pointed out they are unpredictable and not related to dose because even an increase in dose to any amount cannot produce same reactions in other individuals.

On the other hand anaphylaxis is an allergic reaction, that is severe and sudden which may lead to loss of consciousness or even death. Photosensitivity is another type of allergic reaction by some individuals.

II.C *Genetics*: Genotype of particular individual, cause variation in the effects of drugs, hence there is possibilities for ADR. Sometimes to produce the same effect 500% increase in dose may be required for some individuals depend on their genetics. It is because their rate of metabolism differs and we know that rate of metabolism depends on microsomal enzymes which in turn is controlled by genes. Site of action or its sensitivity to drugs also plays an important role in drug's effect which differs due to genotypes.

For example, glucose 6 phosphate dehydrogenase deficiency may lead to haemolysis with Primoquine. Drugs are acetylated in liver during metabolism, if it is slow in some individuals due to genotype; there is possibility of adverse drug reactions for the drugs like procainamide, isoniazid etc.

Differences between Type I and Type II ADR

No.	Type I	Type II
1	Can be predicted	Cannot be predicted
2.	Dose related	Occurs independent of dose
3.	Commonly occurring	It is rare
4.	Not serious, very rarely cause death	It is a serious and may be a fatal reaction
5.	If the dose of drug concerned, is reduced problem is solved.	Requires complete stopping of the drug
6.	Generally identified even before first time marketing of the drug	Occur rarely hence require continuous post marketing surveillance
7.	The effects of this type of ADR are qualitatively normal but quantitatively excess	The effects are unusual unexpected and harmful.

Methods of Detecting and Monitoring ADR

As it is difficult to differentiate between the disease manifestations and the Adverse Drug Reactions, many methods are developed to identify ADR. They are:

1. Case control studies

2. Cohort studies

3. Spontaneous case reports and

4. Vital statistics and record linkage studies

1. **Case Control Study:** In this study group of persons with disease (cases) and groups of persons without disease (control) are compared. Here the disease selected should be due to the drug. Patient's medication histories are collected and compared, if the drug has caused the disease its use among the cases should many times more than the controls.

   This type of study can be conducted quickly and effectively and that too at less cost. But it requires more scientific knowledge to conduct correctly and to interpret the data obtained after the study.

   For example in a study of relationship between lung cancer and cigarette smoking it was found, the disease is 10 to 11 times more in smokers than non-smokers. As the connection between the two depends on the amount of smoking and there is very less scope for chance factor, hence the conclusion drawn from the above study is justified.

2. **Cohort Study:** Cohort is a group of people having approximately the same age and put under same and similar conditions like receiving the same drug. In this study the drug under study is given to the group and watched for varying periods, to find out the ADR. This can be for a short period, say the treatment period plus 1 month. The study is carried out in various places of the country and up to 2000 to 3000 patients are selected.

Usually toxic effects due to excessive pharmacological effects are detected by this method. Delayed effects of the drug can also be detected.

In the long term study lasting for few years more patients up to 20,000 may be followed for detecting adverse drug reactions. Information is collected from the Doctor, Pharmacist and the patient if possible. The problem with this method is drop outs due to migration etc. It is an expensive and difficult method and known as Post Marketing Surveillance.

3. **Spontaneous Case Reports:** If a prescriber suspects some problem with the patient because of drugs usage, he reports it to medical or pharmaceutical journals or to the manufacturer of the drug. This is called spontaneous case repot. Other prescribers are alerted by this method.

Now-a-days ADR reporting agencies are available like the one with World Health Organization (WHO). Once a report is send to them with relevant particulars, they investigate and or report it to all medical practitioners through journals, newsletters and associations etc. It is a cheaper method; however frequency of particular ADR, its correlation with drug and disease etc has to be determined. Also it cannot be claimed to be a complete report.

4. **Vital Statistics and Record Linkage Studies:** All the health care institutions (hospitals and clinics) and local bodies are required to maintain morbidity and mortality data. From these records disease prevailing and causes of death in a particular area can be collected and analyzed.

However, this method is not successful, because of long delay in collecting data, reliability of the data etc. If the data are faithfully entered in records and computerized, it may be useful to collect and analyse them easily in future.

Management of Adverse Drug Reactions – Role of Pharmacists

Irrespective of careful treatment of the patient ADR do happen due to many factors, beyond the control of health care team. In those unfortunate events, pharmacist has the following functions to manage ADR.

First of all, he should review the available literatures regarding the ADR of the particular drug. Any worthwhile point found should be discussed with physicians. Next the pharmacist should check the patient's medication history. He should also review other factors like co-administration of other drugs, stage of disease etc. Therapeutic Drug Monitoring (TDM) should be started immediately, if not started already. Plasma concentration of the drug in the particular patient should be analyzed and weather the reaction is dose dependent or not can be detected. Finally depends on the seriousness of the reaction he can advice to stop the drug. For this he has to analyse the risk/benefit ratio and the availability of substitute drugs.

If pharmacy and therapeutic committee is available in a particular hospital, pharmacist as the secretary of PTC should inform the committee about the ADR occurred. PTC in turn discusses it and advises the treating physician, what to do and how to proceed with further treatment. It monitors the recovery of the patient from ADR and ensures proper treatment thereafter. Pharmacist has to implement the decisions of PTC as its secretary.

All Records of adverse drug reactions should be preserved and reported to suitable higher authorities. These works and model ADR reporting forms are given in chapter No.3.

Causality Assessment Scales

Introduction: An ADR is difficult to identify because of the following factors:

1. It is difficult to distinguish an ADR from disease manifestations. The patient is already affected by the disease and it is expressed by various signs and symptoms. Any extra symptom manifested by ADR, during the course of treatment is also considered as disease manifestation and part of disease.

2. Sometimes the ADR is without symptom and goes unnoticed until very serious complications occur and

3. The patient himself or herself is the best identifier of his or her bodily changes or suffering. Only when they report any such event with seriousness it can be investigated. But most of the time either they don't report or even if they report it is not taken seriously by health care team.

   If it is the case, even to identify the ADR, one can imagine the difficulties in establishing the link between the ADR and the drug caused it.

Problem of Linking ADR and Drug

Though it is difficult to establish the drug responsible for ADR, health care professionals cannot leave it as such. They have the duty and responsibility to investigate, first, for treating the patient affected by it and limit the damage, next for preventing it from occurring in other patients. Hence after much debate and discussions, some methods have been devised and they are known as 'causality assessment scales.' They are for assessing weather an ADR is definitely, probably or possibly due to the drug. Number of approaches or algorithms has been developed, though they are considered to be of little value by a section of health care professionals.

If an ADR occur immediately after the administration of a particular drug, it can be linked to that drug. Stoppage of that drug and receding symptoms of ADR will almost confirm the association between the two. But if an ADR is produced after the administration of multiple drugs – which is often the case – and if it occurs many days or weeks after the drug administration, it may not be possible to establish this link. Hence the following causality assessments scales are used in various countries.

1. WHO method,
2. European ABO system
3. Naranjo scale and
4. French infutation method.

Among these scales WHO method and Naranjo's scale are much used.

WHO scale categorises the assessment into Certain, Probable, Possible, Unassessable, unlikely and conditional. On the other hand Naranjo scale categorises the assessment as definite, probable, possible and unlikely.

The WHO scale of assessment from its website is summarized in the following table and the popular Naranjo scale which is found in many websites including Wikipedia is given next.

Table 35.1 W.H.O Scale of Causality Assessment

Scale or Parameter	Certain	Probable	Possible	Unassessable	Unlikely	Conditional
Event or Lab test abnormality within reasonable time of drug intake	Yes	Yes	yes	Insufficient or contradictory information	Relationship between drug & ADR improbable	yes
Cannot attribute to disease manifestation or other drug	Yes	Yes	Doubtful [may also be due to disease or other drug]	Report cannot be supplemented or verified	No. disease or other drug may be responsible	More data needed
Response to withdrawal of drug	Yes, reasonable	Yes, reasonable	Lacking or unclear	Report cannot be supplemented or verified	----	Additional data under examination
ADR leads to recognizable& definitive medical disorder or phenomenon	Yes	--	--	--	---	---
Re-challenge [restart the drug again]	If necessary	Not necessary	---	---	---	---

Note: The blank columns above indicate uncertainty or unassessability or unverifiable nature of ADR.

Naranjo Scale of Causality Assessment

The Naranjo algorithm, Naranjo Scale, or Naranjo Nomogram is a questionnaire designed by Naranjo *et al.* for determining the likelihood of whether an ADR is actually due to the drug rather than the result of other factors. Probability is assigned via a score termed definite, probable, possible or doubtful. Values obtained from this algorithm are sometimes used in peer reviews to verify the validity of author's conclusions regarding adverse drug reactions. It is also called the Naranjo Scale or Naranjo Score.

Questionnaire

1. Are there previous conclusive reports on this reaction?

   Yes (+1) No (0) Do not know or not done (0)

2. Did the adverse events appear after the suspected drug was given?

   Yes (+2) No (-1) Do not know or not done (0)

3. Did the adverse reaction improve when the drug was discontinued or a specific antagonist was given?

   Yes (+1) No (0) Do not know or not done (0)

4. Did the adverse reaction appear when the drug was readministered?

   Yes (+2) No (-1) Do not know or not done (0)

5. Are there alternative causes that could have caused the reaction?

   Yes (-1) No (+2) Do not know or not done (0)

6. Did the reaction reappear when a placebo was given?

   Yes (-1) No (+1) Do not know or not done (0)

7. Was the drug detected in any body fluid in toxic concentrations?

   Yes (+1) No (0) Do not know or not done (0)

8. Was the reaction more severe when the dose was increased or less severe when the dose was decreased?

   Yes (+1) No (0) Do not know or not done (0)

9. Did the patient have a similar reaction to the same or similar drugs in any previous exposure?

   Yes (+1) No (0) Do not know or not done (0)

10. Was the adverse event confirmed by any objective evidence?

    Yes (+1) No (0) Do not know or not done (0)

Scoring

- ≥ 9 = definite ADR
- 5-8 = probable ADR
- 1-4 = possible ADR
- 0 = doubtful ADR

Reference

Naranjo CA, Busto U, Sellers EM et al. (1981). "A method for estimating the probability of adverse drug reactions". *Clin. Pharmacol. Ther.* 30 (2): 239-45. doi:10.1038/clpt.1981.154. PMID 7249508.

Questions

Short Answer Questions

1. Define ADR.
2. Classify ADR.
3. Discuss the reasons for ADR.
4. How ADR can be reduced?
5. List the differences between two types of ADR.
6. Write a note on Naranjo Scale,

Long Answer Questions

7. Explain the Type I and Type II ADRs in detail with examples.
8. Enumerate various methods of detecting or monitoring ADR.
9. How ADR is managed? Discuss the role of pharmacist.
10. Write in detail about Causality assessment

CHAPTER 36

DRUG INTERACTIONS AND DRUG INDUCED DISEASES

Introduction

Though drug interactions are part of adverse drug reactions it is studied separately, because of its importance. Concurrent administration of many drugs to the patient is a reality and hence the possibility of drug interactions is always there. Invariably almost all the drugs are synthetic chemicals or chemical constituents of natural drugs, and hence the potential for drug interactions is evident. Moreover, these chemicals are administered into the body; where scores of biochemicals are already present and also the chemical drugs given from outside is metabolized to different chemicals inside the body. Thus we mix up lot of chemicals in patient's body and if we ignore this or non-vigilant throughout the course of long treatment, harmful effects cannot be avoided.

Thus, drug interaction is defined as a situation in which the effects of one drug is altered by prior or co-administration of another drug. It also includes drug-food interactions and drug-disease interactions.

Reasons for Drug Interactions

1. *Patients go to many physicians:* Patients are in a hurry to get relief from their disease and hence they go to many physicians and even to many systems of treatment like Ayurveda, Siddha or Homeopathy. Because of this situation, there are chances for adverse drug interactions but usually patients purchase drugs from neighbourhood pharmacy only, and hence pharmacist can counsel such patients.

2. *Simultaneous use of OTC drugs and prescription drugs:* Patients purchase some drugs for their common problems from nearby pharmacies and they continue to use the same along with prescription drugs. They may not reveal it to the physician or pharmacist; hence, questions are asked cleverly using symptoms normally treated with OTC drugs and information collected.

3. **Non-compliance:** Instructions given by doctors or pharmacists regarding the use of drugs are not correctly followed by many patients, which need attention to avoid drug-drug interactions.

4. **Drug's potency:** If potent drugs are used together, chances of harmful effects are more. For example, if antipsychotic, antidepressant and antiparkinsonism agents with anticholnergic activity are used together, dryness of mouth and blurring of vision results.

5. **Drug abuse:** Few patients are abusing drugs knowingly or unknowingly and hence interactions chances increase.

Problems in Detecting Drug Interactions

Patient's disease conditions are too complicated to detect ADR. If something abnormal is detected, it is considered as disease manifestation and not as probable ADR. Sometimes, they are attributed to factors other than drug interaction like tolerance, irregular use of drug etc.

Index of suspicion of many clinicians is low, as they believe nothing will be wrong with their treatment. Only when problem becomes big, they search for earlier reports of ADR of drug used, until then they doubt their own observation of symptoms of ADR.

For many drugs there is no measure for activity similar to antihypertension and hypoglycemic drugs which are measured by blood pressure and blood sugar level respectively. For example, take the case of tranquilizers and analgesics, whose effect potential is not possible to detect.

Above all, if drug interaction in a patient is reported by a physician, he will be in a critical situation that criticism and possible legal actions may result. Hence nobody wants to be in such a bad situation, because of their own reporting.

Uses of Drug Interaction Reports

If interaction between two drugs is known, therapeutic alternatives can be used. For example anticoagulant drug Warfarin interacts with Aspirin, hence it can be given with paracetamol instead of aspirin. Similarly if tetracycline and antacids has to be given together, it can be done with time gap. Thus interacting drugs are given by following adjustments like changing doses or close monitoring of therapy etc.

Some interactions are beneficial so that these interactions can be used for the advantage of patients. For instance, probenecid, if given together with penicillin, the duration of action of the later is increased. Hence the dose of penicillin is reduced.

All, reported drug interactions need not produce the same effect in all the patients. It varies depends on many variables like age, genetics, renal disease, hepatic disorders, drinking habit, smoking, food intake etc. Each of this variables influence the effect of drug, therefore drugs interactions reports should be used depends on the present case. Moreover some interactions are reported based on animal studies; they need not be the same in human body.

It was found that if a person is exposed to DDT pesticide, metabolism of some drugs is affected. Thus even the environment can affect the drug's activity, hence need for dose or therapy adjustment is clear.

Classification of Drug Interactions

Depends on the benefit or otherwise of a drug interaction they are classified into two types:

1. Beneficial interactions and
2. Adverse interactions

1. *Beneficial interactions*: Few drugs on interaction with other drugs produce beneficial effects. Potentiation or synergisms are some of the examples of such benefits. Some drugs are used deliberately to enhance the effect of other drug or minimize the unwanted effect of it. The examples are sulphamethaxozole and trimethaprim combination, and carbidopa and levodopa respectively. There are many formulations in the market using these beneficial effects like estrogen – progestogen combination as contraceptive, ampicillin, cloxacillin combination as potent antibiotic and β.blockers – diuretic combination as hypotensive agents.

Drug interactions can also be used to treat drug over- dose patients, as they nullify or antagonize the adverse effect of overdose drug. Examples are levodopa and vitamin B_6, warfarin and vitamin K, narcotic analgesics and nalorphine.

2. *Adverse interactions:* As newer and newer chemicals are introduced for doctors to treat the patients and multiple drugs are commonly prescribed, possibility for adverse interactions also increase day by day. These adverse reactions can be put under two broad classifications, namely,

   1. Pharmacodynamic drug interactions and
   2. Pharmacokinetic drug interactions

If drug interactions are based on their effect on the body, they are called pharmacodynamic drug interactions, and if they are due to absorption, distribution, metabolism or excretion of the drug, they are referred to as pharmacokinetic interactions.

1. Pharmacodynamic Drug Interactions

These interactions happen when two drugs with same effects are concurrently administered unknowingly. All the beneficial interactions listed above are also based on the activity of drugs only. Some adverse interactions due to drugs activities are listed below.

If hypnotics are given with antihistamines or narcotic analgesics or tranquilizers or alcohol, their effect is increased drastically resulting in unwanted proportions. Hence combinations of CNS depressants should be avoided but sometimes it is overlooked or hidden from prescribers.

Digoxin and quinidine combination is another example for pharmaco dynamic drug interaction. Basic properties of all the drugs prescribed should be remembered by prescribers and pharmacists to avoid such problems.

2. Pharmacokinetic Drug Interactions

These interactions are due to

1. Change in absorption of drugs
2. Alteration in protein binding and distribution
3. Biotransformation changes and
4. Drug elimination problems

(i) *Change in absorption of drugs*: Iron preparations and drugs containing calcium, magnesium and aluminium (antacids) precipitate or chelate tetracyclines, hence its absorption from GI tract is affected. Propanthelene if administered along with digoxin or pethidine its absorption is delayed or reduced.

(ii) *Alteration in distribution*: If chloral hydrate is given with warfarin, trichlero acetic acid, the metabolite of the former displaces the warfarin from its protein binding sites. Hence Warfarin concentration in blood increases to double the quantity. However it is temporary as clearance increases correspondingly.

(iii) *Biotransformation changes*: Some drugs increase the drug metabolizing enzymes, some other decrease it. Hence there are changes in plasma drug concentration and drug's activity which either decreases or increases. If the given drug produces pharmacological activity, it is reduced by induction of enzymes, and if the metabolite is responsible for drug's activity, it is increased. Example is co-administration of phenylbutazone and phenytoin. Here phenytoin effect is increased by induction of enzyme by phenylbutazone. Like this when allopurinol and mercaptopurine are given together metabolizing enzymes are inhibited by Allopurinol, hence, 6 mercaptopurine metabolism is delayed and its toxic effect increased. Dose of 6 mercaptopurine should be reduced in such cases.

(iv) *Drug elimination problems*: Some drugs if administered together compete for elimination via active tubular secretion. As a result each of these drugs eliminates slowly and consequently stays longer inside the body. Duration of action thus increases. One example already given is probenecid and penicillin, another one is salicylates and uricosuric agents.

If we alter the pH of the urine, drug's elimination is affected. This type of drug interaction is used for treating poison cases. For example, if we make urine pH alkaline using sodium bicarbonate, acidic drugs like salicylates and phenobarbitone are eliminated quickly from the body. Similarly if we make urine pH acidic using ammonium chloride alkaline drugs like quinidine is eliminated faster.

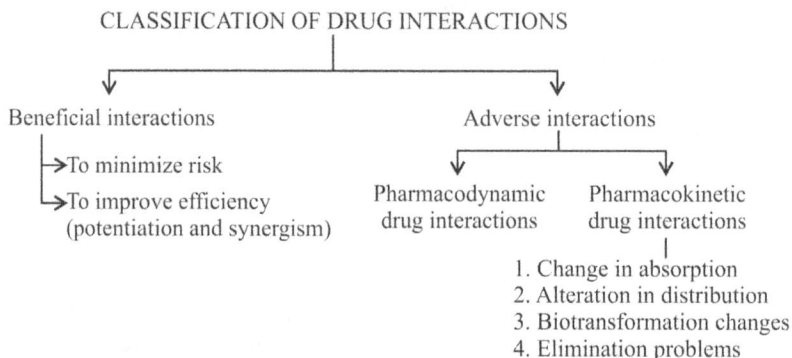

CLASSIFICATION OF DRUG INTERACTIONS

Beneficial interactions
→ To minimize risk
→ To improve efficiency
(potentiation and synergism)

Adverse interactions

Pharmacodynamic drug interactions

Pharmacokinetic drug interactions
1. Change in absorption
2. Alteration in distribution
3. Biotransformation changes
4. Elimination problems

Drug Interaction Examples

I. Analgesics	
1. Aspirin with Alcohol	GI irritation and bleeding
2. Aspirin with Ibuprofen	No superior action
3. Narcotic analgesics with CNS depressants like barbiturates	Excessive depressant action
4. Paracetamol with Metaclopromide	Increased onset of Paracetamol action
II. Cardio Vascular Agents	
1. Digitalis and its preparations with barbiturates	Increase the metabolism of Digoxin hence, more dose may be required
2. Digitalis and its preparations with Diuretics	Potassium depletion, give KCl tablets. If not, heart become sensitive to Digitalis and its toxicity
3. Digitalis and its preparations with Reserpine	Increased risk of cardiac arrest
4. Methyl Dopa with Levodopa	Potentiation, so reduce dose.
5. Propranolol with Insulin, Tolbutamide etc	Increase the action of hypoglycemic agents, results in acute hypoglycemia. Additional danger is that effect is not noticeable till serious stage
6. Anticoagulants Warfarin etc with	
(a) Aspirin	Increased effect
(b) Antacids	Decreased effect
(c) Chloromphenicol	Increased effect
(d) Phenylbutazone and oxyphenbutazone	Increase anticoagulant effect
(e) Phenytoin	Phenytoin effect increases, anticoagulant effect decreases
(f) Vitamin K	Antagonism

Table Contd...

III. GI Agents	
1. Antacids with Bisacodyl	GI irritation due to disintegration of enteric coating in stomach itself.
2. Antacids with Tetracycline	Metal ions in antacids like Ca, Mg, Al form complex with Tetracycline, so poor absorption
IV. Hypoglycemic Agents	
Insulin, Tolbutamide, etc with	
1. Corticosteroids like Prednisolone	Increase the blood glucose level
2. Alcohol	Different effects with various intake quantities, may induce faster hypoglycemia
3. Propranolol	Increase the action of insulin etc
4. Coumarin (anticoagulant)	Increase in action due to decrease in metabolism. Reduce dose.
5. Phenylbutazone	Increase the action, so reduce dose
V. Psychopharmacological Agents	
With alcohol	More CNS Depressant action. Hence avoid it.
1. Antidepressants with	
(a) Coumarin	Increase the effect of anti coagulants
(b) MAO inhibitors	Tremors, convulsions
(c) Reserpine	Contraindicated
2. Antipsychotic agents (chlorpromazine group) with	
(a) Antacids	Magnesium trisilicate decrease plasma level of the drug. Avoid or delay
(b) Anticholinergics	Dryness of mouth, blurring of vision, constipation, and urine detention
(c) Levodopa	Action of Levodopa inhibited
(d) MAO Inhibitors	Increase the action of the antipsychotic drugs
3. Sedatives and Hypnotics with	
(a) Alcohol	Enhanced CNS depression
(b) MAO inhibitors	Enhanced CNS depression so avoid it
(c) Digitoxin	Increase the rate of metabolism of Digitoxin
(d) Griseofulvin	Decrease in action of Griseofulvin
VI. Vitamins	
1. Folic acid with Phenytoin	Development of Folic acid deficiency and reduced Phenytoin level
2. Vitamin B_6 with Levodopa	Antagonism patients under Levodopa therapy should avoid multivitamins
3. Vitamin C with Aspirin	Reduced Vitamin C absorption
4. Vitamin D with Phenytoin	Increase the metabolism of Vitamin D, so Vitamin D deficiency (Rickets, etc)
5. Vitamin K with Coumarin	Antagonism

Drug Induced Diseases

It is a paradox that drugs produced for curing diseases, themselves produce diseases, if misused or abused. As pointed out earlier, drug interactions and ADR, may damage various parts of our body. These damages or diseases caused by prescription drugs are hence known as physician induced diseases or Iatrogenic. Liver and kidney are the major organs usually damaged, though other organs like skin, GI tract and blood may also be affected. Hence the drugs which cause these problems should be used with caution and properly monitored when prescribed by doctors. These problems are:

I. Drug Induced Liver Diseases

Liver may be damaged directly or indirectly by drugs. Direct liver damage is caused by drugs like isoniazid, tetracycline etc. Liver is damaged indirectly due to patient's hypersensitivity to certain drugs like sulphonamides, erythromycin etiolate etc. These damages may suddenly appear (acute) or sustained for a long time (chronic), the former is called acute hepatotoxicity and induced by cimetidine, rifampicin, phenylbutazone, methyl dopa, INH, PAS, erythromycin etc, The later is known as chronic drug induced liver diseases caused by sulphonamides, penicillin, oral contraceptives, alcohol, anabolic steroids etc.

II. Drug Induced Renal Diseases

Kidney is the place from where all toxic materials are eliminated through urine. Hence it is susceptible to damages. In order to eliminate the toxins, kidney breaks toxins-protein complexes and hence there is high concentration of toxins in kidney. Sometimes, pH of urine precipitates certain drugs or their metabolites, similarly the antigen-antibody complexes present in large endothelial area of kidney may cause hypersensitivity reactions. Thus kidney is vulnerable to damages and hence drugs like sulphonamides and allopurinol should be used with caution, as the sulphonamides causes kidney stone and crystals, the allopurinol induces uric acid crystallization.

III. Drug Induced Hematological Disorders

Blood and its composition are affected by many drugs and the resultant disorders are anemia, leucopenia and thrombocytopenia. First two disorders are induced by chloromphenicol, INH, phenytoin, antimalarials, analgesics, phenyl butazone, sulpha drugs etc. Thrombocytopenia is caused by aspirin, ibuprofen, penicillin, alcohol etc. These damages are called disorders not diseases – because they are all temporary and can be corrected by simple corrective measures.

IV. Drug Induced Gastrointestinal Disorders

Constipation, diarrhoea, vomiting and ulceration are the disorders caused by antibiotics, salicylates, ephedrine, furosemide, cimetidine, methyldopa, etc. These disorders also depend on the diet.

V. Drug Induced Dermatological Reactions

They are due to photosensitive reactions, known as phototoxic and/or photo allergic. When the patient is exposed to light (sun or artificial), after the administration of the drug, they develop reactions like reddening of skin, itching, blisters etc. They are sudden and should be treated immediately.

VI. Teratogenicity

In this problem, somatic cells of developing embryo are affected and hence one or other organ system of it is damaged. This effect is known as teratogenicity and the agents causing them are known as teratogens. The common teratogens are thalidomide, tetracycline, diethyl stilbesterol etc. Care should be taken while administering these drugs during the first trimester of pregnant women. The damages caused to the infant are comparable with healthy baby before delivery (pre-natal) and can be seen after delivery (post-natal).

Questions

Short Answer Questions

1. Define Drug - Drug interaction and what are the two types of Drug Interactions?
2. What are the reasons for Drug- Drug Interactions?
3. What are the problems in detecting drug interactions?
4. How can we use the Drug Interaction information?

Long Answer Questions

5. Classify drug interactions. Explain each one of them with examples.
6. What are pharmacokinetic drug interactions? Give examples.
7. Write in detail about drug induced diseases.

CHAPTER 37

PHARMACOVIGILANCE

Definition

W.H.O defines Pharmacovigilance as the science and activities relating to the detection, assessment, understanding and prevention of adverse effects or any other possible medicine related problems.

Need for Pharmacovigilance

It is a known fact that almost all drugs can cause harm if misused or abused. But some drugs produce adverse effects even at normal dose that baffled the health care team. In order to find out those adverse effects and reason for it, everybody involved in the treatment of the patient need to be vigilant, analytical and careful. Thus the need for monitoring drug treatment was felt and it was redoubled after the 'Thalidomide' tragedy of 1960s.

Though the process of introducing new drug was tightened and lengthened after1960s, [see chapter on concept of clinical pharmacy] it cannot be delayed indefinitely. Obviously a new drug cannot be tested on crores of people in a clinical research laboratory. That is possible only after the drug is marketed in various countries with varying population differing in race, ethnicity, environment, customs and habits. The results of use of new drug in risky people like, children, old people and pregnant women also has to be gathered as clinical trials are not done on these people normally. Hence 'Post Marketing Surveillance' [PMS] is the only option available before the drug regulators of the world to detect the ADR and other problems. As this surveillance has to be carried out for many years after marketing of the drug, there arises a need for a program to monitor, collect and document information about ADR pouring in periodically. Also the information is from different countries and with long time gap in between and hence an international agency to do that work was felt by health care professionals. Thus W.H.O started the Pharmacovigilance program by realizing its need and importance.

Origin of Pharmacovigilance

The concept of 'vigilance while using medicines' took concrete shape around the middle of 1960s after the Thalidomide tragedy. In 1965 the 18th World Health Assembly [WHO 18.42] drew attention to the problem of ADR monitoring. It was emphasized subsequently in further resolutions in 1966, 67 and 1970 and by then the International Drug Monitoring program was established. In 2005 there were 78 countries participating in that program. In the last decade many developing countries have enrolled in it. It is now functioning through National Pharmacovigilance Centers in member countries which are all co-ordinated by two WHO centers one at Uppsala, the WHO collaborating center for international drug monitoring, and another pharmacovigilance department of WHO at Geneva.

Aims of Pharmacovigilance

The primary aims of Pharmacovigilance program are,

1. To improve patient care and safety
2. To enhance public health
3. To encourage monitoring understanding and training in pharmacovigilance program thereby alerting health care team and general public and
4. To evaluate drug's benefits, risks and effectiveness and thereby to promote safe and rational use of drugs.

In order to achieve above aims Pharmacovigilance program has to be broad based and its scope should not be restricted or narrower. It has to include all the stakeholders of drug use in this program.

Stakeholders of Pharmacovigilance

Even though drug use is a matter between patient and prescriber, its result has great influence over the society as a whole. The result may be a success or failure, but both impact not only the patient and his family, but also help the community to learn from that experience. Thus there are many stakeholders coming into the picture of pharmacovigilance program. They are,

1. Patients
2. Health care team
3. Hospitals and medical / para medical institutions
4. Government
5. Pharma industry and its regulators
6. Medical and pharmaceutical associations
7. Drug and poison information centers

8. General public [consumers]

9. The media and

10. World Health Organization.

Co-operation between all the above stakeholders is essential for the success of pharmacovigilance program for which governments of all countries should help. Necessary infrastructure for monitoring, documenting and communicating the findings of the program should be provided by all governments. Guidelines and training required for conducting the program will be provided by pioneers of the program or WHO. All the above stakeholders should understand that this is a program for common cause and the information obtained from it will save not only money, time and energy but also the precious lives of patients. Thus the scope of the program is multi dimensional and mutually beneficial.

Scope of Pharmacovigilance

The scope of pharmacovigilance has been widened to include herbal, traditional and complementary medicines, blood products, biological, medical devices and vaccines. According to WHO, many other issues are also of relevance to the science of pharmacovigilance. They are, substandard medicines, medication errors, lack of efficacy, use of medicines for indications that are not approved and for which there is inadequate scientific basis, case reports of acute and chronic poisoning, assessment of medicine-related mortality, abuse and misuse of medicines, and adverse interactions of medicines with chemicals, other medicines and foods and drinks.

This apart the scope of pharmacovigilance also extends from an individual patient to Government to entire society. However let us restrict its application to some important area, so as to understand its significance and opportunities to work with.

1. ***Pharmacovigilance and clinical pharmacy practice***: Therapeutic Drug Monitoring [TDM] and Drug Therapy Review are the important tools in pharmacovigilance program of clinical practice. It has great impact on the quality of health care. The information gathered during this program, if relevant, has to be conveyed to all health care providers, other pharmacovigilance centers and health policy developers. Thus an effective patient care can be ensured.

2. ***Pharmacovigilance and medicine policy***: In order to frame a national drug policy, pharmacovigilance program is of much use to the authorities, as it provides needed information about which drugs are not suitable in community settings and which other drugs can be promoted in national health programs etc. through such policies government can forge links between various partners of pharmacovigilance program such as pharmaceutical industries, universities of health sciences, voluntary social organizations and professional associations who in turn promote rational and safe use of drugs.

3. ***Pharmacovigilance and drugs control:*** Pharmacovigilance program is more helpful to Drugs control department than others as it make their work easier. Drugs control organization is gathering information about spurious drugs, sub-standard drugs, etc, by its own vigilance and intelligence wings. The pharmacovigilance centers by monitoring drug therapy provide much needed information about drug's quality, side effects etc to them. Based on these information and input, drugs regulatory department can start their investigation and weed out any problem drug from the market.

Pharmacovigilance program also emphasize monitoring of clinical trials, medicines of alternative systems and vaccines. Thus it opens a link between all parties who have interest in medicine safety and ensures that they all function in co ordination with each other.

4. ***Pharmacovigilance and public health program:*** Many developing countries are implementing at least few public health programs at the same time. Thus vaccination, T.B, Malaria & Leprosy eradication programs and the famous family planning programs are run concurrently through all primary health centers and sub centers attached to them. Pharmacovigilance program stress the need to monitor these public health programs as many of them are overlapping and can cause ADR, drug interaction etc on the unsuspecting, illiterate and innocent rural masses. This vigilance has to be doubled during national calamities, epidemic attacks and large gathering of people during festivals.

Thus the scope of pharmacovigilance covers range of products and people from allopathic medicines to food and drinks and individual patient to health care providers, drug regulators and the government.

Advantages of Pharmacovigilance

1. It is a cost effective method of detecting and minimizing problems to patients and thereby preventing potential disaster.
2. It function like a safe guard against the undetected use of ineffective, substandard or counterfeit medicines and hence reduce the wastage of resources.
3. It communicates the information on the effectiveness and risks of drugs and thereby educates the health care team and the public.
4. Compare to the cost of ADR causing to a country, the cost of pharmacovigilance program is very less.
5. Overall the pharmacovigilance program ensures safe, rational and effective use of medicines by patients

Pharmacovigilance Practice

Pharmacovigilance program is implemented by various methods of collecting information about ADR and other drug related problems. They are

1. Case-Control study

2. Cohort study

3. Spontaneous case report and

4. Vital statistics and record linkage study.

These are explained in detail in a chapter on ADR [Chapter 35]. However among the above 'spontaneous case report method is given more attention recently as it is fast and the information is given directly by the people involved. In this method the information is either directly obtained from the patient who experience the benefit or harm of a medicine taken or through their health care providers. The health care team also monitor for ADR while treating the patient and report if it occurs to the national pharmacovigilance center. In some countries national reporting system provides for direct patient reporting. In many states of India this is being implemented by offering a toll free telephone number and patients are encouraged to report any drug related problem through this number. This type of facility will be useful when disease specific programs are implemented. The information gathered by any of the above methods are processed by national pharmacovigilance centers and then sent to WHO center for International Drug Monitoring.

Conclusion

Medicines are like double edged weapons and to use it wisely without being hurt, vigilance is needed. If it is assured in the form National Pharmacovigilance program, it

- Increases the confidence and faith of people on medicines and health care providers.
- Provide essential information to Drugs regulatory authorities, so as to function more effectively and
- Educate the health care professionals about the medicine they prescribe, dispense and administer.

Thus pharmacovigilance program take the entire health care sector one step forward towards excellence in their practice.

Questions

Short Answer Questions

1. Write short note on the need for Pharmacovigilance

2. Who are all the stakeholders of Pharmacovigilance program?

3. List the advantages of Pharmacovigilance program

Long Answer Questions

4. Define Pharmacovigilance. What are its aims and scope?

CHAPTER 38

PHARMACEUTICAL CARE

Introduction

Pharmaceutical care is a new concept evolved during the middle of 1970s, after the pharmacists were given the responsibility of monitoring drug therapy in 1960s. It is an extension of Clinical Pharmacy services started towards the end of 1960s and developed into a full scheme of pharmaceutical care. Many of the functions assigned under this concept are new to pharmacists and hence a section of them were reluctant to accept those responsibilities. These works involve not only monitoring, reviewing and documenting the therapy but also taking full responsibility for the result.

Definition

Helper and Strand have defined, "Pharmaceutical care as the responsible provision of drug therapy for the purpose of achieving definite outcomes that improve a patient's quality of life"

FIP adopted the above definition with little modification. They inserted the words 'or maintain' after the word 'improve' and thus the new definition is,

"Pharmaceutical care is the responsible provision of drug therapy for the purpose of achieving definite outcomes that improve or maintain a patient's quality of life"

It is obvious in certain disease conditions like AIDS or Diabetes, improving patient's quality of life is not always possible. Just maintaining it at the present level of quality, without further deterioration, itself considered as significant achievement.

Pharmaceutical care and clinical pharmacy: The above definition looks similar to the definition of clinical pharmacy services. What is the difference between them? Roger Walker says, 'the practice of clinical pharmacy is an essential component in the delivery of pharmaceutical care.' He further elaborates, ' the delivery of pharmaceutical care is dependent on the practice of clinical pharmacy, but the key feature of care is that the practitioner takes responsibility for a patient's drug related needs and is held responsible for that commitment. Thus "pharmaceutical care is a cooperative, patient centered system for achieving specific and positive patient outcomes from the responsible provision of medicines" he concludes. From the above quote, it is clear in pharmaceutical care pharmacist takes direct responsibility for the patient's drug related needs and thereby assures its quality in this care.

Types of Pharmaceutical care: As per the above definition pharmacist takes full responsibility for the drug therapy given to an individual patient under the concept of pharmaceutical care, immediately the question arises who is responsible for the therapy given to the community as a whole under special circumstances. Here too pharmacist should provide pharmaceutical care. In this population based pharmaceutical care, he has to use demographic or epidemiological data for serving the needs of the society. It includes, according to a document published by WHO, establishing hospital formulary, developing and networking pharmacy services, conducting and evaluating drug utilization review, developing and educating drug related policies etc. On the other hand the first type of pharmaceutical care given to individual patient involves monitoring drug therapy and modifying it if necessary. Though pharmaceutical care is provided in co operation with entire health care team, pharmacist alone is responsible for the cost, quality and outcome of pharmaceutical care

Basic Concept of Pharmaceutical Care

1. In pharmaceutical care, first the pharmacist plans an individualized drug therapy for the patient. It aims at specific results and formulated in consultation with other health care professionals and patient.
2. For the above plan evidences are collected, its merits and demerits are studied and then adopted for implementation.
3. Patient is educated about the plan and its method of execution and
4. While the patient is under therapy, the outcomes are constantly monitored and modified if required.

Thus pharmacists in co-operation with other health care professionals and patients, design, implement and monitor a therapeutic plan that produces definite outcomes for the patient. These works are nicely presented by Helper et al in their paper "Opportunities and responsibilities in pharmaceutical care" published in 1990 in American Journal of Hospital Pharmacy.

Pharmaceutical Care, for whom?

Though it is ideal to provide pharmaceutical care for all patients, in practice, it is not possible. Hence patients should be selected on the basis of following situations.

- Patients in critical conditions or disease, that is patients with cardiac problems, hypertension, diabetes, asthma etc, should be given priority.
- Patients whose body conditions are vulnerable to adverse reactions, such as patients with liver or kidney damage, pediatric and geriatric cases etc

- Patients who are given risky drugs which are sure to cause damage, if wrongly used. E.g. Anticancer drugs, Amonoglycosides, anticoagulants etc

- Patients in acute conditions and when the drugs given do not produce desired level of therapeutic action, as in certain infectious diseases and severe diarrhoea.

When provided with pharmaceutical care these risky patients can be saved with the co-operation and efforts of entire health care team. Though pharmacist plan, execute and monitor pharmaceutical care program he has to ensure the support and active participation of full health care team to achieve the definite outcome planned.

Principle and Practice of Pharmaceutical Care

In 1995 American Pharmacists Association [APhA] has published 'the principles of practice for pharmaceutical care' to guide the concept of pharmaceutical care when it was started developing. In that document it is pointed out what is needed to achieve the goal of pharmaceutical care and various steps involved in it. The following are the excerpts from the document:

To fulfill the objectives of pharmaceutical care,

- Pharmacists must establish a professional relationship with patient and maintain it.

- Patient specific medication information must be collected, organized, recorded and maintained

- The above information must be evaluated and a drug therapy plan developed mutually with the patient

- The pharmacist assures that the patient has all supplies, information and knowledge necessary to carry out the drug therapy plan and

- The pharmacist reviews, monitors and modifies the therapeutic plan as necessary and appropriate in concert with the patient and health care team.

Steps Involved in the Practice of Pharmaceutical Care

1. *Data collection:* By medication history interview with the patient, if it is not possible—with the patient's care takers, old medical records, left over medicines etc, patient specific data is collected first. This data must be complete and comprehensive in all aspects. All these data are recorded accurately and confidentially. It is shown to others only with the permission of the patient or if required by law.

2. *Data Evaluation:* After evaluation some decisions can be taken from the above data like opportunity to improve present condition, effectiveness of planned therapy, way to reduce future drug related problem etc. These decisions can be conveyed to the patient, to the extend necessary, in order to make him understand his present condition and future prospects.

3. ***Designing a plan:*** Then the pharmacists should design a plan to treat the patient with specific achievable goal. For this he can consult other health care professionals and enroll their co-operation. Drugs suitable for the patient should be selected next and ways of monitoring its effect has to be identified. The design can also include non-drug treatment, dietary changes etc. It also should be clear about therapeutic end point and monitoring limitations.

4. ***Executing the plan:*** The plan evolved as above should be implemented with care. During this stage the pharmacist requires the support and involvement of other health care professionals, patient attendants and of course patient himself. All the supplies starting from drug to other items in time should be ensured by the pharmacist.

5. ***Monitoring the plan and outcome:*** The pharmacist has to regularly monitor the out come of the treatment to determine whether satisfactory progress is there or not. If it is not satisfactory the plan should be modified and then implemented. While monitoring the therapy patient's vital parameters should be checked using lab tests wherever and whenever necessary. However costly tests should be avoided as far as possible to keep the cost of treatment minimum and affordable to the patient as that is also one of the goals of pharmaceutical care. If positive outcomes are noticed they should be conveyed to other health care professionals to elevate their confidence in the treatment plan. All these developments should be recorded in patient's case diary or record, so that follow up will be easier. Always patient's medical and/or pharmacy records should be kept updated. Communications with other health care providers also should be recorded.

Requirements for Successful Pharmaceutical Care

American Pharmacists Association has listed the important requirements for successful implementation of pharmaceutical care. They are,

1. Knowledge, skill and function of personnel
2. Systems for data collection, documentation and transfer of information
3. Efficient workflow processes
4. References, resources and equipment
5. Communication skills and
6. Commitment to quality improvement and assessment procedures

If all these requirements are in place while implementing the program of pharmaceutical care, better results can be achieved to improve the quality of patient's life.

Evaluation of Pharmaceutical Care Services

Any product or service provided to the society should be evaluated for its quality; pharmaceutical care is not an exemption. The quality of any service including health care services can be assured by evaluating its structure, process and outcome according to Donabedian. On completion of this evaluation short comings if any can be rectified and thus it serve to achieve better patient outcome. The evaluation or quality assurance process starts with the focus on the patient, process and then the result. As described above patient specific plan must be prepared and implemented with the co operation of the team. The result obtained is evaluated in the light of set goals. The quality of pharmaceutical care can be assured if the resources or structure is properly mobilized and the plan correctly executed.

Questions

Short Answer Questions

1. Write a note on principle and practice of Pharmaceutical care.

2. What are the requirements for a successful Pharmaceutical care?

3. List the steps involved in the pharmaceutical care process

Long Answer Questions

4. Define Pharmaceutical care. How it is carried out? Explain.

5. Describe the concept of pharmaceutical care

CHAPTER 39

PATIENT COUNSELLING

Introduction

Counselling is done at the end of long course of treatment just before discharge, but that is not a hard and fast rule. Counselling can also be at the beginning or middle of the treatment depends on the need. During the patient medication history interview, information about the patient is gathered, whereas information is given during counselling. After the diagnosis, the treating physician give some outline about the disease suspected and probable treatment and duration. If more information is required to be given to the patient, counselling is conducted. Similarly during the treatment, in order to ascertain patients feeling about his disease, its severity or comfort, problems in medicine usage etc, counselling session is conducted.

At the end of the treatment just before discharge patient is instructed, about continuation of treatment in home, do's and dont's regarding diet, exercise, repeat visit to hospital etc. This session of counselling will be worthwhile because after discharge, patient looses the supervision by doctor, pharmacist and nurses and hence a careless attitude of the patient may result in relapse of the disease or more complications.

Patients used to hide some facts or mistakes committed by them to the doctor. By counselling, a good counsellor can bring out those hidden truth by winning the confidence of patients. Thus counselling is beneficial to both health care team and patients.

Need for Counselling and Privacy

Counselling involve two way exchange of information between the pharmacist and the patient and hence it is better than written communication. Moreover, legally and morally pharmacists has to give information about the drugs, patients use. It should be in sufficient quantity and in language the patients understands. Hence the need for counselling is obvious. Again if the counselling has to be effective, it should be conducted in a place free from noise, interruption or distractions. If such a privacy is provided, patient will understand the importance given to it and co-operate with counsellor. It improve the image of the pharmacist and he will be recognized as one contributing to his welfare. Generally disease is a private affair of the patient hence he is hesitant to speak about it openly. When such a foolproof privacy is provided, he tends to speak more about his inner problems and feelings.

Thus a fruitful counselling can be conducted when privacy is provided.

Classification

Counselling can be classified into:

1. Direct counselling (face to face) and
2. Distant counselling through phone

Though direct counselling is the one advised, distant counselling can also be useful for the patients who could not visit hospitals or clinics for the reasons of disease, immobility or other problems. In developed countries such services are available for a service fee, patients themselves can opt for it. Usually, out- patients with chronic illness and elderly patients seek these services.

Suitable Person to Give Counselling

Generally doctors, nurses and pharmacists can conduct counselling for the patients. However the first two, do not have required time or environment for such services. As both doctor and nurses need to attend emergency cases at any time, their services remain confined to the ward. Moreover, waiting period, restlessness, anticipation, apprehension and even fear make the patient out of mood to cooperate with counselling by doctors. The smell, fellow patients and their disease complications, administration of different medicine through different route to other patients, various surgical instruments and apparatus present in the hospital ward-surrounding affect patients mind sct, to be counselled by nurses. In these circumstances, pharmacist is more suitable, as he is away from these environment and has no emergency to attend and available at all times. By nature of his job, he is an expert in human relations (HR) and has knowledge about drugs and its side effects. Thus pharmacists can take care of patients need and direct him suitably if needed.

Selection of Patients for Counselling

Routine counselling of all patients is both impossible and unneccessary. Patients are selected according to the need. For others, few minutes of counselling is sufficient and given during regular ward rounds or at the time of administration of drugs. Relatively long counselling sessions are needed for:

A. Patients to be subjected to long term treatment e.g.: Epilepsy cases.

B. Patients with diseases but without severe symptoms e.g.: Prophylactic cases of TB.

C. Patients using drugs with narrow therapeutic index. e.g.: Warfarin.

D. Patients with danger of abrupt stopping of treatment. e.g.: Corticosteroid therapy.

E. Patients with potential for non-compliance, abuse or misuse of drugs. e.g.: Treatment with tranquilizers.

Patient Education and Councelling

Patient counselling is nothing but a form of patient education as majority of information given during counselling is for the purpose of educating the patient. If it is considered as an education, then it need not be restricted to few patients. As many patient as possible should be educated so as to achieve best clinical outcome of the treatment.

American Society of Health System Pharmacists [ASHP] says "Pharmacists should educate and counsel all patients to the extent possible, going beyond the minimum requirements of laws and regulations." ASHP also emphasize, "Pharmacists should encourage patients to seek education and counselling and should eliminate barriers to providing it." Though guidelines are given above to select patients for counselling, pharmacists should try to accommodate as many patients as possible, in the interest of the patient, society and his own profession which earn respect from the patients by these services.

Patient education and counselling can be carried out in all the four types of pharmacy practice, viz, Inpatient care, Outpatient care, Home care and Community care settings. However counselling requires some prior preparation to be useful to the patient and to the institution.

Preparation for Counselling

It differs between the four settings mentioned above. If the counselling is for an inpatient at the time of discharge, needed information about the patient can be obtained from hospital records. However, if counselling is to be carried out at the time admission of the patient or few days after the admission or for outpatient or in community pharmacy settings, pharmacist should gather all relevant information about the patient before starting counselling. If a pharmacist could acquire knowledge about patient's cultures, especially his health and illness beliefs, attitude and practices it goes a long way in dealing with him. If the counselling is done after few days of admission and in the middle of the treatment, counselling has to be in different plain, so as the patient to realize his disease can be cured, if he adheres to the instructions of health care team. After all every patient want to go home earlier after curing their disease, hence getting their co-operation may not be a problem. Small complaints like frequent injections, lab procedures and big bitter tablets they start tolerating if the counselling is effectively done. Similarly outpatients will realize whatever the doctor, pharmacist or nurse told was for their welfare, after a brief counselling. Hence for the counselling to be successful the pharmacist should get himself ready for it.

As there is no effective supervision of patient after discharge, proper counselling is needed to prevent relapse and readmission of the patient. Appropriate learning aids like graphics, anatomical models, medication devices, memory aids, printed pamphlets and audio visual resources should be kept ready in the counselling room. Whichever aid needed must be used to boost the level of understanding of the patient, if necessary by demonstration.

This apart, while getting ready for counselling, pharmacist should review discharge prescription, ensure clear medication list and instruction for discharge. The patient's follow up plan should also be ready. As mentioned above fairly good idea about the patient to be counseled can be collected from hospital records. The patient may be a child or aged patient or mentally ill or terminally ill patient. Depends on the type of patient, pharmacist has to plan his counselling content. For example to counsel a child prior idea about its level of understanding is important. On the other hand an elderly patient may be vision or hearing impaired, a terminally ill patient may not be interested in counselling at all and may not listen and mentally ill may not understand and co-operate with counselling. Before counselling a pharmacist must prepare to face all the above situations.

Scope of Counselling or Contents of Counselling

The scope or purpose of patient counselling is for giving instruction and motivation to patients and monitoring them. The counselling for outpatients differ from counselling for inpatients. To inpatients, certain points like, how to open or administer drugs, timing and amount of dose etc need not be discussed, as they are taken care of by nurses. Those instructions need to be given only at the time of discharge along with storage conditions refill information etc. However all these informations have to be conveyed to outpatients, along with possible side effects, what to do if one or two doses are missed and duration of treatment. For complicated regimen like multiple drug regimen or sophisticated or complex packings, drugs has to be shown to the patient and explained. This, not only make them understand better, but also helps the pharmacist in detection of dispensing or prescription error. A few words about use and importance of each drug will lead to better compliance and consequent success of treatment.

Moreover patients may be interested in knowing expected duration of treatment and expected benefits. They can be briefly mentioned while discussing the importance of adhering to the instructions. Possible drug- drug interaction and drug-food interaction should be informed. Technique of self monitoring of treatment should be taught to the patient. Depending on the patient's disease management and therapeutic plan some education can be given regarding the disease state, its effect on normal life and identification of disease manifestations.

Before closing the counselling session patient may be encouraged to speak his mind regarding the treatment. This is very important because, they have many unanswered questions, misunderstandings and problems which they may not reveal to health care team. In the absence of answers to these problems, they make their own decisions regarding the treatment. Only when they are prompted, they tend to open up and ask questions and share their experiences with treatment.

After clearing patient's doubt pharmacist can ask few questions at the end to estimate the patient's level of understanding and knowledge about counselling points. If required, pharmacist can once again clarify his doubts with materials and demonstrations. At any point time, pharmacist should not assume that patient has understood all the information given and think if there is problem he will contact him. Also he should not assume that some one else in the health care team—doctor or nurse—might have already told everything to the patient while he was in the ward.

Effect or uses of Counselling

DUE to Counselling

1. Knowledge of disease and its treatment among the patients improved.
2. Patient compliance improved.
3. Repetition of drugs already under use or used can be avoided.
4. Pharmacist contribution towards disease documentation increased.
5. Since compliance improved, disease aggravation reduced.
6. Because of it, emergency visit to hospital or hospitalization or subsequent expenses reduced.

Thus counselling plays an important role in disease management. Hence clinical pharmacists should be appointed in all Indian hospitals.

Barriers or Problems in Patient Counselling

Though there are many advantages in patient counselling, in practice it has many barriers or problems. They are,

1. *Hospital Environment*: The hospital ward environment is not always suitable for patient counselling. Unless the patient is admitted in a separate room called special ward, it is not conducive to go for counselling in a crowded general ward where

dozens of patients are admitted in beds close to each other. Thus there is no privacy and hence patient may not openly discuss his or her problems, doubts and observations of their body conditions. Also the noise or sound level in the general ward is distracting and disturbing and it is especially difficult for the patient to raise their voice. The remedy is to take the patient –even on a wheel chair- to a separate counselling room if provided in the hospital. If it is not provided, at least one common room for two wards- the counselling become a ritual.

2. *Language Barrier*: Many patients of Govt. hospitals are from poor families and they are the people actually requiring counselling. But majority of them only know their mother tongue and use of English or other languages and technical terms during counselling make it useless. Hence counselling pharmacist should able to speak in the language the patient understands.

3. *Educational Level*: It is fallout of above situation where the patient's education level is poor. Hence they may not be in a position to read the label or written instructions or information given to them. Even if they read it comprehending or understanding that information is very low.

4. *Disabilities of body*: Many patients are in their advanced age and hence their eye sight and hearing abilities are below normal. Such patients have to be counseled with written materials if they are able to read or with sign language, if they can see it. Repeated instructions during counselling until the patient understand it may be required.

5. *Patient motivation*: It is one of the important factor that any amount of counselling goes waste unless the patient is motivated to listen and learn. If the patient is suffering from chronic illness or not completely cured or has to continue treatment in his home or depressed or at the tail end of their life they tend to show disinterest in counselling. Clinical pharmacist should understand it and conduct counselling according to ground realities. Definitely it is one of the difficult situations in his career.

6. *Inadequate time or training*: Usually senior, experienced clinical pharmacists are assigned the duty of patient counselling. But on some rare occasions or during trainings, juniors may be counselling. That may reflect on the quality of counselling. Sometimes due to lack of time or pressing other engagements Clinical Pharmacists tend to cut short counselling sessions and that also considered as one of the barriers in counselling.

Documentation

Pharmacist should document counselling points in patient's permanent medical record as per the guidelines of hospital or law. If the above medical record is not available for any reason, pharmacist can record it in patient's medication profile or in specially designed counselling record of the pharmacy department of the hospital. In this record pharmacist should note when, where, how and for whom the counselling was given and also the patient specific points discussed including drug-food interaction warnings. He should also record the patient's level of understanding as perceived by him. These records should be safe guarded as patient's confidential personal record till the time it is legally required.

Questions

Short Answer Questions

1. Write briefly about the need for patient counselling.

2. How a pharmacist is suitable to give counselling?

3. What are the scope for counselling?

4. List the uses of counselling.

5. Who are all the patients needed counselling?

6. Write a note on barriers of counselling

Long Answer Questions

7. How will you counsell a patient?

8. Write an essay about patient counselling.

9. Conduct a mock counselling using one of your classmates, document it and submit.

CHAPTER 40

DRUG INFORMATION CENTER AND ROLE OF PHARMACISTS IN EDUCATION AND TRAINING

Introduction

Traditionally, pharmacists used to give just the needed informations like dosage, use and storage about the drugs to the patients visiting hospitals and retail outlets. This traditional role has changed now, from product oriented to patient oriented. He is now expected to provide all informations about drugs and also other related informations like availability, substitute, ADR, Research findings etc. Hence drug information centers are established in all the big hospitals and other places. As the custodian of knowledge bank (Drug Information Center, DIC) Pharmacist is expected to play much larger role as teachers and information provider.

Need for Drug Information Centers

Due to fast scientific developments and consequent research possibilities in the last few decades lot of new drugs and formulations are added daily to the book of drugs, throughout the world. Now the volume of information available about drugs is impossible to manage or remember by an individual, however experienced or educated he may be. Hence some sort of arrangement is needed to collect, edit and arrange such a huge quantity of information. Thus drug information centers become an essential entity.

Moreover, all the informations published are not needed to everybody. For example, for a cancer hospital, information related to its activities are essential, whereas other informations are only of academic interest. Hence someone is needed to collect and edit the needed information and to bring to their attention. This itself a tremendous task as there are few journals and magazines in each sub division of science now-a-days. As the information technology revolution has resulted in flooding of information from every nook and corner of the world, the need for someone or service to sortout those information is felt. Hence Drug Information services become necessary.

A busy practicing physician or surgeon is in need of some information urgently in a complicated situation. He has to put lot of efforts, wasting his precious time and energy to collect such information. If a centre or service is available for ready reference, it will be of great help to him. Moreover even general public can clarify their doubts regarding the drugs they use or diseases they have, by enquiring with Drug Information centres, without much effort or money. If such a centre is not available they have to disturb or depend only the treating physician, for which they are reluctant and hence deprived of even essential information, resulting in complications.

Thus the need for Drug Information Center is evident.

Suitable Person to be Incharge of DIC

In a hospital setup, pharmacist is a member of Pharmacy and Therapeutic Committee, and incharge of hospital library, hence a pharmacist is suitable to be incharge of Drug Information Center.

Usually, informations are provided by drug manufacturers, distributors and their representatives. By nature of his job pharmacist is always in touch with these sources of information. Hence he can collect those informations easily. Moreover these information suppliers are his fellow pharmacists or their employees thus, a natural binding exists between them.

Pharmacists undergo a thorough education about drugs and their physical, chemical, pharmaceutical and pharmacological properties for few years. Hence they are more knowledgeable than others about drugs and that knowledge is useful in critically evaluating all literatures available about the drugs and selecting a correct information. Those informations can be edited by him and passed on to the needed persons. Thus none other than a pharmacist is suitable to be incharge of Drug Information Center.

Establishing D.I.C

To establish a DIC, a pharmacist must give attention to three important aspects. First and foremost is information gathering and storing, second one is information retrieval and the last one is information dissemination.

For information gathering, the sources of information should be approched and the relavant materials purchased. Textbooks, journals and other printed materials are available from the publishers, either they can be purchased or subscribed. Apart from these printed hard copies, database soft copies in the form of CD should also be purchased from the authorities or suppliers concerned. They are priced from few thousand rupees to few lakh rupees each.

Moreover an ideal internet connection with high download speed should be obtained and installed in all Drug Information Centres. In order to supplement the informations thus collected, literatures and booklets, if any, published by pharmaceutical manufacturers, National pharmaceutical and Medical associations should be collected and kept ready for reference. Now-a-days, all the Drug Information Centers and libraries of Universities of Health Sciences and colleges are networked and information can be collected from any of these istitutions.

For information retrieval, DIC pharmacist should establish and maintain a system for quick retrieval from available sources. Retrieval of information from internet sources are explained elsewhere in this chapter. But trieval has to be from hard copies of reference books, pharmacopoeias and journals also. Hence DIC should have a bucca catelogue of them arranged not only topic or subject wise also author and/or publisher wise, just like any public library. Necessary software is available for this and that should be installed in DIC computers and used. While available information can be retrieved quickly, some information may be insufficent, some may be of doubtful in nature.

Unavailable information can be gathered from other sources in the network, which may require little more time. As most of the information sought from DIC may be for immediate adoptation and implementation, pharmacist should get the information as quick as possible. But information or data of doubtful nature requires clarification. Those information has to be passed on to a panel of drug consultants. After their opinion or advice such information can be given to the seeker. Hence DIC needed to constitute a panel of pharmacy experts. Sometimes DIC pharmacist himself has to critically evaluate the drug information and literature before adding them to his collections. This is explained separately.

The third important aspect of DIC is dessimination of information. This requires some systematic approch.

Sources of Information

Based on the origin and nature of information the sources of information can be divided into three. They are:

1. Primary sources
2. Secondary sources and
3. Tertiary sources

1. **_Primary Sources_:** These are the original informations generated by research scholors and scientists and published either in scientific journals and/or presented in conferences, seminars etc. These information are not condensed, interpreted or edited by a second party. Other examples are patent applications, theses, dissertations and technical reports.

2. ***Secondary Sources***: These informations are collected from all or any one of the above primary sources and edited or interpreted by other than original authors. Usually it is done for a specific purpose or audience. Examples are, review articles, hand books, text books, encyclopedias and computerized services like abstracting or indexing services, which are described below.

3. ***Tertiary Sources***: The information derived from both or either of the above sources is known as Tertiary information. Here the information provided, are composite and in diluted version. Examples are, guides, literatures and pamphlets issued by manufacturers etc. Information gathered from people who attended the conferences and seminars are also falling under this category.

It is clear from the above, primary sources of information are reliable, accurate and most current in nature. On the other hand, secondary and tertiary information are less accurate or less recent in nature, because they have passed through several authors or publishers.

Computerized Services

This is one of the secondary sources of information, where details are collected from various sources edited and published as data bases, in CD.ROM format or uploaded in websites or portals of internet. They are further differenciated into indexing services and abstracting services. Both these services are very much useful for libraries and information centers like Drug Information centers, where online searching can be used for searching database of remote locations without networking facilities and for use by single users, on the otherhand CD is used when many people use the same computer.

Abstracting Services: As the name indicates it contains the summaries or abstracts of original reports. It also interpret the original report according to editorial guidelines. Popular examples are

- (a) Drugdex
- (b) International Pharmaceutical Abstract
- (c) Pharmline.

Pharmline database (http://www.pharmline.com) is an abstracting system deals with drugs and professional pharmacy practice. This data base abstracts articles on pharmacy practice and clinical use of drugs from over 100 English pharmacy and medical journals and produced by National Health Service Information specialists.

International pharmaceutical abstracts is produced by American Society of Health System (ASHP) pharmacists. It has abstracts from the articles published in more than 750 pharmacy, medical and other health related journals, published worldwide. This service is there from 1970. It is a paid service, available via http://www.ashp.org/ipal.

***Indexing Services*:** Examples for indexing services are:

1. Medline
2. BIOSIS [Biosciences information service] previews
3. Clinalert
4. Embase
5. IDIS (Iowa drug Information System)

An indexing service is not interpreting the original article but provide only the indexed topic and the original abstract or full text.

1. ***Medline*:** Medical, dental and nursing journals are indexed here which is prepared by US National Library of Medicine from 1966 onwards, some 11 million records from more than 4300 journals are indexed in this service. Important pharmacy journals like "The Pharmaceutical Journal" is not covered. This database is updated daily CD versions like OVID and silver platter are also available. Medline system via internet include 'Pubmed' and 'Biomed net'. They just differ in their presentation and search systems.

2. ***BIOSIS*:** [Biosciences information service] It gives the journal, meetings, books, and patents data we need to prepare research projects, grant proposals and follow trends in the life sciences. BIOSIS research databases provide us with today's most current sources of life sciences information, including journals, conferences, patents, books, review articles and more

3. ***Clinalert*:** It provides pharmacists, physicians and other health care professionals with comprehensive summaries of adverse drug reactions, drug interactions and market withdrawals from over 100 key medical and research journals from around the world

4. ***Embase*:** It is produced by Elsevier science. It is a major database covering pharmaceutical and biomedical journals. More than 4000 international journals are indexed and about 8 million records from 1974 are available.

5. ***Iowa Drug Information Service (IDIS)*** : It is produced by University of Iowa, USA. It covers about 200 important English medical and pharmaceutical journals. Only the articles relating to treatment of human are indexed and they are available in their full version. It is available both in inernet and as CD ROM.

Retrieval of Information

As the database contain millions and millions of informations, retrieval of information require some skill. If you are able to search with precious or correct terms, the retrieval is easier. To do that indexing language of the data base (controlled vocabulary or thesaurus or keywords) should be used. All possible synonyms, if used, make the search easier, on the otherhand if a common language or free text is used, all relevant information may not be obtained. Hence before starting the search, a clear question must be framed. For example, "How effective are ACE inhibitors in the treatment of heart failure?".

The next step is to choose relavant subject headings or key words to include in the search. These can be included in the search question using the Boolean operators (and/or/not) to get relevant citations. Some databases like Medline and Embase, use sub headings like Adverse effects, Use, Diagnosis etc, to direct the search towards the specific question.

Critical Evaluation of Drug Information and Literature

For successful running of a Drug Information Center, pharmacist in charge has to add latest information to his collections. This information is mainly coming from drug manufacturers through their representatives about new formulations introduced in the market by them. Sometimes they claim new indication [use] for existing formulations. Evaluation of this information is not an easy job; as such information is coming almost daily. Pharmaceutical industry is so vast and competitive that one or other new drug is introduced every week.

These drugs bring with them lot of literature claiming that they are superior and the best among the existing formulations and they site some references for this claim in the brochure of the drugs. Many times these references are half truth and inconvenient portion of references will be left out cleverly. Pharmacists have to go through the full text of these references and arrive at a conclusion about it worthfulness and reliability. Pseudo research articles are published in non-reputed Medical/Pharma journals either to promote their products or mudsling competitor's product by some pharmaceutical companies! Few years back editors of reputed medical journals of developed countries have publicly announced that they are pressurized to publish pseudo research papers by big Pharma companies. Good scientists are being bribed to permit to use their names as authors of such research [!] papers. Hence pharmacists should be vigilant while including a literature to his DIC and if necessary, he should consult senior clinicians or research scientists for the purpose.

Most of the busy doctors do not have time to go through all these literatures deeply or patience to cross check the references. Hence unscrupulous Pharma manufacturers find it easy to hoodwink them. It can be illustrated with one example. One smart manufacturer has claimed in his literature and label for a vitamin tonic that it contains Methyl paraben sodium and Propyl paraben sodium and hence patients will be getting much needed sodium ion! All manufacturing pharmacists know these chemicals are added almost in all liquid oral formulations as preservatives. More over these essential ingredients [not sodium ion] are added at a concentration of just 0.18 % and 0.02% respectively and hence the sodium ion available is negligible in the daily dose of the above tonic, compared to body's requirement and its availability via food. Still these people try to cheat doctors and public by such literatures. One must be vigilant such dubious claims are more in manufacturer's propaganda materials. If a Pharmacist points out such tricks to doctors they appreciate the services of pharmacist and DIC.

Hence pharmacist must critically evaluate all drug information and literature coming to his notice. Critical evaluation is the ability to judge the scientific value of literature or drug information sent to him. This he must do before adding them to DIC and dissipating to information seekers. In order to perform that function successfully he must ask the following questions and get satisfactory answer for them:

1. Weather the drug claimed in the literature has new molecule?
2. If so, is it approved in the country of origin and in other countries?
3. Weather it is approved by Govt. agencies and listed in Pharmacopoeia or Drug Index or purchase list of those Governments?
4. Weather scientific reference quoted in support of the drug is by reputed authors and published in reputed journals?
5. Is those references are readily available fully for verification? Is it worth including after verification?
6. Is their any conditional approval for the product? If yes, what are those conditions?
7. Weather any important information is partial, hidden or left out?
8. Is there any ADR reported anywhere in the world because of the drug?
9. Is the particular drug is still sold in the country of origin? If stopped the reason for it.
10. Weather the drug is exorbitantly priced?

These questions are almost the same asked during the process of including a drug in Hospital Formulary. No wonder, the efforts of DIC and PTC are identical to provide and promote safe drugs to the patient. Unsafe and doubtful drug and its propaganda material have no place in hospital and DIC.

Evaluation of Sources of Information

Drug information is also collected from many primary, secondary and tertiary sources mentioned elsewhere in this chapter. Among them secondary and tertiary sources are less reliable as they are just collected by third parties from primary sources of information. The primary sources of information are the original research articles, patent applications etc. Most of the time a pharmacist administering the DIC need not critically evaluate these primary research articles, as these works are normally carried out by research scientists, reviewers or editorial board experts of scientific journals before publication. Hence a pharmacist of DIC who receive publications from reputed journals and magazines need not burden him with such difficult tasks. However these are the duties of Clinical Pharmacists hence they should learn it. That is why the method of 'Critical Evaluation of Biomedical Literature' is separately given in another chapter.

Systematic Approach in Answering Drug Information Queries

Drug information queries cannot be answered casually, just like that in any customer care centre or public relations office as it involve life saving drugs. In order to give, correct, vital and needed information, drug information centre pharmacist has to approach it in a systematic manner. Watanabe and Conner have described well, such a approach for answering DI queries in their paper 'Principles of Drug Information services' [Drug Intell Publ, Hamilton IL: 15,1978].Incorporating those suggestions, before answering the question DIC pharmacist should ask the following counter questions either to the enquirer or himself. They are,

1. Who is enquiring?
2. What is his purpose?
3. What is the background information?
4. What category the query belongs to?
5. How to retrieve the answer quickly?
6. Is the answer retrieved worth disseminating?
7. How best the answer can be provided?
8. What is the feed back?

Let us analyze the answers to the above questions in detail.

1. *Identity of the person enquiring:* It is required to decide to what extend answer can be given to him. If he/she is a health care professional, detail scientific information can be given which he/she can understand. On the other hand if a member of a general public asks the question, needed information in short, in the manner she understands should be provided. If a research scholar enquires about something, elaborate answer may be needed. Thus length of answer depends on the person enquiring the DIC.

2. *Purpose of query:* Depends on the answer from DIC, a patient may start, continue or stop his treatment! Some people may misuse the information for commencing self medication. Still some others may adorn the role of doctor and start treating their children or other dependents. On the other side Clinicians may require some information to clear their doubt, or refresh their memory or even to commence, continue or change the course of treatment. Hence the genuine purpose of query must be ascertained from the person contacting DIC. Depends on the answer received, appropriate reply can be prepared and supplied.

3. *Background information:* Often vague questions are asked with DIC. From these questions neither the purpose nor the core of answer to be given can be ascertained. Hence DIC pharmacist has to enquire background information like patient's profile, stage of disease or treatment etc. Patient's profile includes patient's age, sex, diagnosis, allergy, current therapy etc. These details help the pharmacist to determine what is actually needed by the enquirer. It is obvious

that, without these details a vague answer for a vague question will not serve any purpose. This is especially true in the case of drugs with multiple uses. Simple example is Aspirin and its use. We know it can be used as analgesic, antipyretic and in angina. Without knowing the background what for it is used, how can a pharmacist answer its dose or side effects? Hence pharmacist must gather background information with minimal questions, without offending the caller.

4. *Category of question*: From the above information pharmacist can understand which category the question belongs to and thereby where to look for the answer. Usual questions like dose, indication, contra indication, possible side effects can be put under general category and can be answered from Drug Index book like, 'Pharmacist's Drug Hand Book' by ASHP, CIMS, MIMS, IDR TRIPLE I, etc, whereas questions like possible interaction between two drugs has to be categorized as 'Drug Interaction' query and answered after thorough reference to available resources. Similarly more probing questions like symptoms of ADR, Toxic manifestations of drugs has to be classified as 'Serious query' and answered after full checking of literatures available.

5. *Quick retrieval of answer*: In order to prepare answer in a short and reasonable time, step 4 above will be much useful. Reference sources should be classified before hand as indicated above into various categories and that make the information retrieval easier and quicker. As we know, if we search something in internet, thousands if not, lakhs of citations are listed. To get the needed information, proper key word should be used in advanced search options. Such key words can be obtained only by above category wise classification of questions. By experience will come to know where to look for answer in the jungle of information. His burden is reduced larger extend by modern databases mentioned in the beginning of this chapter under resources. DIC pharmacist should familiarize with those resources to get correct information as early as possible and he should not forget to record the source of information for future reference.

6. *Evaluation of answer*: Before delivering answer to the questioner, pharmacist must evaluate the answer he has retrieved. It should be co-related with answers obtained in previous steps like, person, purpose, background etc. Only after his full satisfaction about answer, pharmacist must disseminate it to the questioner. If he feels the answer obtained is insufficient or self-contradicting he must try to answer the question after taking needed time. Occasionally, there may be contradiction between multiple answers he got for a single question. Then he should present the facts with detail and also his opinion about the correct answer. He should be able to provide reason for his selection of that particular answer among the multiple answers. Thus skills of evaluation of literature become part and parcel of his professional duty which is elaborated below separately.

7. ***Best Way of Presenting Answer***: The answer given by the DIC must be acceptable to physicians, research scholars and other health care professionals. Even the answer given to the general public must convince them and clarify their doubt in a best possible manner. In these days of communication explosion and availability of internet everywhere, even in hand held devices like mobile phones, those who are enquiring DIC themselves can search the net and get the answer. Hence there should be 'professional touch' to the answer provided by the pharmacist and that should show the difference between professional and non-professional getting drug information.

8. ***Feed back and follow up***:_DIC pharmacist must encourage his clients to send feed back after his answer is used by them. As it is not always forth coming, he should follow up deserving cases on his own. Usually patient specific questions to the DIC can be persuaded and their response recorded. Only through such follow up exercises, pharmacist can evaluate his own service weather it was sufficient, and satisfactory or not, In-time or not, good or bad, and useful or not useful. That gives him an opportunity for course correction or perfection. Actually, DIC's services if evaluated using feed back leads to quality assurance of Drug information services.

Preparation of Written and Verbal Reports

Throughout his career as drug information provider, pharmacist has to supply that information either verbally or by written report. To prepare good report pharmacists need to have a best communication skill which is elaborated in a separate chapter.

With his basic understanding and knowledge of the subject, pharmacist can easily prepare written reports which can be given to information seekers. A good written report should have a basic format which helps in organized presentation. It should start with the question asked or information sought, followed by its purpose as told by the enquirer. These information helps to evaluate, weather the answer given is appropriate or not. Then the elaborate or short answer, as the case may be, given in a clear language with the interpretation of technical terms, if necessary. It depends on the patient enquiring. Wherever necessary, the source of information or reference can be given, so that, the receiver can cross check it or search for more information. The report can be concluded with the name and signature of pharmacist answering the query.

Verbal reports on the other hand, are given either directly to the patient or his care takers in the ward or via phone to the information seeker. Needless to point out verbal report should be in clear tone and in simple language, so that the questioner can comprehend and understand the answer given to him. At the end of verbal report, pharmacist should ask few questions, to ascertain weather the important points of information given are understood by him or not. Also the information seeker can be encouraged to seek clarification of his doubts about the verbal report. This is more important because verbal report cannot be verified later, if it is not recorded. In order to avoid future complications pharmacist must develop good verbal and written communication skills.

The duties of DIC pharmacist not ends with the above reports given to the questioners. He has to record it for his own and higher authority's reference in future. The format for recording is given below. These records not only helps to evaluate the Drug Information services, but also useful to prepare the budget of DIC, by providing which resources were often used and hence a 'must purchase' in the forth coming years. It is also useful as defense in cases of liability and court proceedings.

Model Drug Information Enquiry Record

ABC Drug Information Center Chennai

Enquiry No.........   Date................

Query received by .... On (Date) ....Time.................

Section A : Details about Person making Enquiry

Name:

Profession: Doctor / Nurse / Pharmacist / Patient / Others

Address: ....

Phone No:..

Section B: Nature of Request

Drugs identification	ADR
Dose	Drug Interaction
Use	Pharmaceutical aspects
Side effect	Pharmacology
Availability	Clinician comment
Substitute	Others

Section C: Sources of Answer

Literature:...

Martindale/Pharmacopoeia:..

Reference Book:...

Abstract Service:..

Others:..

Section D: Time taken to Answer

Less than 15 minutes

15 minutes to 1 hour

1 hour to 3 hours

1 day

Others

Not answered

Section E : Method of Replying

Personal

Letter

Telephone

Others

Patient Details: Name, Age, Sex, Diagnosis, Drug History etc.

Question Asked and Answer given (separate sheet, preferably copy of written report given to the questioner, enclosed)

Sd/ ....

Signature of Pharmacist Answering

Summary of Functions of Drug Information Center

1. Establishing and maintaining a system for getting information about drugs.

2. Providing information to Inservice training or continuous education programmes.

3. Answering queries from Research Scholors, PG students, Poison information center etc.

4. Answering questions from physicians regarding drugs and therapy.

5. Preparation and distribution of periodical Drug Information bulletins to doctors, nurses, pharmacists and students of these courses.

6. Helping in the preparation and maintainence of Hospital Formulary or Drugs list.

7. Critical analysis of pharmacy literatures and filing them with comments and opinions.

8. Above all, clearing the doubts and answering the enquiries of general public regarding their treatment.

9. Producing educational materials for Mass Education Programs.

10. Co-ordinating with outside agencies relating to Drug Informations, in serving the community at large and.

11. Maintaining a record of all enquiries.

Role of Hospital Pharmacist in Education and Training

Introduction: As the graduate and post graduate pharmacists are educated and trained in almost all aspects of drug, they are experts in the field of their specialization--drugs. They not only study about the pharmacological properties of drugs, but also about its physical, chemical and pharmaceutical properties. Thus their knowledge about a drug is almost complete and hence pharmacists are well qualified to teach about drugs. They can teach student nurses, pharmacists and medical students and House surgeons about practical aspects of drugs usage. Pharmacists can also educate social workers, general public and of course patients.

Teaching Hospital Staff and Students

By nature of their job nurses are not given extensive coverage of pharmacology during their course of study, except the basics. Hence any addition to that knowledge is welcome. Study materials can be prepared by the teaching pharmacists and specific topics can be taught and discussed in classes specially arranged for them.

Similarly, seminars can be arranged for medical staff and graduate nurses on topics like hospital formulary, prescription errors, incompatibilities in IV admixture, new drug regulations and drug drug interactions. Needless to mention, the importance of showing slides, short films and other audio visual materials to the audience, in these seminars in addition to printed literature, brochures etc. These materials can be procured from WHO or pharmaceutical manufacturers, or prepared from internet by using drug information center attached to the hospital.

New drugs or new sophisticated packings of old drugs can also be shown to the participants in order to disseminate hands-on practical knowledge. Continuing education programs for working pharmacists or health care team is an ideal example for teaching for staff.

Teaching Patients and/or their Attendants

It may not be possible to teach patients while they are sick and still undergoing treatment, however, they can be educated at the time discharge. Majority of the patients are given some medicines and lot of instructions at the time of discharge. Unless they are openly educated via counselling, the disease may relapse. Hence a suitable program can be drown to educate the patients as well as their care takers to monitor the post discharge medications and symptoms. Instructions of general nature, such as, how to identify adverse drug effects can be given to group of patients via short lectures or closed circuit television programs.

Teaching the Community

Pharmacists can accept outside lecture assignments on general or specific topics and educate general public. They can participate in seminars and lectures arranged by social service organisations like Lions club, Rotary club etc. Pamphlets and posters can be prepared by pharmacists to educate the general public in large numbers at a time. If possible they should organise such programs for rural masses, where the poor and illiterate people are starving for information and hence, have lot of superstitions and bad practices about diseases and their treatments. Audio visual method of communication is more suitable for rural peoples and hence cinema, drama and other art forms like street corner short plays are used to educate them. Pharmacists can wirte scripts for these methods of education. Drug abuse prevention program is also one of the area where a pharmacist can contribute his knowledge and experience. Above all pharmacists can write general article about topics like dangers of antibiotic resistance, misuse or abuse of drugs, self medications etc in professional and news journals and magazines.

Training

Suitable training program should be drawn for student pharmacists, by hospital/ community pharmacists. The students should be trained in all aspects of stores and dispensary managements apart from usual dispensing practices. Starting from drug purchase procedure to storage, distribution and accounting, they should be trained by chief or senior pharmacists. At the end of the training they should be evaluated for adequate knowledge and certified. Similarly student nurses and doctors can also be trained in specific aspects of proper methods of use, storage and disposal of dangerous and other important drugs.

Questions

Short Answer Questions

1. Write briefly about the need for Drug Information Center.

2. How pharmacist is suitable to manage DIC?

3. What are the sources of Drug Information?

4. List the function of Drug Information Centre?

5. How will you answer a drug information query?

6. Write short note on written report by Drug Information Center

Long Answer Questions

7. Write in detail about secondary source of information including computerized sources.

8. Discuss the role of pharmacist in education and training.

9. How a Drug Information Center is established?

10. How will you evaluate a Drug information or literature before adding to the collection of DIC?

CHAPTER 41

POISON INFORMATION CENTER AND TREATMENT OF POISON CASES

Importance of PIC

Poisoning can be intentional or accidental and occur at anytime. Obviously, if not treated immediately, it may be fatal. Hence there is always urgency in providing needed information. Almost all enquiries are through phone and the reply must be given then and there at once. As it is a matter of life and death Poison Information Centers must be open round the clock for all the 24 hours and all the days of the year without any holiday. Thus, it differs from Drug Information Center, where the enquiries are not always urgent except for rare occasions.

Sources of Poison

There are many sources of poison ranging from natural sources to synthetic sources. Natural sources include plants, animals or minerals; whereas synthetic sources are cosmetics, house hold items and pharmaceuticals.

Most of the time chemicals including drugs are used as poisons. Chemicals usually available for a common man are from agricultural or horticultural sources. Rarely laboratory chemicals cause poison. Next source of poison common to majority of Indian population is poisonous plants of wild growth. Fungi, cosmetics and house hold items like disinfectants; acids or even diamond is used to commit suicide. Children accidently swallow anything comes to their hand. Thus the sources of poison are vast and unimaginable.

Information about Poisons

In order to treat the poison cases effectively and immediately all the information about the poison must be available. Hence the data should be collected, before hand and kept ready. But in practice there are number of problems in treating poison cases. Most of the time, what substances caused the poisoning, is not known, because the patient may not be in a position to reveal it. The persons accompanying or admitting the patients must bring the container, box, tube or paper found near the patient to the treating hospital, from which many times poisons can be identified. Next important problem is the quantity or dose of poison consumed by the patient, which has to be just guessed.

The third problem is the composition of the product consumed. For drugs and formulations, they are completely declared in labels whereas for other industrial products, it is not known. Hence that information for at least commonly used poisons should be collected from manufacturers, antidotes found and kept ready to use them in emergency situations. Even after this, some problems like, conversion of raw material to the finished product and its nature is not known, as only raw material used is revealed by the manufacturer. Sometimes manufacturers are reluctant to disclose their secret formula, when compelled by law for the purpose of treating poisons, they reveal it and that should be kept confidential. In few instances manufacturers change the composition without declaring it in labels. Thus treatment of poison cases is very difficult and most of the time only symptomatic treatment is given.

However, a poison information center should collect poison information as much as possible from as many sources as well. Usually reference books available are,

1. Chemical toxicology of commercial products – By Glason, *et al.*
2. Treatment of common acute poisoning – clinical – By Mathew. H. *et al.*
3. Hand Book of poisoning – By Driesbach
4. Extra pharmacopoeia
5. Merck Index etc.

Storage of Information

Information collected as above should be arranged in such a way that, they should be retrieved as quickly as possible. In olden days they were arranged alphabetically in written cards and handled manually. Now-a-days, computer is used to store and retrieve information in a fraction of second.

In order to have as much information as possible about each poison, the following format can be followed.

1. Name of the poison
2. Synonym
3. Source: Synthetic / plant / animal / mineral
4. Family (In case of plant or animal poison)
5. Description of external characters (macroscopy)
6. Habitat

7. Minimum lethal dose

8. Toxic effects

9. Symptoms

10. Pharmacokinetic properties

11. Treatment including antidotes

12. Supportive therapy

13. Prognosis

14. Any other relevant points and

15. References

Providing Information

It is not just a mechanical work to be carried out by any non-health care professional. It requires expertise in providing needed information with all professional details in shortest possible time. For this one need to have understanding of basic principles of poison treatment. That is why a brief outline of treatment of poison cases is given below (The purpose ends with that, at the maximum a pharmacist can give first aid to such cases and should not attempt to give treatment to poison cases)

Depends upon the time and weather first aid has been given to the patient or not, information to be given varies. Hence that should be enquired first, for that, the detail about the person enquiring must be asked. Professional or clinical information are required for doctors, nurses and other health care professionals, but general public need to know what is the first aid and what to do next. Advice them accordingly and instruct them to contact later after taking the patient to a nearby hospital or clinic. More information, if required, can be provided during the second call.

As far as possible, detailed information should be given directly to the doctor, not to the third party. All these conversations depend on pharmacist's discretion and skill. Details of each enquiry should be properly recorded in registers (Model record is given in the previous chapter: DIC).

Follow up: Job of pharmacist of Drug Information Center is not over with providing information in the poison cases. He has to follow it up and relevant details obtained from the treating physician or nurses or relatives of the patient, should also be recorded. These details may be useful for future cases and appreciated by physicians.

Treatment of Poison Cases

Introduction: Virtually all materials are used to poison living things. It ranges from high doses of comparatively harmless drugs to cosmetics like nail polish, shaving lotion, etc.

Hence poison is defined as any substance which when consumed in any form, causes toxic effect on the body. Scientific study of poisons is known as Toxicology.

Identification of poison in poison cases is very difficult. Hence in poison cases, only the patient has to be treated, not the poison. That is to say, while treating, measure and monitor, all vital parameters of the patient and his symptoms and treat accordingly.

Poisoning may be acute or chronic. In acute poisoning the effect of poison is immediate and severe. If not treated quickly, death may result. The symptoms are, vomiting, diarrhoea, convulsions, unconsciousness and coma. The poison may be detected in vomiting, stool or urine. In the case of chronic poisoning, the effect may be rather slow, gradual, less severe and for a long period. Environment or habits may be the reason for this type of poisoning, hence, if removed or stopped the causes, symptoms disappear. The symptoms are chronic ill health, repeated GI Irritation or disturbances, weakness etc.

Classification

Poisons can be classified according to origin or mechanism of action. Synthetic poison or natural poison is the major divisions, in the classification according to origin and natural poison may be of vegetable, animal or mineral origin.

Depending on the mechanism of action poisons can be classified as follows:

(a) *Irritants*: They may be of inorganic, organic or mechanical irritants. Inorganic substances are either metallic or non metallic. Phosphorous, Chloride, Iodine, Bromine are the examples of non-metallic poisons; lead, mercury, copper etc are the metallic poisons. Organic poisons are either animal origin, like venoms of snake, scorpion and insects, or vegetable origin like Ergot, Aloe, Capsicum, and Castor seeds. Sometimes powdered glass or diamond is used as poison which is examples for mechanical irritants.

(b) *Corrosive Poisons*: Strong acids and alkalies are the example for corrosive poisons. They destroy the internal organs, especially GI tract when taken orally by their strong corrosive property. Hydrochloric acid, sulphuric acid, and sodium hydroxide are usually misused to kill self or others.

(c) *Neurotic Poisons*: They act on the central nervous system and cause toxic effects. They may act on Brain, Spinal cord or on peripheral nerves. Sedatives, hypnotics, insecticides and cocaine are the example for the brain poisons, Nux vomica act on spine and curare alkaloids act on the peripheral nerves.

(d) *Cardiac Poisons*: Digitalis, stropanthus and aconite are the examples for cardiac poisons.

(e) *Respiratory Depressants*: Poisonous gases like carbon monoxide and coal gas depress respiratory organs and the patient dies due to poor oxygen supply.

(f) *Other Poisons*: Drugs like analgesics, antipyretics, antihistamines and antidepressants if consumed in higher doses, produce many toxic effects and finally results in death of the patient.

General Treatment of Poison Cases

It is obvious that poison cases should be treated as early as possible, otherwise poisons get absorbed into the systems and start damaging vital organs one by one and finally the patient collapses.

It is better to identify the poison, before the treatment is started. However in majority of the cases it is not possible to identity the poison hence the plasma analysis has to be carried out without delay which may require time to reveal the result. The treating physician need not wait till the result of analysis; he can start the following general treatment at once:

1. Removal of unabsorbed poison from the body to prevent further absorption.
2. Excretion of absorbed poison.
3. Treating general symptoms of the patient and
4. Maintaining patient's general condition.

After identifying the poison, specific treatment can be started with specific antidotes. However the above line of general treatment need not be stopped.

1. Removal of Unabsorbed Poison

Poison might have gone through various routes of the body. Depends on the route; various measures should be adopted to remove the poison from the body. If it is an inhalant poison through the nose, first of all, patient should be taken to fresh air for respiration, followed by artificial respiration in hospitals. Poisons entered through skin, eye or wound can be removed by washing them with plain, warm water. If specific antidote is available they are used to neutralize the poison. Sometimes poisons like venoms of snakes, scorpion, insects etc are administered by them by sting or injection; such poisons are removed by making incision at the site of bite and contaminated blood drained out. More blood with poison can be removed by suction.

Poison by oral route is the very common method of poisoning. It is removed by following methods:

1. Inducing vomiting by giving Ipecac or Apomorphine.
2. Stomach washing or Gastric Lavage by forcefully administering lot of water through mouth of the patient which dilute the poison and induce vomiting.
3. *Purgation or Catharsis*: If considerable time is passed after oral ingestion of poison, purgation should also be induced with strong cathartics, like Sorbitol, Magnesium sulphate or Sodium sulphate

4. Inert substances like activated charcoal are given orally at a dose of 50 gm in 300 ml of water to adsorb the poison. The dose should be repeated every 4th hour

2. Excretion of Absorbed Poison

If considerable time, say about 6 hours, is elapsed after poisoning, poison might have entered intestine and absorbed in considerable amount. Hence, inducing vomiting or stomach washing is not useful. The following methods of excreting absorbed poison can be tried.

(a) Use of Diuretics: Chlorothiazide and/or mannitol are administered intravenously to eliminate the poison through urine.

(b) Cathartics: Strong cathartics are used to induce purgation.

(c) Hot bags are used to increase sweating.

(d) Haemodialysis is used to eliminate some poisons like salicylates, barbiturates, thiocyanates and bromides. Peritoneal dialysis is done on children if salicylates poison is diagnosed.

3. Treating General Symptoms of the Patient

When the poison is not identified, only option available is treating patient according to symptoms. For example if too much pain is there morphine is given, if circulating failure is expected, cardiac stimulants are used, similarly for respiratory problems, artificial respiration is given. Patients showing symptoms of dehydration is treated with electrolyte infusions.

4. Maintaining Patient's General Health Conditions

Along with treatment for poisoning, general therapy is given to maintain or improve patient's general condition. To prevent upper respiratory tract infection in unconscious patients, prophylactic antibiotics are given. Hypotension and hypothermia (low body temp) are taken care off. Thus intensive supportive therapy is essential to save the patient. Acid base balance, low sugar, low potassium etc are monitored in the blood plasma and suitable corrective actions taken.

Treatment of Specific Poisonings and Antidotes

As mentioned earlier, if the poison is identified with certainty specific treatments with specific measures like use of antidotes can be undertaken.

For example if narcotic agent poison is confirmed intravenous naloxane is given, it dilate the constricted pupil. Similarly IV Flumazenil produces arousal in benzodiazepine poison cases. Thus specific antidotes help in quick neutralization of poisons.

There are four types of antidotes; physical antidote, chemical antidote, physiological antidote and universal antidote.

Physical Antidotes

Inert, harmless substances are administrated to poison cases, just to physically absorb the poison and then to eliminate from the body. They do not react with any poison to neutralise them. Sometimes absorption of poison is inhibited or delayed using substances like egg albumin, fat or oil. Banana is given to absorb and bind the glass pieces. Activated charcoal is used to absorb alkaloidal poisons; care should be taken not to administer oil or fat to phosphorous poison cases, because they are soluble in it.

Chemical Antidotes

These are chemical substances which react and neutralize the chemical poisons. They form nontoxic products as precipitate or soluble compounds inside the body. For instance acids are neutralized with magnesium oxide or calcium oxide, lead is precipitated with potassium sulphate or sodium sulphate. Other examples are administration of tannins to alkaloid poison cases and lime water to oxalic acid poison.

Physiological Antidotes

Substances which act against poison and produce just the opposite effects are used to counteract toxic effects. They are called antagonists. Up to which extent they counteract the poison and effects produced by antagonist themselves are the point of concern. Examples are given below separately.

Universal Antidotes

If the identity of the poison is not known with certainty the universal antidote is used. They neutralize the acids, absorb alkaloidal poisons and chelate metals etc. The composition of universal antidotes is as follows:

Magnesium	– 1 part
Activated charcoal	– 2 parts
Tannic acid	– 1 part

It is administered at the dose 20 to 30 gm in 200 ml of water and given once or twice only. *Various poisons and specific Antidotes with doses are given below:*

Poison	Antidote	Dose
Iron Salts	Deferroxamine	15 mg/kg/hr
Lead	Calcium EDTA	50 to 75 mg/kg/day IM or IV in divided doses for a maximum of 5 days
Arsenic, Gold and Mercury	BAL. (Dimercapol)	3 to 5 mg/kg/4 hourly IM for 2 days followed by 2 5 mg to 3 mg/kg/6 hourly for 7 days
	Penicillamine	1 gm orally daily 4 divided doses before meals.

Table *contd...*

Poison	Antidote	Dose
Narcotic drugs like Morphine	Naloxane	1 to 2 mg or more IM or IV or SC.
Barbiturates	Coramine	Coramine IV at a dose of 5 ml increased to 10 ml in 15 minutes followed by 20 ml every 30 minutes till reflexes return.
Paracetamol	Acetyl cysteine	Loading dose 140 mg/kg. Then 70 mg/kg orally every 4 hours until serum level of paractamol is zero
Cardio tonic drugs like Tricyclic antidepressants Quinidine etc	Sodium bicarbonate	1 to 2 mg/kg. Care should be taken as antidote may produce heart failure.
Physostigmine	Atropine	Test dose of 1 to 2 mg until symptoms of atropinism like Tachycardia, dilated pupil appear. Repeat the dose every 10 to 15 minutes until secretions stop.
Organo phosphorous compounds like Insecticides	Atropine followed by Parlidoxime	After cholinergic symptoms are controlled by atropine, parlidoxime can be given in doses of 1 gm IV. Repeat every 3 to 4 hours if necessary or give 250 to 400 mg/hour by infusion
Thallium	Prussian blue	--

Questions

Short Answer Questions

1. Write briefly about the importance of PIC.
2. What are the sources of Poison?
3. Classify poisons.

Long Answer Questions

4. Explain how information about poison is provided in a poison information center.
5. Write an essay about general treatment of poison cases.
6. What are antidotes? Classify and give examples.

CHAPTER 42

COMMUNICATION IN PHARMACY AND PRESENTATION OF CASES

Introduction

To be successful in life, fluency in communication is essential for everybody, pharmacists cannot be an exemption. Already by nature of his job, pharmacist has to communicate more to the patients, now clinical pharmacy services has increased this requirement by many fold, because of varieties of new functions assigned to him.

Clinical pharmacist has to conduct useful interview with the patient to get his medication history, he should able to communicate effectively with doctors during ward round participation, he should conduct one or more counseling sessions with each patient, and also he has to provide drug information to the variety of people. All these require effective communication skill.

However many pharmacists find it difficult to communicate effectively as there are few chances for him during his education to develop language skills. Professional college students are not taught languages like arts and science students during their course of study and hence, a pharmacist has to develop it on his own.

Aim and Process of Communication

In order to develop communication skill, one must understand what is communication, what are its aims and what are the processes involved in communication.

Communication is nothing but passing on information to someone. It is a connecting passage or channel between people. It may be via oral (voice) or print or visual media. However oral communication is the commonly and widely used method of communication. It involves not only spoken words but also body language.

One can communicate even without speaking a single word. Communication between a deaf and dump and others is a classical example for this. Hence communication is both an art and science. What is more important is what you are communicating must reach the other party. Important aim or goal of communication is understanding by the receiving party. Hence one should not use doubtful or double meaning words during communication, only the words with single common meaning must be used.

How a communication is processed by our brain? The process of sending message is known as encoding, the process of understanding is after decoding. Response or reply to the message is another encoding or feedback. This gives the sender of message an opportunity to clarify and correct any misunderstanding. Thus the entire communication process consists of repeated encoding and decoding only.

Having seen the importance and need for communication the next questions arises are what to communicate, how to communicate and to whom to communicate etc. These questions are answered below:

What to communicate?

In these days of internet, information spread within seconds through out the world. It is not only fast, the volume of which is unimaginable and beyond human capacity to go through all those content in websites, social media, magazines, news papers, professional journals and data bases. Nevertheless, a pharmacist or his team in charge of collecting and passing information must shift through content and pick up the essential information. To do that effectively first there should be clear idea of what we are going to communicate.

Therapeutics, toxicology, drug interactions, new drugs , new uses for old drugs, resistance developed for drugs are some of the topics which can be communicated to health care team. Trends in research, new findings of research etc can be included in these communications. Similarly new rules and regulations or announcements or amendments to the act by state or central governments can be communicated, if they are useful to the health care professionals.

How to communicate?

There are many methods of communication like voice, visual and print communications. Among them printed communication occupy a lion's share as it is somewhat permanent, easy to carry and use. Hence hospital pharmacy communications are through print media where bulletins, news letters or reviews are published to send the information to the staff of the hospital.

Communication during Drug Administration or Dispensing

While giving drugs to the patient, pharmacists must communicate effectively with him. His voice must be clear, louder and understandable. Pharmacists should make the patient to understand the instructions. Improper and half hearted communication results in grave error. This is doubly so when Polypharmacy is practiced, that is, when multiple drugs are given to the patients. Also it is more important to communicate effectively in simple language in our country where a large number of people with low literary level are using government hospitals and community pharmacies for their treatment. Because of this and other reasons like patient's condition, age and literacy level, we may have to use written communication also. Diagrams of tablets and capsules may have to be drawn to indicate the number of doses per day. This helps in reducing errors by the patient.

A pharmacist must be thorough with the common terms (medical and non-medical) used in the clinical practice of the hospital. He should also understand the abbreviations used by medical staff in prescriptions and other records, so that he can communicate effectively with colleagues and patients.

Sometimes, pharmacists are not communicating enough with the patients due to various reasons like work load, fatigue and surrounding noise and other disturbances. However it is a law in USA and other developed countries that pharmacists must communicate with patients to review the drug use and offer counselling. He must discuss the following with each patient:

1. Name and description of medicine he dispenses.
2. Dosage form, dose, routes of administration and duration of drug therapy.
3. Special directions and precautions for preparation, administration and use by the patient.
4. Side effects, adverse effects or interaction and contraindications of the drug he gave and ways of avoiding them, action required if they occur.
5. Technique of self monitoring of drug therapy.
6. Proper storage
7. Prescription refill information
8. Action to be taken if a dose or two is missed and
9. Instruction regarding the use of medical/surgical appliances and
10. Disposal of unused medicines, if any.

Communication during Medication History Interview

Clinical pharmacist has to obtain an accurate medication history from the patient. This is not an easy task, due to various reasons like, patient's physical and mental conditions. He is sick, nervous and in an excited mood and also the questions asked during this interview is mostly personal in nature and hence they are reluctant to disclose the full truth. So it requires great communication abilities on the part of the clinical pharmacists to put clever questions without offending the patient's feelings. Once, you are able to convince the patient about your intention and usefulness of information in diagnosis and treatment, some sort of friendship start developing between you and the patient, resulting in successful interview.

Communication during Monitoring of Therapy

The primary duty of a clinical pharmacist is monitoring of drug therapy. To do this effectively patient's understanding of instructions given to him must be checked. Only the correct understanding leads to proper compliance with the instructions, hence by communicating with the patient, pharmacist has to verify it. This leads to the identification of patient's practices during the course of treatment. Corrections can be made in those practices. By close interaction with the patient, pharmacist can identify any side effect, ADR and / or drug interactions. All these works point to the need of good communication skills.

Communication during Patient Counseling

It is common knowledge, to counsel somebody you need to have empathy, consideration and above all good communication skills in order to make the patient to accept and follow your advice. Patients are counseled either during treatment or after discharge or on both occasions. The former counseling leads to the identification of factors that reduce compliance and the later counseling leads to the prevention of any chance of non-compliance after discharge. During counseling the pharmacist must identify and deal with information deficiency, patient emotions and functional limitations to ensure that patients understand and carryout the instructions. All these require better communication and its importance is evident.

Communication during General Practice

In the course of general pharmacy practice, a pharmacist has to communicate with medical or sales representatives for the purchase of drugs and other items, which require negotiating skill to avail maximum benefit and profit. Similarly during hospital pharmacy practice, pharmacist has to communicate with doctors, nurses and other health care professionals, to offer consultation, advice etc, about selection of formulation, its benefit risk ratio and administration. In drug information centers, pharmacist has to provide information to research scholars, doctors and public. To each of these groups of people, he has to use varying degree of professional terms and as such his communication should be beneficial to them.

Types of Communication

Apart from person to person oral communication, there are few other types of communications like interdepartmental communication and audio-visual communication.

In the inter-departmental communication, pharmacists are expected to write letters to other departments. These official letters are written in a particular manner, format and language. Pharmacist should learn it, though it may sound like a clerical job. During his professional practice, he has to write to other departments requesting services or products or instruments and equipments.

Moreover, a pharmacist, especially who is in charge of drug information centre, has to pass on information to other departments via memos, notices to be displayed in notice boards etc. He may have to prepare news letters or journals in which he should give information about new drugs introduced into the market, proceedings of PTC, general news etc. How to prepare the news letter is discussed below:

NEWS LETTER

Introduction

Communication is an essential part of human life, without which humankind and civilization could not be what it is to day. It acquires more significance in a hospital pharmacy set up as it requires communicating very important information to the life saving team working in a hospital.

In olden days notices with information used to be pasted in pharmacy department notice boards or sent manually to the people concerned. However, with an advent information explosion and its volume and availability, a modern hospital pharmacy can play a more active and productive role in dissemination of data concerning drugs and related topics. It can prepare and send news letter in printed hard copy format for ready reference by health care team.

Preparation of News Letters

Once it is decided to go for a printed communication, the preliminary decisions to be made are about its frequency, format, content and distribution. Frequency is about interval between two issues of news letter. It can be a monthly, quarterly, half yearly or annual publication depends on the facilities and availability of news, infrastructure and finance.

Once frequency is decided the next important aspect is its content. Apart from usual editorial, it should have prominent place for new development in the health care world. It could be new drug introduced in the market or new indication for old drug or adverse drug reaction reported elsewhere. This apart important decisions or resolutions of PTC or other committees can be conveyed to the staff of the hospital. One or two articles written by leaders or forerunners of the health care industry can be included.

Drug profiles, market regulation etc can be published in few pages. Some interesting 'Tidbits' about Pharma or medical or nursing sector can be included in the general section to make the news letter interesting to the readers. If the volume of the content is known, the format and number of pages can be determined for the first issue and the same format can be followed for subsequent issues of news letter. Finally its distribution depends on to whom we are indent to communicate through the news letter.

Distribution of News Letters

The hospital pharmacy news letter is obviously for internal circulation of the hospital concerned. Hence they are distributed to the following category of health professionals and staff.

1. All the members of medical staff.
2. All the members of nursing staff.
3. All the members of pharmacy staff.
4. Staff library.
5. Drug information centre.
6. Reading rooms of students, nurses and house surgeons hostel
7. Clinical lab.
8. Dietician
9. Administrative office and
10. Higher authorities.

Conclusion

Pharmacist by nature of his job is dealing with lot of information about drugs through medical representatives, wholesalers and even retailers. Hence he is the opt person among the health care team to prepare and circulate Hospital Pharmacy News letter. By performing this duty effectively he can earn the goodwill of fellow professionals who are not in a position to gather this information by the very nature of their job and work load.

Hence news letter is not a burden on the pharmacist but a mean to achieve respect and reputation in a hospital set up. So pharmacists should develop the skill of delivering oral and written reports which is discussed in the chapter on Drug Information Center also. Oral communication skill is also required while presenting case details to fellow health care professionals which are detailed below:

PRESENTATION OF CASES

Introduction

A case presentation in clinical settings is a formal communication between health care professionals like doctors, pharmacists, nurses, physiotherapists and lab technologists regarding a patient's clinical condition while under treatment or after discharge. It is the language that health care team use to communicate with each other in their day to day practice. A student in clinical pharmacy or pharmacy practice has to learn the art and science of case presentation for the following reasons.

Need for Clinical Case Presentation

1. As the treatment for patients is a team work, effective communication between the team members is essential.

2. A clinical pharmacy student is expected to express what he learned in wards in the form of case presentation to his teacher or to members of health care team or to classmates.

3. It is required even after he is fully qualified and appointed as clinical pharmacist. There may be occasions when a clinical pharmacist has to hand over the cases to other clinical pharmacist or has to send the patient to other specialty or has to get opinion from experts to proceed with the patient care or explain the case to higher authorities. On all these circumstances he is expected to present the case fully, with out confusion and in the manner his listeners understand even the finer points.

4. Case presentation give the students some opportunities to access patient information, detect drug related problems, methods of solving them and ultimately to take decisions and recommendations which he should able to defend or justify.

5. If a case presentation is effective it stimulates the listeners to facilitate patient care and help to identify the learning needs of individual as well as the team and

6. Case presentation is the tool to access the clinical competence of a clinical pharmacy student.

Hence clinical pharmacy and pharmacy practice students are expected to learn the technique of presenting a case by observation and practice.

Guidelines for Case Presentation

- Student must have worked or involved in the case before presenting it. Obviously then only he can present the case with first hand knowledge and point out his role or contribution in the treatment.

- All the team members as well as the students of the class must be present for case presentation. A brief summary or background information about the case can be given to the participants before presentation, so that an effective discussion can be held.

- Most of the time an oral presentation is sufficient. If the presenter so desire and if it is necessary audio-visual equipments can be used.

- The presentation must be short and to the point, so that it can be of 10 to 15 minutes duration. Another 15 to 20 minutes can be allotted for questions and discussions on drug related topics.

- A well organized format should be followed for case presentation, a model of which is given below. The student or presenter can modify or alter it, if required and permitted by teacher or trainer.

Case Presentation Format

1. Patient information [Name, Age, sex, Race, etc]
2. Reason for admission [Present complaint]
3. History of present illness [circumstances that lead to present problem]
4. Past medical history [diseases treated, medicines taken in the past]
5. Past surgical history [any surgery done, its result, complications etc]
6. Present medical conditions and medications
7. Relevant history about family, social, allergy and compliance
8. Results of physical examination [pulse, Heart beat, Temp,injury,eye, etc]
9. Results of Lab tests [including imaging, biopsy etc]
10. Description of hospital events and its management after admission in chronological order with dates
11. Identification of drug related problems [DRP]and patient care plan
12. Present condition of DRPs and therapeutic outcome.
13. Alternate therapeutic plans[after studying cost,contraindication,efficacy, side effects, etc]
14. Suggestion of one patient specific therapeutic plan from the above with justification and implementation method]
15. Monitoring above plan [parameters, person, duration etc]
16. Causes of success or failure of the treatment so far.

The format given here is just a suggestion, it can vary depends on the need. For example if the case presentation is after an ADR or other events it can be elaborated so that similar problem can be avoided or restricted by the health care team in future. Similarly all the 16 points listed above can be explained depends on the need, allotted time or even mark in the examination. Thus case presentation enriches the knowledge of not only the participants, also the presenter himself, if a sincere attempt is made to present a useful presentation.

Other Types of Communications

Communication can also through audio visual methods. They are more effective because, people are able to see with their own eyes apart from hearing about it, at the same time. Hence they understand better than mere voice communication. Nature of illness, the way medicine acts or to be administered, what to do, what not to do during the treatment, results of non-compliances and bad practices, can be shown to the patient in audio visual format. They include still photographs, filmstrips and cinema, video or audio cassettes, CDs etc. Though it is not possible always to go for visual communication, it is found to be very effective communication without doubt.

Conclusion

From the foregoing pages it is very clear that without proper communication nothing can succeed. It is especially so in clinical set up where not only the cost involved is high but also the consequences. As treatment of sick involves the life and death of a human being, effective communication skills must be learned by clinical pharmacist at any cost. Once acquired, this communication skill helps in making pharmacist and his profession a highly esteemed one with the patients.

Questions

Short Answer Questions

1. What is communication?
2. Write a note on audio visual communication.
3. Write a note an interdepartmental communication.
4. What are the processes of communication?
5. What are the contents of hospital pharmacy news letter?
6. List the need for case presentation
7. What are the guidelines for case presentation?

Long Answer Questions

8. Explain the importance of communication in pharmacy.
9. What is the indicator of successful communication? What are its aim and process?
10. What are the points a pharmacist has to communicate during dispensing? Add a note on types of communications.
11. How Hospital Pharmacy news letter is prepared?
12. Explain the salient features of case presentation

CHAPTER 43

CRITICAL EVALUATION OF BIOMEDICAL LITERATURE

Introduction

Critical evaluation is the ability to judge the scientific value of a literature. This has to be done in a systematic manner, so that all the information given in the biomedical literature is verified without oversight or bias. A clinical pharmacist has to evaluate biomedical literature about clinical trials or review papers or papers describing inventions or therapeutic guidelines developed by hospitals and other institutions.

As the concept of evidence based medicine [EVM] has gained popularity in recent years, he needs to evaluate the evidences presented in those papers critically, so that health care team can be assured of its value. All the above are primary literature but pharmacist needs to evaluate even the secondary and tertiary sources of information. Hence they are also discussed below.

Selection and evaluation: Lakhs of biomedical literatures are published every year which make it impossible to verify each one of them. Hence we need to carefully select the literature for full evaluation. But selection of literature itself requires evaluation. Thus selection and evaluation are inter-dependent in that evaluation requires selection and in turn selection requires evaluation. By careful preliminary evaluation biomedical literatures are selected, fully evaluated and then interpreted. Information obtained from it is applied for patient care problems. Dividing the biomedical literature into various components help to select and evaluate them correctly.

Evaluation of Tertiary Literatures: As described earlier, tertiary literatures are the collection of information from secondary and primary sources. Hence there is always possibility of error, bias and insufficiency of information. However these tertiary sources of information too needed as it make the job of information gatherer easy. With proper evaluation of these sources, a DIC pharmacist can decide, how far they can be relied upon for giving answer to DIC queries. The following are the questions to be asked to select a tertiary literature for evaluation.

1. Who are the authors or editors of the literature?
2. What are their credentials?
3. How much recent are those literatures?
4. Does the literature have single or multiple authors?
5. Is it supported by references?
6. Are the references are easily available for verification? and
7. Is the cost worth of material?

Positive answers to these questions determine selection of such literatures for evaluation and subsequent addition to the collection of DIC.

Evaluation of Secondary Literatures: Secondary literatures are those in which information is indexed or abstracts presented. As it represent huge volume of resources, they are now-a-days published as soft copy in CDs, rather than printed form. Soft copy format made it easy to go for full text of the biomedical literature which are also included along with index and abstract by enterprising publishers of these secondary literatures. However to select these literatures too some basic questions needs to be asked for evaluation of its worth, which are given below:

1. How many journals are covered for indexing or abstracting?
2. How much time has gone between date of original publication and indexing?
3. Weather this secondary literature covers only drugs or secondary literature also?
4. What is the cost?

These resources are marketed as data-bases and periodically updated for which the buyer [DIC] needs to subscribe annually. Though costlier they are worth investing as it make the job of DIC pharmacist more easier, compared to manual search of literatures which is both time consuming and tiresome. If the information is available in computer system, comparison, selection and evaluation can be easily done. However procurement of these costly resources depends on number of users and type of information sought.

Evaluation of Primary Literatures: Primary literature has to be evaluated part by part or component after component, only then, pharmacist can determine its applicability in practice settings. The components of the primary literature are;

- Introduction: Reasons and objectives of the study.
- Materials and methods: Subjects [patients], study design and test methods
- Results: data and its statistical analysis
- Discussion: Conclusions drawn.

The evaluation of these components is discussed below:

Introduction: In this part of biomedical literature, the author usually describes the reason or rational for conducting the study and then the aims or objectives, he proposes to achieve through this research. A careful analysis of this part gives the reader some confidence that the author[s] have defined a valuable course of investigation. The rational for the study also indicates that the investigators have taken up a task of solving some problem which does not have answer at present. Also the aim mentioned in the introduction gives an opportunity to the evaluator to verify weather it is achieved at the end or not.

Materials and methods: It is the more important part of the literature in that it describes how the research was carried out. While evaluating this part the critical points to be noted are the sample, study design and the test method. In biomedical studies the samples included are patients. Next number of patients selected for the study and how far they are representative of the population the study proposes to apply, criteria for their inclusion are to be thoroughly evaluated. Inclusion of patients require many factors to be considered like their age, sex, severity of disease, physical fitness etc. How far these factors have been accommodated should be verified. Many papers on these factors such as the one by young MJ et al [Ann Int Med 99:248, 1983] and Mc Larty JW [Clin Pharm 7.694:1988] are available and they should be consulted.

Next component to be evaluated in materials and method section is study design. Ann B.Amerson of university of Keorucky has proposed, controls, blinding and randomization are the three elements to examine the study design. He elaborates 'controls provide for comparison, the most common being groups of subjects who receive placebo or another standard treatment. The difference in each subject's performance can be compared on the regimens. Blinding and randomization are the two techniques used to reduce bias both on the part of investigators and subjects. Randomization also generally tends to balance treatment groups according to certain prognostic factors, e.g. age, length and severity of disease. Incorporation of these three elements is usually indication of good study design' Ann B Amerson concludes.

Once study design is evaluated as above, then the test methods are evaluated. Needless to mention the tests conducted on the subjects should be uniform and reproducible. Here usually many biochemical lab tests are carried out, apart from physical examination, x-ray, microbiological and pathological investigations. All these tests should be sensitive enough to detect the activities of test and standard drugs. They should give same results when repeated. The investigator of the study should have taken care to establish and standardize the tests. That is what verified by evaluating this part of the literature.

Results: In this section all the data collected during the study is summarized. They are then statistically analysed. Before verifying statistically analysed data, it should be checked for completeness, correctness and relevance to the study design. It should be first verified weather results of all patients enrolled in the project are given, if not, reason for drop out or omission. If graphs are included how far they are integrated with the data and how well they are presented should be evaluated. Next weather all the data given in the test, table, and graph are agree with each other and subjected to statistical analysis has to be verified. Finally the entire process of statistical analysis and the result interpreted from it has to be fully investigated.

Discussion: The last section of biomedical literature is the discussion section in which conclusions are drawn. We have to check weather these conclusions are in conformity with the aim/ objectives mentioned in the introduction section. If not the study design has to be once again evaluated weather it gives needed data to come to this different conclusion. Conclusions should be fully supported by data obtained and there should not be any extrapolation.

Role of Editorial Boards of Biomedical Literatures: In order to critically evaluate biomedical literatures guidelines are developed and published in biomedical journals by their editorial boards. Detail evaluation methods are sent to outside reviewers or evaluators of these journals or their own editorial board members for evaluating the articles received by these journals for publication. The editors of these journals published from various countries form committees to frame and update such guidelines as and when required. Those guidelines are published in these journals itself and students are advised to go through them. This is especially required for clinical pharmacists who are in-charge of DIC, as they are expected to have these skills to perform effectively.

Questions

Short Answer Questions

1. Briefly discuss evaluation of secondary sources of literature.

2. How a tertiary source of literature is evaluated?

Long Answer Question

3. Explain the process of evaluation of biomedical literature.

CHAPTER 44

MEDICATION ERRORS

Introduction

Despite care and vigilance by medical and para medical staff medication errors do occur. Though there are many reasons for these errors as described below, the health care team from treating physician to pharmacist to nurses is very much concerned with such developments. In order to minimize these errors hospitals have framed polices rules and regulations and strict adherence to these rules will definitely help to manage the problem.

Definition: "The administration of wrong medicine or dose of medicine, diagnostic agent or chemical or treatment requiring use of such agents to the wrong patient or at the wrong time in the wrong manner is known as medication error."

Classification of medication error: Medication error can occur at any point of time in the treatment chain, starting from prescription writing by the doctor to dispensing by pharmacist or administration of drugs by nurses or patient's care takers. Medication errors are very common in out-patients than in-patients for the obvious reason that, out-patient's compliance to instructions by the health care team is not supervised by them and it is completely left to the patient or his care taker who may be illiterate, or negligent. However as out patients are usually treated for few days, due to the very nature of their disease or condition, we need to pay more attention to the patients requiring long time treatment, mainly in-patients and few groups of out-patients with diseases requiring long time treatment like T.B, Asthma, Diabetes, Leprosy, Hypertension etc. Thus medication error can be classified as follows:

I. Errors in Drug Administration

A. *Wrong dosage form*: In this type of errors, for instance, tablet might have been given instead of injection and vice versa. Depends upon the patient's condition oral dosage may produce, nausea, vomiting or stomach irritation, apart from delaying onset of action by the drug. On the other hand, needless injection raises the cost of treatment.

B. *Unordered drug given*: Drug not repeated in the prescription is not noted and previous day prescription is routinely followed and thereby unordered drug may be administered to the patient. Not only patient looses the benefit of drug written in the prescription but also their agony is prolonged. Similar to starting of drugs at right time, stopping of it at appropriate time is also important. Without noticing such decision, administering previous day's drug may complicate the treatment.

C. *Wrong time*: If any drug is given half an hour before or after the time specified it is considered as administration of drug at wrong time. Commonly it happens because of basic lethargic attitude towards punctuality and interference by factors in the ward atmosphere. It may seem to be a simple error but in some critical cases it may lead to drug-drug interaction, if the required dosing interval is not followed between drugs.

D. *Wrong administration*: If a drug is given through different route than the one mentioned in the prescription it is known as wrong administration of drug. One has to be careful while reading the label. Some injections have to be given only through I.M not by I.V. Many health care professionals think all injections can be administered via IM or IV depends on emergency. It is a wrong conception as the excipients of injections differ depends on many factors, hence wrong route may cause local irritation, swelling and dispersal problems at the site of injection.

II. Errors in Dose of Drugs

A. *Omission of any dose*: If a drug is not administered by the time the next dose is due, it is called omission of dose. Nurses may fail to administer a drug, forgetfully or due to other emergencies in the ward, till the time of next dose. If not for all drugs, for few drugs like Digoxin and antibiotics this may lead to complications.

B. *Wrong Dosage*: Correct quantity of the dose written in the prescription should be administered to the patient. Any dose above or below 5% of correct dose is considered as wrong dose, hence a careful measuring, counting and double reading of prescription is a must to avoid complaints of wrong dose.

C. *Extra dose:* Sometimes patient may be given an extra dose of the prescribed medicine without checking weather the drug has been already given or not. This usually happen when it is not recorded in the medication charts immediately or during change in duty staff at the end of working hours [shift].

Reasons for Medication Error

1. *Engaging non-professionals*: Medication error occurs when the members of health care team is not able to find out while the error is being committed. Usually it happens when non-professionals are involved in professional works where professional judgment is required. For example if a non-pharmacist dispenses drugs, he is not able to find out incompatible drugs prescribed or how to instruct the patient about the use of those drugs without interaction. For example when enteric coated tablets are prescribed with alkaline drugs they have to be taken with minimum of half an hour gap, otherwise the enteric coating breaks in the stomach itself instead of intestine, and releases drug in the stomach which may irritate the stomach or become useless for the patient. Thus any one who can read the prescription cannot dispense the prescription as claimed by few vested interests in the field.

2. *Inadequate labeling*: Insufficient information on the label leads to medication error. All the necessary information like dose, route of administration, expiry date, storage etc should be mentioned in the label, otherwise patients tend to assume things and consume the drugs as they presume. Important points like 'Poison' 'caution' or 'warning' has to be highlighted in labels. They are printed in red or different colour to attract the attention of the patients or auxiliary labels has to be affixed on the containers. This information is very much important and useful even to nurses in the ward who are in a hurry or hard pressed for time. Sometimes, 'pictograms' [pictures] are fixed on the containers to help the illiterate patients.

3. *Non-reporting of medication error*: Majority of the people try to hide their mistake, health care team is not an exemption. Thus any medication error or untoward incidence is not reported to the hospital administration to take remedial measures immediately. Many people think it is an unnecessary headache to report such errors, even it occurs due to some other reason than their fault. Thus prevention, treatment, correction and subsequent benefits are denied to the patient for that inadequate hospital policies have to be blamed. Correct policies encourage people to be truthful, so as to report incidents in wards. An incident is any happening which is not consistent with routine operation of hospital or the routine care of the patient. It may be an accident or situation which might result in an accident. If an incident is not reported it goes uninvestigated and thereby the chance for detecting its real reason is diminished. Thus without knowing the root cause, the team looses foresight if it occurs at another time for the same patient or other patient. Hence this time and every time they fail in preventing similar medical error. Thus absence of proper education and policies by hospital administration, inculcated to health care team, is one of the reasons for medical error.

Minimizing Medication Error

Medication error can be prevented to a maximum extend, but it is difficult to eliminate altogether. Though the aim is to have zero error in all treatments, errors do creep in due to human factors. But its frequency can be reduced. The reasons for medication errors are listed above, if the shortfalls pointed out in those reasons are corrected medication errors can be avoided to a larger extend. Thus engaging only pharmacists for handling drugs, good dispensing practices by way of adequate labeling and faithful reporting of errors etc help the hospital administration to minimize medication errors.

Apart from the above pharmacists and nurses can help to avoid medication error by their co-ordinate works. Pharmacists – if appointed in wards – can prepare patient medication profile card for each in-patient in which he can record list of drugs given, allergy, possible drug-drug interaction, precautions to be followed etc, which can be viewed by nurses before administering drugs. Similarly nurses while preparing to administer drugs to the patient should

1. verify whether the medicine was already given
2. collect the drug from the cub board read the label 2 or 3 times and check the content for physical stability
3. discard any balance left over medicines and
4. check whether the previous medicine or dose is incompatible with the present one.

During the administration of medicine nurses should once again verify all the information. The medicine should be prepared just few minutes before administration. Patient should be properly identified and she should wait until the administration of medicine is completed [except LVP]. Then she should write 'given' on the medication card against the name and time of the drug and put her initials.

If the above regulations are followed sincerely medication errors can be reduced to very minimum and the patient who is already suffering from his disease can be saved from unnecessary trouble and problems.

Questions

Short Answer Question

1. Classify medication errors

Long Answer Question

2. Define medication error. What are the reasons for it? How it can be minimized?

CHAPTER 45

CLINICAL TRIALS

Introduction

"A Clinical Trial is a research study in human volunteers to answer specific health questions". In other words "Clinical Trials are a set of procedures in medical research and drug development that are conducted to collect safety and efficacy data for health interventions". It requires more time and money and conducted by Contract Research Organizations (CRO) or by clinical trials unit of the academic sector. Some pre-conditions are to be satisfied by the organisations which conduct the clinical trials. First of all they should have completed animal studies on the test product and obtained approval from the ethics committee formed for the purpose. It may be conducted in single centre in one country or in multiple centres in many countries.

Reasons for Conducting Clinical Trials

Primarily clinical trials are conducted to test whether a new drug or new device is safe and efficient for people to use. Other reasons are to develop newer methods of treatment, even though old method works. It helps in betterment of old ways of treatment or to replace it with new one. The new method must be better in efficacy or cost or duration of treatment and/or with decreased side effects.

One more reason for conducting clinical trial is to use the old standard treatment on patients for whom the treatment was not given previously. For example treatment given to adults is to be tried on children as well.

Sometimes old drugs are tested for new indications (diseases) for which the drug is not already approved. If various methods of treatment are already available for a particular disease, they are compared by clinical trials and merits and demerits of each one of them is determined. The comparison need not be between two methods of treatment or dose or device, it can be between 3 or 4 methods also. Moreover clinical trials are used to test a hypothesis, and monitored carefully, thus they are considered as application of scientific method especially the experimental part of it, to understand the human biology.

Phases of Clinical Trials

Clinical trials for new drugs are conducted in 4 phases. It takes several years to complete all the 4 phases. However approval for marketing the new drug is given after successful completion of first 3 phases. The fourth phase is conducted after marketing of the drug and known as post marketing surveillance.

Phase I

It is usually started only after completing preclinical trials conducted *in vitro* (Test tube or cell culture) or *in vivo* (animal) with a range of doses. Once the drug under test is proved to be worth to undertake further studies, they are taken to Phase I trial, here, the drug is given to 20 to 100 healthy volunteers and its safety, tolerability, pharmacokinetics and pharmacodynamics are determined. These trials are usually conducted in clinics attached to Contract Research Organisations (CRO) where the volunteers are monitored for 24 hours for a particular period, say one month, at least. Gradually the dose administered to the volunteers is increased until it near the toxic level; but well below the 50% lethal dose (LD_{50}) determined in animals. Volunteers are paid for this study.

Phase I trials are conducted by varying the dose by single administration or multiple administration and/or after or before the food. Thus the pharmacokinetic and pharmacodynamic variations are collected and evaluated to arrive at a correct dose and dosage interval.

Phase II

If the safety of the drug is confirmed in Phase I trial, they are taken to Phase II trial, where the drug is tested on more number of volunteers and patients say 100 to 300. Here the safety of the trial drug is established on more people. If a trial drug fails, it occurs usually at this stage when they do not work as expected or show unexpected toxic effects.

Phase II studies are used to confirm the dose and efficacy of the drug. Some Phase II trials are designed to demonstrate activity and safety of the drug in selected group of persons and other Phase II trials are known as randomized clinical trials where volunteers receive the drug/device and others receive placebo or standard treatment. In this randomized study less number of volunteers is used than the next one under Phase III.

Phase III

It is carried out in many centers and is known as randomized controlled study. It is carried out on 300 to 3000 patients or even more depends on the disease or conditions for which the drug/device is used. It almost confirms the efficacy of the drug and compared with standard treatment. Because it is carried out on large number of patients and in multicenter, it take long time to complete and also obviously, expensive.

It is continued, even after submitting the data for Government approval for two reasons. One is to provide the drug to the trial patients until it is approved for marketing and available for purchase and two is to find out possible other indications. During this extended study, additional safety data or points for better marketing can be obtained.

The results of Phase III trials are submitted along with all other full particulars about the drug, its formulation, manufacturing procedure, shelf life etc to the Drugs control authorities for verification and review. If the drug is to be marketed in many countries, the details are sent to authorities of those countries also.

Phase IV

As mentioned earlier, the Phase IV trial is known as post marketing surveillance. Pharmacovigilance program on the new drug is undertaken by the manufacturing company with the help of practicing doctors and other health care professionals. Only during this phase, the drug is administered to patients with widely differing conditions than the patients participated in earlier three phases. For example, drug interactions studies are usually not carried out during the earlier phases, whereas, now it is possible as different patients with different diseases and treatment will use the new drug. Moreover now the drug may be prescribed for pregnant ladies also and the safety or otherwise can be found out, as they are usually not enrolled during the first three phases. Delayed on set of adverse drug reactions can be identified during this post marketing surveillance. If such effects are discovered during this phase, the drug is withdrawn from the market.

Guidelines Governing Clinical Trials and
Good Clinical Practice (GCP)

"It is a standard for clinical studies or trials that encompasses the design, conduct, monitoring, termination, audit, analysis, reporting and documentation of the studies. It ensures that the studies are implemented and reported in such a manner that there is public assurance that the data are credible, accurate and that the rights, integrity and confidentiality of the subjects are protected. GCP aims to ensure that the studies are scientifically authentic and that the clinical practice of the investigational product is properly documented". Thus the guidelines for clinical trials define the GCP. It was issued by Central Drugs Standard Control Organisation [CDSCO] and formulated and approved by Drugs Technical Advisory Board (DTAB) of Government of India.

The documents deal with the subject is in great length (about 100 pages) and covers all the aspects of clinical trial. It starts with definition of all terms related to clinical trials. The following are the topics explained in the guidelines document.

1. **Prerequisite for the Study**

   It is further classified into three sections

   (i)   Investigational pharmaceutical product

   (ii) Preclinical Supporting Data and

   (iii) Protocol

   Protocol is a document that states the background, objectives, rational, design, methodology and statistical considerations of the study. It also states the condition under which the study shall be performed and managed.

2. **Responsibilities**

   This section describes the responsibility of various peoples involved in the clinical trials. It starts with the responsibility of sponsor, followed by Monitor and Investigator. While the responsibility of sponsor include, compensation to participants, confirmation to ethics, information about safety, ADR etc and audit, responsibility of other two categories of people deal with their qualification and compliance with protocol.

3. **Record Keeping and Data Handling**

   It deals with documentation and its validation regarding the clinical trials. The responsibility of investigator, monitor and sponsor in record keeping is also mentioned here.

4. **Quality Assurance**

   "The sponsor is responsible for the implementation of a system of quality assurance in order to ensure that the study is performed and the data is generated, recorded and reported in compliance with protocol, GCP, and other applicable requirements. Documented standard operating procedures (SOP) are the prerequisite for quality assurance". The guidelines also specify that all observations and findings should be verifiable and the verification processes must therefore be specified and justified.

5. **Statistics**

   This section deals with role of biostatistics, study design and statistical analysis. Study design includes randomisation study and blinding study.

6. **Special Concerns**

   This final section of guidelines for clinical trials describes the procedure to be followed for special products other than drugs. They are vaccines, contraceptives, surgical procedures or medical devices, diagnostic agents including x-ray and radioactive materials, and herbal remedies and medicinal plants.

   This apart, the guidelines describe other requirements like format for submission, essential documents and investigator brochure in its appendices.

Ethics in Clinical Research

As it is obvious that getting volunteers for clinical trials is difficult, because of people's fear of untoward effects of unknown drugs, investigators and sponsors try to hide many facts and risks involved in clinical trials. They lure the uneducated and innocent people into the clinical trials as volunteers by offering money or promises like giving job in their organization etc.

Thus ethics in clinical trials are pushed to the background and false documents are prepared and submitted to the authorities. The rule of "Informed Consent" to trial is available only in paper than in practice. Hence governments of many countries including India have brought in legislations and guidelines to control the clinical trials in their country.

According to these guidelines, an Independent ethics Committee (IEC) has to be formed in all clinical trials organizations. The composition and functions of such committees are specified in the guidelines. The composition of ethics committee may be as follows:

1. Chair person
2. One or two basic scientists (preferably one pharmacologist)
3. One or two clinician from various institutes
4. One legal expert or retired judge
5. One social scientist or representative of non-governmental voluntary agency
6. One philosopher/ethicist/theologian
7. One lay person from the community and
8. Member secretary

There should be adequate representation of age, gender, community etc in the committee, to safeguard the interest and welfare of all sections of the society. The IEC members should be made aware of their role and responsibilities as committee members. They are outlined below:

1. Ethics committee should review every research proposal on human subjects.
2. For this the clinical trial organisation should submit an application to the committee with all relevant details.
3. Ethics committee should take decisions regarding the proposal in its meeting attended by adequate number of members (Quorum).
4. IEC can undertake interim review of trial, if the circumstances or developments warranted.
5. It can stop the clinical trial, if anything goes wrong with trial or if its objectives are fulfilled.
6. All documents and communications of the committee should be numbered and filed.

7. All the proceedings of the committee meetings must be recorded in minute book and signed by Chair person and members present.

8. Under special circumstances like enrolment of children, pregnant women and lactating mothers in clinical trials extra care and considerations should be paid by the committee. Moreover issues related to commercialisation of research and international collaboration should also be closely monitored.

9. The committee should also maintain the confidential nature of the trial and subjects involved in the study. Unless compelled by court of law or highest controlling authorities of government it should not be revealed to anybody.

Questions

Short Answer Questions

1. What are the reasons for conducting clinical trials?

2. What is post marketing surveillance?

Long Answer Questions

3. Write in detail about various phases of clinical trial.

4. Explain the guidelines for conducting clinical trials.

5. Explain the ethics in clinical research.

APPENDIX - I

WHO MODEL LIST OF ESSENTIAL MEDICINES

Anesthetics

General anesthetics and oxygen

Halothane, Ketamine, Nitrous oxide, Oxygen, Thiopental

Local anesthetics

Bupivacaine, Ephedrine, Lidocaine, Lidocaine + epinephrine

Preoperative medication and sedation for short-term procedures

Atropine, Diazepam, Morphine, Promethazine

Analgesics, antipyretics, non-steroidal anti-inflammatory medicines, medicines used to treat gout and disease modifying agents in rheumatoid disorders

Non-opioids and non-steroidal anti-inflammatory drugs (NSAIDs)

Acetylsalicylic acid (aspirin), Ibuprofen, Paracetamol (acetaminophen)

Opioid analgesics

Codeine, Morphine

Medicines to treat gout

Allopurinol

Disease modifying agents used in reheumatoid disorders (DMARDs)

Chloroquine, Azathioprine*, Methotrexate*, Penicillamine*, Sulphasalazine *

Antiallergics and medicines used in anaphylaxis

Chlorphenamine, Dexamethasone, Epinephrine (adrenaline), Hydrocortisone, Prednisolone

Antidotes and other substances used in poisonings

Non-specific

Activated carbon

Specific

Acetylcysteine, Atropine, Calcium gluconate, Deferoxamine, DL-Methionine, Methylthioninium chloride (methylene blue), Naloxone, Penicillamine, Potassium ferric hexacyanoferrate(II) (Prussian blue), Sodium calcium edetate, Sodium nitrite, Sodium thiosulphate

Anticonvulsants/antiepileptics

Carbamazepine, Diazepam, Ethosuximide, Magnesium sulphate, Phenobarbital, Phenytoin, Valproic acid, Sodium valproate

Anti-infective medicines

Anthelminthics

Intestinal anthelminthics

Albendazole, Levamisole, Mebendazole, Niclosamide, Praziquantel, Pyrantel

Antifilarials

Diethylcarbamazine*, Ivermectin, Suramin sodium *

Antischistosomals and antitrematode medicine

Oxamniquine*, Praziquantel, Triclabendazole

Antibacterials

Aquaflavine emulsion

Beta Lactam medicines

Amoxicillin, Ampicillin, Benzythine benzylpenicillin, Benzylpenicillin, Cefazolin, Cefixime, Ceftazidime*, Ceftriaxone*, Cloxacillin, Co-amoxiclav (amoxicillun + clavulanic acid), Imipenem/Cilastatin (Imipenem + Cilastatin) *, Phenoxymethyl-penicillin, Procaine benzylpenicillin

Other antibacterials

Azithromycin, Chloramphenicol, Ciprofloxacin, Clindamycin*, Co-trimoxazole (sulfamethoxazole + trimethoprim), Doxycycline, Erythromycin, Gentamicin, Metronidazole, Nitrofurantoin, Spectinomycin, Sulfadiazine*, Trimethoprim, Vancomycin *

Antileprosy medicines

Clofazimine, Dapsone, Rifampicin

Antituberculosis medicines

Amikacin*, p-Aminosalicylic acid*, Capreomycin*, Cycloserine*, Ethambutol, Ethionamide*, Isoniazid, Isoniazid + Ethambutol, Kanamycin*, Ofloxacin*, Pyrazinamide, Rifampicin, Rifampicin + Isoniazid, Rifampicin + Isoniazid + Ethambutol, Rifampicin + Isoniazid + Pyrazinamide, Rifampicin + Isoniazid + pyrazinamide + Ethambutol, Streptomycin

Antifungal medicines

Amphotericin B*, Clotrimazole, Fluconazole, Flucytosine*, Griseofulvin, Nystatin, Potassium iodide*

Antiviral medicines

Antiherpes medicines

Aciclovir

Antiretrovirals

Nucleoside/ nucleotide reverse transcriptase inhibitors

Abacavir (ABC), Didanosine (ddI), Emtricitabine (FTC), Lamivudine (3TC), Stavudine (d4T), Tenofovir disoproxil fumarate (TDF), Zidovudine (ZDV or AZT)

Non-nucleoside reverse transcriptase inhibitors

Efavirenz (EGV or EFZ), Nevirapine (NVP)

Protease inhibitors

Indinavir (IDV), Lopinavir + Ritonavir (LPV/r), Nelfinavir (NFV), Ritonavir, Saquinavir (SQV)

Combination drugs

Efavirenz + Emtricitabine + tenofovir, Emtricitabine + Tenofovir, Stavudine + Lamivudine + Nevirapine, Zidovudine + Lamivudine, Zidovudine + Lamivudine + Nevirapine

Other antivirals

Ribavirin

Antiprotozoal medicines

Antiamoebic and antigiardiasis medicines

Diloxanide, Metronidazole

Antileishmaniasis medicines

Amphotericin B*, Meglumine antimoniate, Pentamidine*

Antimalarial medicines

For curative treatment

Amodiaquine, Artemether, Artemether + lumefantrine, Artesunate, Chloroquine, Doxycycline, Mefloquine, Primaquine, Quinine, Sulphadoxine + Pyrimethamine

For prophylaxis

Chloroquine, Doxycycline, Mefloquine, Proguanil

Antipneumocytosis and antitoxoplasmosis medicines

Pentamidine*, Pyrimethamine, Sulfamethoxazole + Trimethoprim

Antitrypanosomal medicines

African trypanosomiasis

Eflornithine, Melarsoprol, Pentamidine, Suramin sodium

American trypanosomiasis

Benznidazole, Nifurtimox

Antimigraine medicines

For treatment of acute attack

Aspirin, Paracetamol

For Prophylaxis

Propranolol

Antineoplastic, immunosuppressive and medicines used in palliative care

Immunosuppressive medicines

Azathioprine*, Ciclosporin*

Cytotoxic medicines

Asparaginase*, Bleomycin*, Calcium folinate*, Chlorambucil*, Cisplatin*, Cyclophosphamide*, Cytarabine*, Dacarbazine*, Dactinomycin*, Daunorubicin*, Doxorubicin*, Etoposide*, Fluorouracil*, Mercaptopurine*, Methotrexate* Procarbazine*, Vinblastine*, Vincristine*

Hormones and antihormones

Dexamethasone*, Hydrocortisone*, Prednisolone*, Tamoxifen*

Antiparkinsonism medicines

Biperiden, Levodopa + Carbidopa

Medicines affecting the blood

Antianaemia medicines

Ferrous salt, Ferrous salt + Folic acid, Folic acid, Hydroxocobalamin

Medicines affecting coagulation

Heparin sodium, Phytomenadione, Protamine sulfate, Warfarin

Blood products and plasma substitues

Plasma substitutes

Dextran 70

Plasma fractions for specific use

Human normal immunoglobulin*, Factor VIII concentrate*, Factor IX complex (II, VII, IX, X concentrate)

Cardiovascular medicines

Antianginal medicines

Antenolol, Glyceryl trinitrate, Isosorbide dinitrate, Verapamil

Antiarrhythmic medicines

Atenolol, Digoxin, Epinephrine, Lidocaine, Procainamide*, Quinidine*, Verapamil

Antihypertensive medicines

Amlodipine, Atenolol, Enalapril, Hydralazine (for acute, severe pregnancy-induced hypertension only), Hydrochlorothiazide, Methyldopa, Sodium nitroprusside*

Medicines used in heart failure

Digoxin, Dopamine, Enalapril, Furosemide, Hydrochlorothiazide

Antithrombotic medicines

Acetylsalicylic acid, Streptokinase*

Lipid-lowering agents

Simvastatin

Dermatological medicines (topical)

Antifungal medicines

Benzoic acid + Salicylic acid (see also Whitfield's ointment), Miconazole, Selenium sulfide*, Sodium thiosulfate

Anti-infective medicines

Methylrosanilinium chloride, Neomycin sulphate + Bacitracin, Potassium permanganate, Silver sulfadiazine

Anti-inflammatory and antipruritic medicines

Betamethasone, Calamine lotion, Hydrocortisone

Astringent medicines

Aluminium diacetate

Medicines affecting skin differentiation and proliferation

Benzoyl peroxide, Coal tar, Dithranol, Fluorouracil, Podophyllum resin, Salicylic acid, Urea

Scabicides and pediculicides

Benzyl benzoate, Permethrin

Diagnostic agents

Ophthalmic medicines

Fluorescein, Tropicamide

Radiocontrast media

Amidotrizoate, Barium sulphate, Iohexol, Meglumine iotroxate*

Disinfectants and antiseptics

Antiseptics

Chlorhexidine, Ethanol, Povidone iodine

Disinfectants

Chlorine base compound, Chloroxylenol, Glutaral

Diuretics

Amiloride, Furosemide, Hydrochlorothiazide, Mannitol, Spironolactone

Gastrointestinal medicines

Antacids and other antiulcer medicines

Aluminium hydroxide, Ranitidine, Magnesium hydroxide, Omeprazole

Antiemetic medicines

Metoclopramide, Promethazine

Anti-inflammatory medicines

Hydrocortisone*, Sulphasalazine

Laxatives

Senna

Medicines used in diarrhea

Oral rehydration

Oral rehydration therapy salts, RESOMAL

Medicines for diarrhea in children

Zinc sulphate

Antidiarrheal (symptomatic) medicines in adults

Codeine

Hormones, other endocrine medicines and contraceptives

Adrenal hormones and synthetic substitutes

See section 3 Antiallergics and medicines used in anaphylaxis

Androgens

Testosterone*

Contraceptives

Oral hormonal contraceptives

Ethinylestradiol + Levonorgestrel, Ethinylestradiol + Norethisterone, Levonorgestrel

Injectable hormonal contraceptives

Medroxyprogesterone acetate, Medroxyprogesterone acetate + Estreadiol cypionate, Norethisterone enantate

Intrauterine devices

Copper-containing IUD

Barrier methods

Condoms, Diaphragms

Implantable contraceptives

Levonorgestrel-releasing implant

Estrogens

Ethinylestradiol

Insulins and other antidiabetic agents

Glibenclamide, Insulin injection, Intermediate-acting insulin, Metformin

Ovulation inducers

Clomifene*

Progesterones

Medroxyprogesterone acetate*, Norethisterone

Thyroid hormones and antithyroid medicines

Levothyroxine, Potassium iodide, Propylthiouracil

Immunologicals

Diagnostic agents

Tuberculin

Sera and immunoglobulins

Anti-D immunoglobulin, Antitetanus immunoglobulin, Antivenom immunoglobulin, Diphtheria antitoxin, Rabies immunoglobulin

Vaccines

Bacillus Calmette-Guerin vaccine (BCG) for tuberculosis, Cholera vaccine, Diphtheria vaccine, Hepatitis A vaccine, Hepatitis B vaccine, Haemophilus influenzae type b vaccine, Influenza vaccine, Japanese encephalitis vaccine, Measles vaccine, Meningococcal meningitis vaccine, Mumps vaccine, Pertussis vaccine, Pneumococcal vaccine, Poliomyelitis vaccine, Rabies vaccine, Rotavirus vaccine, Rubella vaccine, Tetanus vaccine, Typhoid vaccine, Varicella vaccine, Yellow fever vaccine

Muscle relaxants (peripherally-acting) and cholinesterase inhibitors

Alcuronium, Neostigmine, Pyridostigmine*, Suxamethonium, Vecuronium

Ophthalmological preparations

Anti-infective agents

Aciclovir, Gentamicin, Tetracycline, Ganciclovir

Anti-inflammatory agents

Prednisolone

Local anesthetics

Tetracaine

Miotics and antiglaucoma medicines

Acetazolamide, Pilocarpine, Timolol

Mydriatics

Atropine, Epinephrine*

Oxytocics and antioxytocics

Oxytocics

Ergometrine, Mifepristone-misoprostol*, Misoprostol*, Oxytocin

Antioxytocics

Nifedipine

Peritoneal dialysis solution

Intraperitoneal dislysis solution*

Psychotherapeutic medicines

Medicines used in psychotic disorders/diseases

Chlorpromazine, Fluphenazine, Haloperidol

Medicines used in mood disorders

Medicines used in depressive disorders

Amitriptyline, Fluoxetine, Sertraline, Bupropion

Medicines used in bipolar disorders

Carbamazepine, Lithium carbonate, Valproic acid

Medicines used in generalized anxiety and sleep disorders

Diazepam

Medicines used for obsessive compulsive disorders and panic attacks

Clomipramine

Medicines used in substance dependence programs

Methadone*

Medicines acting on the respiratory tract

Antiasthmatic and medicines for chronic obstructive pulmonary disease

Beclomethasone, Epinephrine, Ipratropium bromide, Salbutamol

Other medicines acting on the respiratory tract

Caffeine citrate

Solutions correcting water, electrolyte and acid-base disturbances

Oral

Oral rehydration salts (see 17.5.1 Oral rehydration), Potassium chloride

Parenteral

Glucose, Glucose with sodium chloride, Potassium chloride, Sodium chloride, Sodium hydrogen carbonate, Sodium lactate

Miscellaneous

Saline solution for injection/rehydration

Vitamins and minerals

Ascorbic acid, Calcium gluconate*, Ergocalciferol, Iodine, Nicotinamide, Pyridoxine, Retinol, Riboflavin, Sodium fluoride, Thiamine

Notes

*Indicates the medicine is a complementary item, that is one which enhances the action of another item on this list.

References

1. "WHO Model List of Essential Medicines 15th edition (March 2007)" (PDF). World Health Organization. March 2007. Retrieved 2007-07-01.

2. "WHO Model Lists of Essential Medicines

3. "WHO Model List of Essential Medicines, 16th edition (March 2009)" (PDF). World Health Organization. March 2009. Retrieved 2009-12-11.

4. "WHO Model List of Essential Medicines for Children, second edition (March 2009)" (PDF). World Health Organization. March 2009. Retrieved 2009-12-11.

5. "WHO Model List of Essential Medicines, 17th edition (March 2011)". World Health Organization (WHO). March 2011. Retrieved 2011-07-03.

6. "WHO Model List of Essential Medicines for Children, third edition (March 2011)". World Health Organization (WHO). March 2011. Retrieved 2011-07-03.

REFERENCE BOOKS

1. Remington's 'Pharmaceutical Sciences'. 18th edition.

2. 'Hospital Pharmacy' by Willian E. Hassan. 4th edition.

3. 'Clinical Pharmacy and Hospital Drug Management' by David H. Lawson and Michael E. Richard.

4. Oxford's 'Textbook of Clinical Pharmacology and Drug Therapy, by D.S. Graham Smith and J.K. Armson.

5. 'Clinical Pharmacokinetics Concepts and Applications' by Malcolm Rowland and Thomas N. Tozer.

6. British National Formulary.

7. 'Textbook of Biopharmaceutics and Clinical Pharmacokinetics' by Sartaray Hiage.

8. 'The Pharmacological Basis of Therapeutics' edited by Louis S. Goodmann and Alfred Gilmann.

9. 'Clinical Pharmacokinetics and TDM' Article by S.B. Bhise, *et al.*, IJPE, Sept 1998.

10. 'A Textbook of Hospital Pharmacy' by S.H. Merchant and J.S. Qadry.

11. 'Biopharmaceutics and Clinical Pharmacokinetics' by Gibaldi M. 4th edition.

12. 'Basic Clinical Pharmacokinetics' by Winter M.E.

13. 'Avery's Drug Treatment' 3rd Edition – edited by Trevor M. Speight.

14. 'Textbook of Therapeutics' by Herfindal and Gourley – 6th edition.

15. 'Materials Management' by C.B. Agarwal.

16. 'Pharmaceutical Practice' by Richard and Winfeild.

17. 'Medical Pharmacology' by K.D. Thirupathi.

18. 'A Textbook of Clinical Pharmacy Practice' edited by G. Parthasarathi, *et al.*

19. 'Clinical Pharmacy and Therapeutics' by Roger Walker *et al.*, 4th edition.

20. 'Remington: The Science and Practice of Pharmacy'—19th Edition & 22nd Edition.

21. 'The Merck Manual'– 15th edition. MSD Research Lab, N.J.

22. 'Pharmacist's Drug Hand Book' –American Society of Health System Pharmacists.

23. 'Clinical Pharmacy and Therapeutics' 4th Edition – Eric T.Herfindal, et al, Wolters Kluwer, NY.

24. 'Biochemistry' 4th Edition – U. Satyanarayana, et al, Elsevier.

25. 'Practical Medical Microbiology'—J.K.Collee et al, Churchill Livingstone, New York.

26. "Microbiology in Clinical Practice' II Edn. D.C. Shanson, Wright, London.

27. 'Practical Microbiology' 3rd Edition —Dr. R.S. Gand, et al, Nirali Prakashan.

REFERENCE WEBSITES

1. www.who.int

2. www.ncbi.nlm.nih.gov

3. www.mun.ca

4. www.fda.gov

5. www.ajhp.org

6. www.en.wikipedia.org

7. www.student.bmj.com

8. www.lifetechnologies.com

9. www.medilexicon.com

10. www.guideline.com

11. http://quizlet.com

12. http://.nih.gov

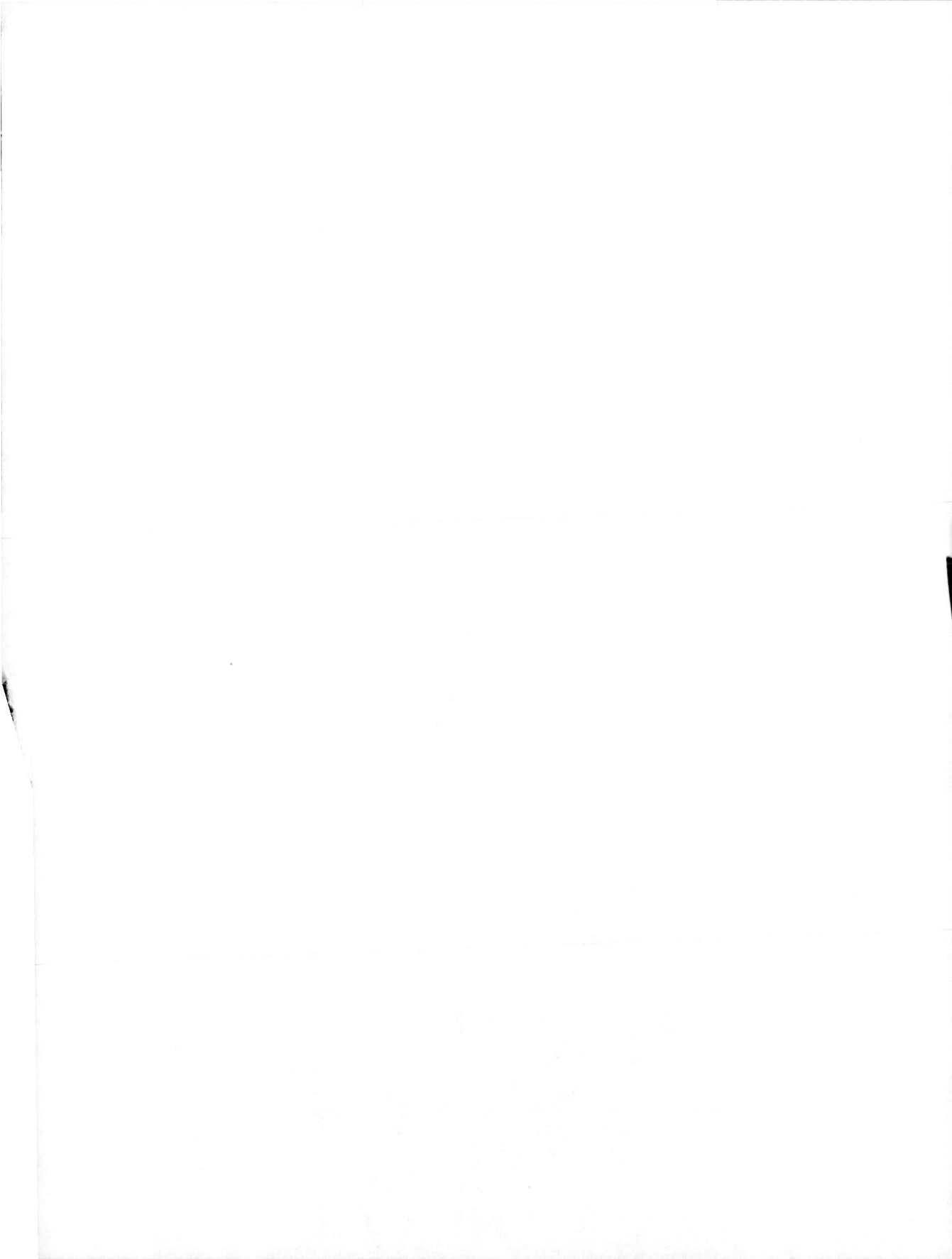

www.ingramcontent.com/pod-product-compliance
Lightning Source LLC
Chambersburg PA
CBHW061924190326
41458CB00009B/2649

* 9 7 8 9 3 8 5 4 3 3 4 6 7 *